CONTROVERSIES IN SCHIZOPHRENIA

Vol. I (33rd Meeting): *Trends of mental disease.* Joseph Zubin (Introduction), 1945.*

Vol. II (34th Meeting): *Current therapies of personality disorders.* Bernard Glueck (Ed.), 1946.

Vol. III (36th Meeting): *Epilepsy.* Paul H. Hoch and Robert P. Knight (Eds.), 1947.

Vol. IV (37th Meeting): *Failures in psychiatric treatment.* Paul H. Hoch (Ed.), 1948.

Vol. V (38th Meeting): *Psychosexual development in health and disease.* Paul H. Hoch and Joseph Zubin (Eds.), 1949.

Vol. VI (39th Meeting): *Anxiety.* Paul H. Hoch and Joseph Zubin (Eds.), 1950.

Vol. VII (40th Meeting): *Relation of psychological tests to psychiatry.* Paul H. Hoch and Joseph Zubin (Eds.), 1951.

Vol. VIII (41st Meeting): *Current problems in psychiatric diagnosis.* Paul H. Hoch and Joseph Zubin (Eds.), 1953.

Vol. IX (42nd Meeting): *Depression.* Paul H. Hoch and Joseph Zubin (Eds.), 1954.

Vol. X (43rd Meeting): *Psychiatry and the law.* Paul H. Hoch and Joseph Zubin (Eds.), 1955.

Vol. XI (44th Meeting): *Psychopathology of childhood.* Paul H. Hoch and Joseph Zubin (Eds.), 1955.

Vol. XII (45th Meeting): *Experimental psychopathology.* Paul H. Hoch and Joseph Zubin (Eds.), 1957.

Vol. XIII (46th Meeting): *Psychopathology of communication.* Paul H. Hoch and Joseph Zubin (Eds.), 1958.

Vol. XIV (47th Meeting): *Problems of addiction and habituation.* Paul H. Hoch and Joseph Zubin (Eds.), 1958.

Vol. XV (48th Meeting): *Current approaches to psychoanalysis.* Paul H. Hoch and Joseph Zubin (Eds.), 1960.

Vol. XVI (49th Meeting): *Comparative epidemiology of the mental disorders.* Paul H. Hoch and Joseph Zubin (Eds.), 1961.

Vol. XVII (50th Meeting): *Psychopathology of aging.* Paul H. Hoch and Joseph Zubin (Eds.), 1961.

Vol. XVIII (51st Meeting): *The future of psychiatry.* Paul H. Hoch and Joseph Zubin (Eds.), 1962.

*This volume was published by King's Crown Press (Columbia University). Volumes II through XXVI were published by Grune & Stratton. Volumes XXVII through XXXI were published by The Johns Hopkins University Press. Volumes XXXII through XXXIX were published by Raven Press. Volume XL was published by The Guilford Press.

Vol. XX (53rd Meeting): *Psychopathology of perception.* Paul H. Hoch and Joseph Zubin (Eds.), 1965.

Vol. XXI (54th Meeting): *Psychopathology of schizophrenia.* Paul H. Hoch and Joseph Zubin (Eds.), 1966.

Vol. XXII (55th Meeting): *Comparative psychopathology—Animal and human.* Joseph Zubin and Howard F. Hunt (Eds.), 1967.

Vol. XXIII (56th Meeting): *Psychopathology of mental development.* Joseph Zubin and George A. Jervis (Eds.), 1968.

Vol. XXIV (57th Meeting): *Social psychiatry.* Joseph Zubin and Fritz A. Freyhan (Eds.), 1968.

Vol. XXV (58th Meeting): *Neurobiological aspects of psychopathology.* Joseph Zubin and Charles Shagass (Eds.), 1969.

Vol. XXVI (59th Meeting): *The psychopathology of adolescence.* Joseph Zubin and Alfred M. Freedman (Eds.), 1970.

Vol. XXVII (60th Meeting): *Disorders of mood.* Joseph Zubin and Fritz A. Freyhan (Eds.), 1972.

Vol. XXVIII (61st Meeting): *Contemporary sexual behavior: Critical issues in the 1970s.* Joseph Zubin and John Money (Eds.), 1973.

Vol. XXIX (62nd Meeting): *Psychopathology and psychopharmacology.* Jonathan O. Cole, Alfred M. Freedman, and Arnold J. Friedhoff (Eds.), 1973.

Vol. XXX (63rd Meeting): *Genetic research in psychiatry.* Ronald R. Fieve, David Rosenthal, and Henry Brill (Eds.), 1975.

Vol. XXXI (64th Meeting): *Evaluation of psychological therapies: Psychotherapies, behavior therapies, drug therapies, and their interactions.* Robert L. Spitzer and Donald F. Klein (Eds.), 314 pp., 1976.

Vol. XXXII (65th Meeting): *Hormones, behavior, and psychopathology.* Edward J. Sachar (Ed.), 325 pp., 1976.

Vol. XXXIII (66th Meeting): *Psychopathology and brain dysfunction.* Charles Shagass, Samuel Gershon, and Arnold J. Friedhoff (Eds.), 399 pp., 1977.

Vol. XXXIV (67th Meeting): *Critical issues in psychiatric diagnosis.* Robert L. Spitzer and Donald F. Klein (Eds.), 355 pp., 1978.

Vol. XXXV (68th Meeting): *Stress and mental disorder.* James E. Barrett (Ed.), 310 pp., 1979.

Vol. XXXVI (69th Meeting): *Psychopathology in the aged.* Jonathan O. Cole and James E. Barrett (Eds.), 332 pp., 1980.

Vol. XXXVII (70th Meeting): *Anxiety: New research and changing concepts.* Donald F. Klein and Judith G. Rabkin (Eds.), 440 pp., 1981.

Vol. XXXVIII (71st Meeting): *Treatment of depression: Old controversies and new approaches.* Paula J. Clayton and James E. Barrett (Eds.), 352 pp., 1983.

Vol. XXXIX (72nd Meeting): *Childhood psychopathology and development.* Samuel B. Guze, Felton J. Earls, and James E. Barrett (Eds.), 320 pp., 1983.

Vol. XL (73rd Meeting): *Psychotherapy research: Where are we and where should we go?* Janet B. W. Williams and Robert L. Spitzer (Eds.), 436 pp., 1984.

Controversies in Schizophrenia
Changes and Constancies

Edited by Murray Alpert

PROCEEDINGS OF THE 74TH ANNUAL MEETING OF THE AMERICAN PSYCHOPATHOLOGICAL ASSOCIATION, NEW YORK CITY, MARCH 1–3, 1984

THE GUILFORD PRESS
New York *London*

A Division of Guilford Publications, Inc.
200 Park Avenue South, New York, N.Y. 10003

Printed in the United States of America

LIBRARY OF CONGRESS CATALOGING IN PUBLICATION DATA

American Psychopathological Association. Meeting
(74th : 1984 : New York, N.Y.)

Controversies in schizophrenia.

Includes indexes.
1. Schizophrenia—Congresses.
I. Alpert, Murray. II. Title.
[DNLM: 1. Schizophrenia—congresses. W3 AM632 74th 1984c / WM 203 A5125 1984c]
RC514.A633 1985 616.89'82 83-25310
ISBN 0-89862-657-9

Contents

CONTROVERSIES IN SCHIZOPHRENIA

SECTION ONE

CONCEPTUAL ISSUES

1

The Concept of Schizophrenia

SEYMOUR S. KETY
National Institute of Mental Health, Bethesda, Maryland

The syndrome of schizophrenia is the most venerable and one of the most important of the phenomenological clusters that describe the mental disorders. Progress in all of the branches of medicine including psychiatry has depended upon accurate and perceptive observations with the tools at hand, and an intellectual process similar to that which developed in other areas of science for the recognition of common features or unifying concepts and the formulation and evaluation of hypotheses of etiology and pathogenesis. Before gross, microscopic, or chemical pathology were able to differentiate morbid processes, and microbiology, biological chemistry, toxicology, or epidemiology had advanced sufficiently far to specify causal factors, a groundwork had been laid by phenomenological syndromes defined simply on the basis of common course and symptoms and the presumption that this suggested of common features in the underlying pathology. Many of the descriptions of these syndromes are among the classics in medicine and have made further progress possible as new methods of observation were developed.

In psychiatry, the concept of schizophrenia had its inception in the closing years of the last century, when Emil Kraepelin observed that syndromes previously described as hebephrenia, paranoia, and catatonia had enough important features in common to permit their conceptualization as parts of a single and broader syndrome which he called dementia praecox. Recognizing that "there is in the domain of psychic disorders no single morbid symptom which is thoroughly characteristic of a definite malady," he emphasized that "the composition of the *entire picture* made up its various individual features, and especially also the changes which it undergoes in the course of the disease . . . " were necessary for its differential diagnosis and ultimate understanding (Kraepelin, 1913/1919, p. 257). He described in conscientious detail the major features and more than 50 individual symptoms which together characterized the syndrome.

Eugen Bleuler, a contemporary of Kraepelin who maintained cordial relations with him, was quick to recognize the importance of Kraepelin's contribution, elaborating upon it and giving it a new name—schizophrenia. He was careful to point out that the whole idea originated with Kraepelin and that almost exclusively to his work was to be attributed the grouping and description of the separate symptoms. He could not, however, "shirk the uncomfortable duty of coining a new name for this disease . . . the present one seems to be awkward" (Bleuler, 1911/1950). In their separate textbooks and monographs they described the chronic course with few and incomplete remissions, the "fundamental" and "accessory" features, that is, the characteristic and the nonspecific manifestations, which several generations of psychiatrists throughout the world found useful in recognizing the syndrome and differentiating it from others, particularly manic-depressive illness. The differentiations, it is true, were imperfect, but not notably more so than those among many medical syndromes when they had to depend only on clinical observation. Neither of the originators thought they were describing a single disease, but a syndrome of probably heterogeneous etiology (Bleuler called it "the group of schizophrenias"). They assumed, however, the existence of common "morbid processes" that could account for the characteristic clinical features.

Because of a recent tendency to neglect them, it would be well to review the symptoms of the syndrome that Kraepelin and Bleuler described. The syndrome was described as "a specific type of alteration of thinking, feeling and relation to the external world which appears no where else in this particular fashion." Among the characteristic symptoms were "weakening of judgment, of mental activity and of creative ability, the dulling of emotional interest and the loss of energy . . . loosening of the inner unity of intellect, emotion and volition in themselves and among one another." In their further characterization, they described disorders of association, incoherence or blocking of thought and speech, impoverishment of affect, inappropriate affect, inability to establish affective relationships with others, a tendency to divorce oneself from reality, bizarre and tangential thinking, stereotypy, mannerisms and tics of various sorts. An insidious onset in adolescents and young adults with various premorbid difficulties was noted in a large majority of cases, as was a prolonged course and evidence of dementia, or at least a failure to return to earlier levels of intellectual integration. Particular types of auditory hallucinations and delusions were described and their frequency pointed out, although both Bleuler (1911/1950, p. 204) and Kraepelin (1913/1919, p. 248) emphasized that hallucinations and delusions were present in many psychoses and were not of special importance in diagnosing the presence of schizophrenia. Recent studies (Carpenter, Strauss, & Bartko, 1973; Pfohl & Winokur, 1982) that took into account manifestations of schizophrenia as described by Kraepelin and Bleuler found them to be reasonably consistent and effective in differentiating that syndrome from manic-depressive illness and other types of psychosis.

Over the past 50 years, two trends have developed around or within the original concept of dementia praecox. On the one hand, syndromes were found that resembled the classical syndrome only in certain characteristics and these were appropriately designated by terms that expressed both their similarity to and separation from the classical syndrome. These have included "schizophreniform psychosis," "schizoaffective disorder," and "schizoid personality." Sometimes terms were adopted that assumed a relationship to schizophrenia that had not been established, such as "pseudoneurotic," "acute," or "good prognosis" schizophrenia. A serious epistemological infraction, however, occurred when Kurt Schneider (1959) altered the concept of schizophrenia rather drastically but retained its original name. He specifically rejected features regarded by both Kraepelin and Bleuler as fundamental and specific (impoverishment of affect, disturbances in personal contact and rapport, ambivalence, lack of volition, depersonalization, and stereotypy) because they were difficult to epitomize, and established one of the first "operational" diagnoses of schizophrenia, one that was restricted, in the interest of reliability, to particular types of hallucinations and delusions that Bleuler and Kraepelin had regarded as accessory and nonspecific. No attempt was made originally to demonstrate that Schneider's "First Rank Symptoms" successfully and more economically described the original syndrome and, where that crucial assumption has been tested more recently in several studies, the First Rank Symptoms have not been shown to be very characteristic or discriminating. In a study soon to be published (McGuffin, Farmer, Gottesman, Murray, & Reveley, 1984), in which the Maudsley Twin Series was reexamined using operational criteria of various authors for schizophrenia, the concordance rate using the First Rank Symptoms was higher in dizygotic than in monozygotic twins. The nonspecificity of Schneider's criteria has led some to disparage the value of schizophrenic symptoms altogether (Pope & Lipinski, 1978) but the symptoms in question were largely Schneider's rather than those described by Kraepelin and Bleuler, who alone had the right and the responsibility to define the characteristics of the syndrome they had delineated and named.

Because of the accretions to the original syndrome, parochial differences in emphasis or interpretation of the symptoms as originally described, and a willingness on the part of some to accept entirely different criteria for diagnosis, there has emerged a need to establish some minimal standardized description of the syndrome and putative subtypes. In doing so it has been relatively easy to measure reliability or agreement between raters and, by specifying very concrete and obvious symptoms, to enhance that reliability. Establishing the validity of these more parsimonious descriptions, however, is much more difficult. In the case of a syndrome based entirely on clinical phenomenology, the most appropriate procedure would be to test the specificity and sensitivity of such operational diagnoses against diagnoses made by Kraepelin and Bleuler or, in the absence of that ultimate validation, by careful attention to their descriptions of the syndrome and to tenets they established in their writings. That has rarely been done; instead, the usual practice is to use a consensus of psychiatric opinion. Because that varies over time and from one school of psychiatry to another, the standardized operational concepts of schizophrenia have also varied, sometimes in contradiction of emphatic caveats by the original founders of the syndrome. Bleuler anticipated that problem 70 years ago: "Naturally nothing is gained thereby except another symptomological picture which is then called a disease and which moreover is misleadingly defined by the same terms as the qualitatively and quantitatively quite different Kraepelinian concept" (p. 278). A number of operational definitions of schizophrenia have recently been applied to the same group of 272 patients with sobering results. The number of those patients selected as "schizophrenic" varied from 4 to 68 (Strauss & Gift, 1977). Other comparison studies carried out subsequently have produced similar wide disparities (Endicott, Nee, & Fleiss, 1982). The value of standardized operational diagnostic strategies lies mainly in the economy they offer in description and communication. The description of the syndrome that each provides is necessarily arbitrary and incomplete and offers little reason for assuming that any one of them defines "true" schizophrenia. From the point of view of research, there is also the danger that, by emphasizing the lowest common denominator, the truncated description that will emerge will lose much information that may be of value in arriving ultimately at more homogeneous subgroups.

The DSM-II definition of schizophrenia encompassed the descriptions of Kraepelin and Bleuler but deviated in including "acute schizophrenic reaction," characterized mainly by hallucinations and delusions, despite Bleuler's admonition that these are "partial phenomena of the most varied diseases [whose] presence is often helpful in making the diagnosis of a psychosis, but not in diagnosing the presence of schizophrenia" (Bleuler, 1911/1950, p. 204). Our study of schizophrenic adoptees and their biological and adoptive relatives (Kety, Rosenthal, Wender, Schulsinger, & Jacobsen, 1975) used global diagnoses based on DSM-II and Bleuler's descriptions. Although milder but chronic schizophrenia-like disorders (latent and uncertain schizophrenia) were found to be concentrated in the biological relatives of chronic schizophrenic adoptees, this was not the case for acute schizophrenia. These results would have been anticipated by Kraepelin and Bleuler (Kety, 1980).

DSM-III recognizes the fundamental schizophrenic symptoms of Kraeplin and Bleuler and attaches considerable importance to them in its narrative description of the characteristic features of schizophrenia, while giving them less weight in the minimal required criteria than a number of accessory symptoms. By removing "acute schizophrenia" and recognizing a chronic course and deterioration from a previous level of functioning it has come closer than DSM-II to Kraepelin's original concept, but has also removed "simple schizophrenia," which both Kraepelin and Bleuler had recognized as a subtype of schizophrenia, including it along with Bleuler's "latent schizophrenia" under the rubric of "schizotypal personality disorder."

The DSM-III criteria and the earlier Research Diagnostic Criteria have recently been subjected to the crucial test of validity by applying them to patients described and diagnosed by Kraepelin (James & May, 1981) and have stood up reasonably well, especially in the case of the more typical chronic schizophrenics or manic-depressives. Where characteristic features of both schizophrenia and major affective disorders are present, DSM-III would make a diagnosis of schizophrenia if the schizophrenic manifestations preceded those of affective disorder or were of longer duration. Bleuler (1911/1950) would have gone even further in rejecting the significance of affective symptoms: "All of the phenomena of manic-depressive psychosis may also appear in our disease; the only decisive factor is the presence or absence of schizophrenic symptoms" (p. 304).

In a landmark paper, Guze, Cloninger, Martin, and Clayton (1983) presented the results of a well-designed and exhaustive follow-up and family study of 422 outpatients of the Washington University Psychiatry Clinic intitially evaluated between 1967 and 1969. They found that the diagnostic criteria for schizophrenia originally used, "very similar to those of Feighner *et al.* and DSM-III, were very good at identifying patients who would receive the same diagnosis, although with varying degrees of confidence, at follow-up" (p. 1275). Their blind diagnoses on interviewed relatives led to some conclusions of pertinence to the present discussion:

> The data indicate clearly once again that schizophrenia is a familial disorder. The diagnostic criteria used selected cases whose first-degree relatives experienced the same disorder approximately five times more frequently than did the first-degree relatives of probands who neither at index nor at follow-up were suspected of any schizophrenia-like illness. (p. 1275)

The original criteria for schizophrenia were found to have high specificity; their sensitivity

> proved to be lower, however, failing to identify or even suspect about one third of the cases recognized at follow-up. The fact that many of these latter patients had, at index, received diagnoses of primary unipolar affective disorder, and that two thirds of patients considered schizophreniform at index later received schizophrenia diagnoses at follow-up strongly suggests that the diagnostic bias at index was against schizophrenia in doubtful and borderline cases. (pp. 1275–1276)

They go on to state:

> The results indicate unequivocally, and confirm other reports, that patients with chronic schizophrenia often experience episodes of depression that symp-

> tomatically resemble those seen in primary affective disorder. That these depressions are symptomatic and not the same as primary depression is shown by the absence of any familial increase of affective illness. Thus, the criteria of Feighner et al. need to be modified so as to permit the diagnosis of schizophrenia in patients with intercurrent depressions. (p. 1276)

That recommendation holds as well for DSM-III.

Despite these deviations from specific notations and caveats of Kraepelin or Bleuler, the DSM-III has shown its usefulness in arriving at a standardized, if somewhat arbitrary, definition of schizophrenia and some less-severe syndromes that may be related to or subtypes of schizophrenia. This has apparently been done with sufficient consistency to permit further examination and the possibility of revision.

Our global, blind diagnoses based on transcripts of psychiatric interviews with the biological and adoptive relatives of 34 DSM-II schizophrenic ("index") and 34 control adoptees in the Copenhagen sample (Kety *et al.*, 1975) revealed a significant concentration of chronic and of latent schizophrenia and an even greater and more significant prevalence of what we called "uncertain schizophrenia" in the biological relatives of the schizophrenic adoptees (i.e., genetically related to them), when compared to all the other relatives (biological control and all adoptive relatives) who were not genetically related to the schizophrenic adoptees. This appeared to confirm Bleuler's impression of a milder schizophrenia-like syndrome which he found more frequently in the relatives of his patients than schizophrenia itself. In an attempt to learn what were some of the explicit criteria that characterized that syndrome, which our results suggested was genetically related to schizophrenia, we secured the cooperation of Drs. Robert Spitzer and Jean Endicott and sent them all of the interviews on which we had made diagnoses of latent or uncertain schizophrenia (plus six that we had diagnosed as schizoid or inadequate personality) and an equal number of interviews on which we had made diagnoses outside the schizophrenia spectrum or which we felt to have no psychiatric disorder. By comparing the two groups of interviews, Spitzer, Endicott, and Gibbon (1979) found eight symptoms that appeared capable of distinguishing the schizophrenia spectrum from the nonspectrum subjects. These eventually became the eight characteristics of schizotypal personality disorder in DSM-III.

More recently, Kendler, Gruenberg, and Strauss (1981) independently made DSM-III dignoses on all the interviewed relatives of the Copenhagen schizophrenic and control adoptees. Their results, compared with our DSM-II diagnoses on these relatives are presented in Table 1. The narrower DSM-III criteria yielded fewer diagnoses of schizophrenia than did the DSM-II diagnoses of chronic schizophrenia, but there was a significant concentration of both in the biological index relatives. Our schizophrenia-related diagnoses included latent and uncertain schizophrenia, the only ones that significantly

Table 1. Prevalence of Classical Schizophrenia and Marginal Syndromes in the Biological Relatives of Schizophrenic and Control Adoptees

	Percent prevalence in the interviewed biological relatives of		
Diagnosis in relatives	Adoptees with broadly defined schizophrenia[a]	Control adoptees[b]	Adoptees with narrowly defined schizophrenia
Chronic schizophrenia (DSM-II)	4.3 (.019)[e]	0	7.1[c] (.004)
Schizophrenia (DSM-III)	2.9 (.080)	0	5.7[d] (.040)
Latent or uncertain schizophrenia (DSM-II)	16.1 (.002)	4.3	17.1[c] (.003)
Schizotypal P.D. or paranoid P.D. (DSM-III)	14.3 (.000)	2.2	20.0[d] (.001)

Note. Diagnoses of relatives made blindly from English transcripts of comprehensive interviews. From data of Kety, Rosenthal, Wender, Schulsinger, and Jacobsen (1975), Kendler, *et al*. (1981, 1982), and Kendler and Gruenberg (1984).

[a] 34 adoptees with global diagnosis of chronic, latent, or acute schizophrenia as defined by DSM-II.

[b] 34 adoptees with no record of hospitalization or psychiatric evaluation for mental illness

[c] 16 adoptees with global diagnoses of chronic schizophrenia (DSM-II), independently confirmed by RDC diagnosis of chronic schizophrenia.

[d] 13 adoptees with DMS-III diagnosis of schizophrenia.

[e] Values in parentheses are *p* values (one-tailed Fisher's exact probability) for the difference in prevalence between index and control relatives.

discriminated the group genetically related to the schizophrenic adoptees from the remaining relatives who were not so related, whereas schizotypal personality disorder and paranoid personality disorder were the only diagnoses that did so for the Kendler group. Because both studies were carried out on the same population sample using the same interviews, the results should be viewed as a comparison between DSM-II and DSM-III diagnoses for sensitivity and specificity, rather than independent observations bearing on the strength of genetic factors. In the case of each diagnosis, DSM-III appeared to possess greater specificity by finding a lower prevalence of the diagnosis in the genetically unrelated group.

The genetic relationship of these marginal syndromes to classical schizophrenia can best be examined by their respective prevalence in the biological relatives of adoptees whose disorder is as close as possible to the syndrome described by Kraepelin and Bleuler. This is seen in Table 1 for the two independent groups. Sixteen of our 17 diagnoses of chronic schizophrenia among the 34 index adoptees were confirmed by Spitzer and

Endicott using Research Diagnostic Criteria, whereas Kendler and Gruenberg agreed on a diagnosis of DSM-III schizophrenia for 13 index probands. It is apparent that both studies reveal in the biological relatives of classical schizophrenic adoptees a significantly high prevalence of syndromes resembling schizophrenia but of lesser severity, confirming Bleuler's concept of "latent schizophrenia" and indicating its genetic relationship to the more severe syndrome.

If, as appears likely, both schizophrenia and major affective disorder are syndromes of heterogeneous etiology and pathology, the occurence of some cases that have characteristics of both is not surprising, and assigning them to one or the other syndrome on the basis of clinical symptoms alone will necessarily be arbitrary. The existence of pure forms of the two syndromes, however, suggests that there are different malfunctioning systems or processes in the brain that are involved in each, resulting from different or even the same etiological factors. In the case of numerous medical and neurological disorders, a particular etiological process may affect different organs, systems, or processes, resulting in different symptomatic syndromes, pure or mixed, depending on the degree and complexity of involvement. Where we add to this the recognition that different etiological factors may affect the same system producing similar symptomatic pictures, the distance we must travel between describing the syndromes and elucidating the underlying etiologies and pathologies becomes apparent. The numerous and often arbitrary redefinitions of the clinical picture of schizophrenia that have taken place in the past 75 years have not reduced that distance appreciably. There is reason to hope, however, that new information coming from well-designed and carefully executed family studies and new findings obtainable by recently developed approaches in genetics, immunology, morphology, biochemistry, physiology, pharmacology, and psychology, insofar as they are able to associate clinical features with underlying processes, may bring us closer to that goal. In fact, some progress based on each of these disciplines is now apparent.

REFERENCES

Bleuler, E. (1950). *Dementia praecox or the group of schizophrenias* (H. Zinkin, Trans.). New York: International Universities Press. (Original work published 1911)

Carpenter, W. T., Jr., Strauss, J. S., & Bartko, J. J. (1973). Flexible system for the diagnosis of schizophrenia. *Science*, *182*, 1275–1278.

Endicott, J., Nee, J., & Fleiss, J. F. (1982). Diagnostic criteria for schizophrenia: Reliabilities and agreement between systems. *Archives of General Psychiatry*, *39*, 884–889.

Guze, S. B., Cloninger, C. R., Martin, R. L., & Clayton, P. J. (1983). A follow-up and family study of schizophrenia. *Archives of General Psychiatry*, *40*, 1273–1276.

James, R. L.,& May, P. R. A. (1981). Diagnosing schizophrenia: Professor Kraepelin and the Research Diagnostic Criteria. *American Journal of Psychiatry*, *138*, 501–504.

Kendler, K. S., & Gruenberg, A. M. (1982). Genetic relationship between paranoid personality disorder and the "schizophrenia spectrum" disorders. *American Journal of Psychiatry, 139*, 1185–1189.

Kendler, K. S., & Gruenberg, A. M. (1984). An independent analysis of The Danish Adoption Study of Schizophrenia. VI The relationship between psychiatric disorders as defined by DSM-III in the relatives and adoptees. *Archives of General Psychiatry, 41*, 555–564.

Kendler, K. S., Gruenberg, A. M., & Strauss, J. S. (1981). An independent analysis of the Copenhagen sample of the Danish adoption study of schizophrenia. *Archives of General Psychiatry, 38*, 973–977, 982–984, 985–987.

Kendler, K. S., Gruenberg, A. M., & Strauss, J. S. (1982). An independent analysis of the Copenhagen sample of the Danish adoption study of schizophrenia. IV The relationship between major depressive disorders and schizophrenia. *Archives of General Psychiatry, 39*, 639–642.

Kety, S. S. (1980). The syndrome of schizophrenia: Unresolved problems and opportunities for research. The 52nd Maudsley Lecture. *British Journal of Psychiatry, 136*, 421–436.

Kety, S. S., Rosenthal, D., Wender, P. H., Schulsinger, F., & Jacobsen, B. (1975). Mental illness in the biological and adoptive families of adopted individuals who have become schizophrenic: A preliminary report based on psychiatric interviews. In R. Fieve, D. Rosenthal, & H. Brill (Eds.), *Genetic research in psychiatry* (pp. 147–165). Baltimore: Johns Hopkins Press.

Kraepelin, E. (1919). *Dementia praecox and paraphrenia* (R. M. Barclay, Trans.), 8th German edition of the *Text-book of psychiatry: Vol. 3, Pt. 2. Endogenous dementias*. Edinburgh: E. & S. Livingstone. (Original work published 1913)

McGuffin, P., Farmer, A. E., Gottesman, I. I., Murray, R. M., & Reveley, A. M. (1984). Twin concordance for operationally defined schizophrenia. *Archives of General Psychiatry, 41*, 541–545.

Pfohl, B., & Winokur, G. (1982). Schizophrenia: course and outcome. In F. A. Henn & H. Nasrallah (Eds.), *Schizophrenia as a brain disease* (pp. 26–39). Oxford & New York: Oxford University Press.

Pope, H., & Lipinski, J. (1978). Diagnosis in schizophrenia and manic-depressive illness. *Archives of General Psychiatry, 35*, 811–828.

Schneider, K. (1959). *Clinical psychopathology* (M. W. Hamilton, Trans.). New York: Grune & Stratton.

Spitzer, R. L., Endicott, J., & Gibbon, M. (1979). Crossing the border into border line personality and border line schizophrenia: The development of criteria. *Archives of General Psychiatry, 36*, 17–24.

Strauss, J. S., & Gift, T. E. (1977). Choosing an approach for diagnosing schizophrenia. *Archives of General Psychiatry, 34*, 1248–1253.

2

Current Status of Schizophrenia as a Disease Concept

C. ROBERT CLONINGER
Washington University School of Medicine and the Jewish Hospital

RONALD L. MARTIN
University of Kansas Medical Center

SAMUEL B. GUZE
Washington University School of Medicine and the Jewish Hospital

PAULA J. CLAYTON
University of Minnesota

INTRODUCTION

Much controversy about disease concepts in psychiatry can be avoided by recognizing that there are several levels in the validation of any clinical phenomena such as a disease. In particular, it is useful to distinguish the concepts of a *clinical syndrome* as a correlated set of symptoms, a *discrete clinical disorder* as a unified set of syndromes with a predictable interrelationship, and a natural *disease entity* with a specific pathophysiology. The criteria that are required in the validation of a disease have a natural progression that is shown in Table 1.

Heinz Häffner (1981) has recently reviewed the historical development of disease concepts in psychiatry, and the historical progression of ideas about disease closely follows the increasingly restrictive requirements of criteria 1 through 9 shown in Table 1.

The first step in the scientific specification of a disease is the observation and description of a set of signs and symptoms that distinguishes individuals with the disease from others (criterion 1). Any specific combination of symptoms could be suggested to define a syndrome, but Sydenham (1676/1979) required that these must tend to occur together in the same individual. That is, the characteristic features should be correlated with one another (criterion 2). In addition, the clinical picture should tend to be homogeneous

Table 1. Levels in the Validation of a Disease

Levels of disease concept	Criteria for validation
I. Clinical syndrome	1. Characteristics are distinguishable from other syndromes. 2. Intercorrelated group of symptoms. 3. Consistent clinical picture (stable and homogeneous correlational structure of symptoms).
II. Discrete clinical disorder	4. Explicit inclusion and exclusion rules. 5. Predictable progression of interrelated syndromes as a unit. 6. Rarity of intermediate or combined cases (discrete boundaries from other disorders).
III. Pathophysiologic entity	7. Identification of biosocial risk factors. 8. Pathophysiologic explanation of symptoms, syndromes, and course. 9. Specification of pathway from risk factors to disturbed pathophysiology.

across individuals and stable over time. If there is much heterogeneity among those with the syndrome, then there would be little consistency in the clinical picture of the same individual at different times or of different individuals at the same time. In other words, are the correlations among the characteristics similar in the same group of individuals at different times (stability) and in different subpopulations of those individuals with the syndrome (homogeneity) (criteria 3a & 3b)?

The second major level of disease concept is that of a discrete clinical disorder. Such a disorder may involve more than one syndrome, such as the manic and depressive syndromes of affective disorders and the "positive" and "negative" syndromes in schizophrenia. In schizophrenia, positive symptoms (such as hallucinations and delusions) tend to be positively correlated with one another. Similarly, "negative" symptoms, such as blunting of affect, poverty of speech, and social withdrawal, tend to be positively correlated with one another, but not with the syndrome of positive symptoms (Andreasen & Olsen, 1982; Crow, 1980; Lewine, Fogg, & Meltzer, 1983; Pogue-Geile & Harrow, in press). There should be explicit diagnostic criteria (criterion 4) and a predictable natural history of interrelated syndromes (criterion 5). In the second edition of his textbook, Kraepelin (1887) emphasized the importance of disease units (*Krankheitseinheit*) in which there were a predictable cycle or progression of syndromes. In this way he rejected the idea of a continuum of psychotic features with a uniform or unimodal distribution. Kraepelin emphasized the need to distinguish relatively discrete disease units for purposes of description, treatment, and etiological study. More recently, Kendell (1982) has emphasized the importance of demonstrating that there are discrete natural boundaries between the putative

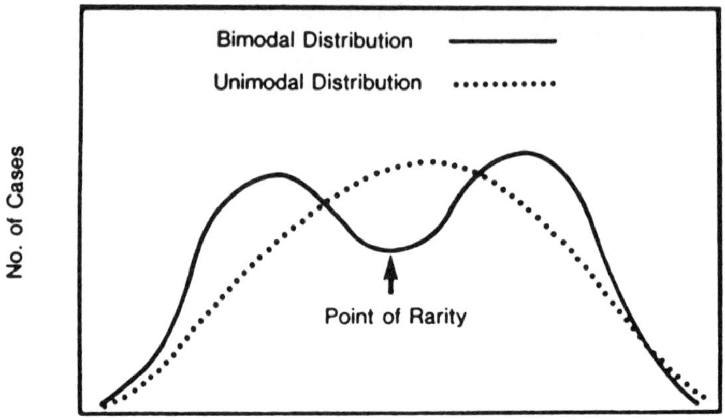

Figure 1. Bimodal versus unimodal distribution in a linear variable measuring symptoms in a group of individuals. (Adapted from Kendell, 1982).

Kraepelinean disease units, by showing the relative rarity of intermediate or combined cases compared to the "pure" cases. In other words, it is necessary to show that the distribution of scores on a variable distinguishing two putative disease units is bimodal with a "point of rarity" (antimode) in the middle rather than unimodal (Figure 1). Thus, criterion 6 requires that there should be such a natural boundary or discontinuity between schizophrenia and other syndromes, such as affective psychosis, in regard to either clinical picture and/or course of illness.

The final level of the disease concept involves the identification of the underlying biosocial risk factors (criterion 7) and explanation of the syndromes and their course in terms of the intervening pathophysiological mechanisms (criteria 8 and 9). Both neurobiological and psychosocial risk factors need to be understood in order to define the pathogenetic process underlying the discrete clinical disorder (Gottesman & Shields, 1982). Of course, it often if found that there is much heterogeneity underlying what appears to be a discrete clinical entity (Cloninger, Reich, & Yokoyama, 1983). Multiple genetic and environmental risk factors may interact and influence a common pathophysiologic pathway that leads to the same clinical phenotype.

In this article we will review recent data about schizophrenia from a prospective follow-up and family study of psychiatric outpatients that has been conducted at Washington University in St. Louis since 1967 (Cloninger, Martin, Guze, & Clayton, 1985; Guze, Cloninger, Martin, & Clayton, 1983). Information about clinical variation over a 6- to 12-year interval and about familial resemblance will be used to assess the current status of schizophrenia in terms of the levels of disease concept described in Table 1. We will address each of the first 7 criteria to evaluate whether or not schizophrenia is a discrete clinical disorder.

METHODS

Selection and Description of Subjects

The subjects are 1,749 individuals in 500 nuclear families (parents, sibs, and children) ascertained through random sample of psychiatric outpatients attending the Washington University Psychiatry Clinic. The procedures for the selection and assessment of the 500 index subjects and their 1,249 first-degree relatives have been previously described in detail (Guze *et al.*, 1983). Briefly, there were three independent phases of the study: the index interviews from 1967 to 1969, the family interviews from 1969 to 1973, and the follow-up interviews of the index subjects from 1973 to 1979. The same structured interview schedule was used in all three phases of the study, but the interviews in each of the phases were carried out independently and by different investigators. Diagnoses were made according to explicit criteria and independently of the results of the other phases of the study. That is, this was a "blind" prospective follow-up and family study.

Data about the location and interviewing of the 500 probands are summarized in Table 2. Some demographic and clinical variables about the probands and relatives are presented in Table 3. The 1,749 subjects represent the full range of variation observed in the general population, and so are well suited for evaluating features that are diagnostic of schizophrenia (Cloninger *et al.*, 1985).

Diagnosis of Schizophrenia

The diagnostic approach to schizophrenia has been detailed previously (Cloninger *et al.*, 1985; Guze *et al.*, 1983). Altogether there were 89 definite or probable schizophrenics and 1,660 other subjects.

Table 2. Location and Assessment of 500 Subjects in 6- to 12-Year Follow-Up

	N	%
Location of subject		
Located and living	453	90.6
Certified as dead	41	8.2
Not found	6	1.2
	500	100.0
Assessment of living subjects		
Complete interview	406	89.6
Partial interview	16	3.5
Refusal or uncooperative	31	6.9
	453	100.0

Table 3. Demographic and Clinical Features at Follow-Up

Variables	Probands (N = 500) %	Relatives (N = 1249) %
Male sex	35.2	44.3
White race	67.0	65.9
Occupational status		
Unskilled	64.6	49.3
Semiskilled	17.2	26.9
Skilled	15.2	19.2
White collar	3.0	4.6
Age, years		
< 20	0	6.9
20–39	45.4	37.2
40–59	38.6	37.4
⩾ 60	16.0	18.5
Psychiatric hospitalization		
None	55.8	92.4
Only one	18.4	4.2
Two or more	25.8	3.4
Diagnosis		
Schizophrenia	11.6	2.5
Bipolar disorder	5.0	0.3
Primary depression	14.0	3.2
Other disorders	68.0	38.8

Statistical Analysis

Discriminant function analysis was used to identify variables that distinguished schizophrenics from others (Nie, Hull, Jenkins, Steinbrenner, & Bent, 1975). The stepwise solution method was used to select variables that minimize Wilks's λ (F value for inclusion, 3.0; F value for deletion, 1.0; tolerance level, .0001). In other words, we maximized the explained variance between schizophrenics and nonschizophrenics. Using the selected variables, Fisher's linear classification method was used to classify subjects with equal prior probability of assignment to each group. We did not use information on the actual probability of schizophrenia in our sample so that the same function would be applicable to samples with different prevalences of schizophrenia.

Analyses were carried out to determine whether the distribution of the canonical coefficient scores generated by the discriminant analysis was better described by a mixture of two or more normal components than by only one normal distribution. This is called an admixture analysis. We used the approach of MacLean, Morton, Elston, and Yee (1976), also described in detail elsewhere (Cloninger *et al.*, 1985).

Kendall's Tau-B was used to measure strength of association for ordinal data (Nie *et al.*, 1975). Tetrachoric correlations (± standard errors) were computed from 2 × 2 contingency tables to measure strength of association between dichotomous variables under the assumption of underlying bivariate normality (Dixon *et al.*, 1981). Strength of association in contingency tables was measured by Pearson's χ^2 statistic. In these and other tests, results were considered significant only if their probability of occurring by chance was less than 5%.

RESULTS

Features Distinguishing Schizophrenics and Others

To identify what clinical features characterize schizophrenics (criterion 1), we used discriminant analysis to identify the variables that distinguish schizophrenics from all others regardless of diagnosis. We divided the 1749 subjects into two samples by random assignment of each family after stratifying them according to the sex and race of the proband. This produced two samples of 250 families each, with 888 and 861 individuals respectively. The large size of each sample allowed us to carry out all analyses in a criterion group (Sample 1, N = 888) and then test the robustness of the findings in the replication group (Sample 2, N = 861).

Seven variables were identified that distinguished schizophrenics from others (Table 4). Five of these were types of hallucinations and delusions. The other two were affective symptoms. Seven other variables were considered but were rejected. The rejected variables were ideas of reference,

Table 4. Psychotic and Affective Symptoms Distinguishing Schizophrenics and Others (Criterion Sample)

Variable	Discriminant function value	Variable means of each group	
		Schizophrenics (N = 49)	Others (N = 839)
Persecutory delusions	+0.57	0.76	0.04
Delusions of control	+0.37	0.37	0.01
Firmly fixed delusions	+0.55	0.45	0.06
Auditory hallucinations	+0.39	0.73	0.08
Grandiose delusions	+0.11	0.35	0.05
Manic spending sprees	−0.44	0.22	0.08
Number depressive symptoms	−0.09	4.82	2.64
Total function score		+4.02	−0.23

Table 5. Classification Accuracy of Schizophrenia Scale

Scale score[a]	Number of subjects	Schizophrenic diagnosis %	Sensitivity %	Specificity %
< 1	1494	1	—	—
+ 1	160	12	90	90
+ 2	55	53	69	98
> 2	40	80	36	99

[a] The schizophrenia scale score is the sum of the following five variables at the time of last information: + 1 if persecutory delusions are present, + 1 if delusions of control, + 1 if firmly fixed delusions, + 1 if auditory hallucinations, and − 1 if spending sprees have occurred.

nonauditory hallucinations, unmarried, number of somatic complaints, current occupational status, sex, and number of psychiatric hospitalizations.

Four of the five hallucinations and delusions contributed positively and nearly equally to increased risk for schizophrenia: three were delusions of persecution, delusions of control, firmly fixed mood-incongruent delusions, and auditory hallucinations. Grandiose delusions had a positive but small influence. Affective symptoms contributed negatively; spending sprees with marked elation had much greater weight than the number of depressive symptoms. More details are presented elsewhere (Cloninger *et al.*, 1985).

The classification accuracy of the discriminant function was about 95% in both the criterion and replication sample. No other diagnostic group was associated with or predicted diagnosis of schizophrenia.

A simple clinical scale was derived as the sum of the following five variables: +1 if persecutory delusions were ever present, +1 if delusions of control, +1 if firmly fixed mood-incongruent delusions, +1 if auditory hallucinations, and −1 if spending sprees have occurred. This "schizophrenia symptom scale" correlated .98 with the full seven-variable discriminant function. Spending sprees with marked elation were characteristic of the manic syndrom, whereas delusions of control, persecutory delusions, firmly fixed delusions, and auditory hallucinations were characteristic of schizophrenia.

As scale scores increased, the proportion of subjects who were diagnosed schizophrenic at follow-up increased nonlinearly with an abrupt increase between +1 (12%) and +2 (53%). The sensitivity and specificity at different levels of scale score is summarized in Table 5. The best overall accuracy was achieved by classifying those with scores of 2 or more as schizophrenic and those with lesser scores as nonschizophrenic. This dichotomy had a sensitivity of 69%, a specificity of 98% and overall classification accuracy of 97%, which was comparable to the full discriminant function. Thus the scale satisfies criterion 1.

Homogeneity of Correlational Structure

The tetrachoric correlations of the five variables in the schizophrenia symptom scale with one another were computed in both split halves in order to evaluate the correlational structure of the scale. Persecutory delusions, delusions of control, and auditory hallucinations are a syndrome or cluster of strongly positively correlated variables ($r \geqslant .68$ in each split half). Spending sprees with marked elation were relatively weakly related to this core syndrome ($r \leqslant .42$ in Sample 1 and $r \leqslant .30$ in Sample 2). Fixed delusions is highly correlated with spending sprees ($r = .93$) but more strongly correlated with the three core symptoms in both samples. Thus, persecutory delusions, delusions of control, and auditory hallucinations represent a syndrome of positive schizophrenic symptoms, satisfying criterion 2. Spending sprees with marked elation and fixed delusions represent manic psychosis. Thus fixed delusions are heterogeneous, regularly occurring in mania, but more often indicating schizophrenia in the absence of mania.

The similarity of the correlational matrices in the two split halves (Cloninger *et al.*, 1985) supported the homogeneity of the clinical picture represented by these symptoms in different samples (criterion 3a).

Stability of Schizophrenia Symptoms Scale Scores

The relationship between scale scores at index and at 6- to 12-year follow-up is shown in Table 6. The product–moment correlation between scores was .60, which indicated substantial association ($p < .001$). Scale score at index was predictive of the diagnosis of schizophrenia at follow-up (Table 7). As the index scale score increases the proportion of affective disorder patients decreases and the proportion of schizophrenics increases. The tetrachoric correlation for the dichotomy of scores most characteristic of schizophrenia (+2 or more versus +1 or less) was $.80 \pm .06$ ($\chi^2 = 105.30$, $p < .001$). This indicates that scale scores were moderately stable over time, satisfying criterion 3b.

Table 6. Relationship of Scale Scores at Index and Follow-Up

	Score at follow-up[a]		
Score at index	<1	+1	>1
<1	249	44	21
+1	27	10	15
>1	5	6	29

[a] Correlation between scores 6 to 12 years apart substantial ($p < .05$).

Table 7. Scale Score at Index Interview and Diagnosis at Follow-Up

Score at index	Number of probands[a]	Diagnosis at follow-up: Schizophrenia row %	Diagnosis at follow-up: Affective disorder row %
−1	6	0	83.3
0	308	4.2	22.1
+1	52	17.3	30.8
+2	17	47.1	11.8
+3	18	72.2	16.7
+4	5	80.0	0

[a] Only the 406 probands with complete follow-up interview (from Cloninger, Martin, Guze, & Clayton, 1985).

Bimodal Distribution of Schizophrenic Symptoms

The distribution of the schizophrenia discriminant function was better described by the admixture of two components than by only one (Cloninger *et al.*, 1985). This was true in both the criterion and the replication sample even with transformation of scale to allow for skewness, as described in detail elsewhere. The observed distributions for discriminant scores are shown in Figure 2. The distributions of scores for primary depressives, manics, and schizophrenics were examined separately and were also found to be bimodal. This indicates that schizophrenics tend to have scores beyond the antimode of the bimodal distribution, that is, scores greater than +1.

Familial resemblance for schizophrenia symptom scale scores is described in Table 8. Association between proband's and relatives' scores was significant for the dichotomy characteristic of schizophrenia (greater than +1 or not) ($\chi^2 = 5.45$, $p < .02$), but not for lower levels of dichotomy (less than +1 or not). Probands with scores of +1 had no excess of relatives with scores greater than +1, and probands with scores of greater than +1

Table 8. Familial Resemblance for Schizophrenia Scale Score

Proband's scale score	Number of subjects	Scale score of relative: +1 Row %	Scale score of relative: >1 Row %
< 1	858	6.8	1.4
+ 1	191	5.8	0.5
> 1	200	5.0	3.5[a]

[a] Association between proband's and relative's scale scores is significant for dichotomy of > 1 or not ($\chi^2 = 5.45$, $p < .02$), but not for lower levels of dichotomy or the full 6-point scale score (from Cloninger, Martin, Guze, & Clayton, 1985).

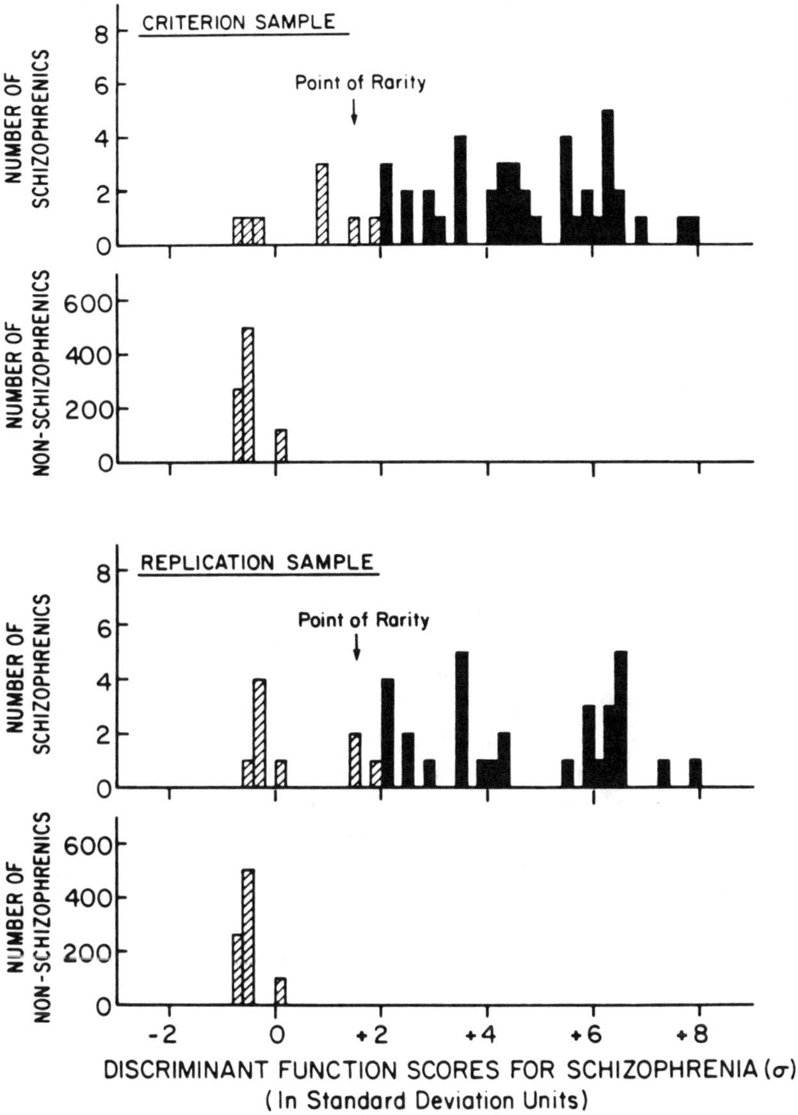

Figure 2. Bimodal distribution of schizophrenia-discriminant function in schizophrenics and nonschizophrenics in both criterion and replication samples. (Adapted from Cloninger, Martin, Guze, & Clayton, 1985.)

had no excess of scores of +1 or less. This indicates that only scores in the discrete component characteristic of schizophrenia were familial. This confirms the hypothesis that schizophrenia is a discrete clinical disorder (criterion 6). It also indicates that familial factors are important in the pathogenesis of schizophrenia (criterion 7).

DISCUSSION

Data from our blind prospective follow-up and family study indicate that schizophrenia is a discrete clinical disorder. Our findings are summarized in Table 9. Persecutory delusions, delusions of control, firmly fixed mood-incongruent delusions, and auditory hallucinations constitute a syndrome of positively correlated symptoms that is moderately homogeneous across individuals and moderately stable over time.

Spending sprees with marked elation are characteristic of the manic syndrome and relatively uncharacteristic of the schizophrenic syndrome. The combination of information on these two syndromes defines the six-point Schizophrenia Symptom Scale. Scale scores were computed as the sum of the four symptoms with positive weights and the one symptom with negative weight. More than 68% of schizophrenics had scores greater than +1, whereas this occurred in fewer than 2% of nonschizophrenics.

Two observations indicated schizophrenia is a discrete disorder. First, the distribution of scores was bimodal: individuals were relatively rare who received scores of +1, which is intermediate to the higher scores of typical schizophrenics and the lower scores of typical nonschizophrenics. Second, there was familial resemblance for the presence or absence of schizophrenia, but no additional resemblance for number of schizophrenic symptoms.

Table 9. Current Status of Schizophrenia as a Disease Concept

Level of disease concept	Criteria	Status of schizophrenia
I. Clinical syndrome	1. Distinct clinical features	Yes
	2. Correlated features	Yes
	3. Stable and homogeneous correlational structure	Yes
II. Discrete clinical disorder	4. Explicit clinical criteria	Yes
	5. Predictable natural history	Yes
	6. Discrete natural boundaries	Yes
III. Pathophysiologic entity	7. Risk factors identified	Partially
	8. Pathophysiologic explanations	Questionable
	9. Specific pathogenesis	No

The six-point scale that we derived to distinguish schizophrenics from others proved to be a valuable adjunct to the categorical diagnosis of schizophrenia. The scale score provided additional information about the certainty or stability of the diagnosis of schizophrenia and about prognosis. The scale was originally derived from symptom data and diagnoses from the follow-up interview, which was blind or independent of all information obtained at the index evaluation 6 to 12 years earlier. It was a priori uncertain whether variables measured at index would predict later diagnoses and outcome. In fact, individuals diagnosed as schizophrenic who had high scores were more likely to retain that diagnosis at follow-up and to have a chronic psychotic course without remission than those with lower scores. Conversely, individuals diagnosed as having nonschizophrenic disorders who had low scores were more likely to have full remission and other nonpsychotic outcomes. Most importantly, among individuals who were *not* chronic schizophrenics at index, scale scores predicted the risk of chronic schizophrenia 6 to 12 years later.

Further attention to the syndrome of negative symptoms is needed, but even without this it is clear that schizophrenia is a discrete disorder or group of clinically homogeneous disorders. This should encourage further work to characterize the pathophysiologic basis of schizophrenic disorders.

ACKNOWLEDGMENTS

This work was supported in part by USBHS grants MH-31303 and Research Scientist Development Award MH-00048 from the National Institute of Mental Health. Eunice Henry and Sue Mattern assisted in coding data. Jonathan Goldberg assisted in computer programming. Norman Sartorius, MD, PhD and Irving I. Gottesman, PhD commented on this work.

REFERENCES

Andreasen, N. C., & Olsen, S. (1982). Negative versus positive schizophrenia. *Archives of General Psychiatry*, *39*, 789–794.

Cloninger, C. R., Martin, R. L., Guze, S. B., & Clayton, P. J. (1985). Diagnosis and prognosis in schizophrenia. *Archives of General Psychiatry*, *42*, 15–25.

Cloninger, C. R., Reich, T., & Yokoyama, S. (1983). Genetic diversity, genome organization, and investigation of the etiology of psychiatric diseases. *Psychiatric Developments*, *3*, 225–246.

Crow, T. (1980). Molecular pathology of schizophrenia: More than one disease process? *British Medical Journal*, *280*, 66–68.

Dixon, W. J., Brown, M. B., Engelman, L., Frane, J. W., Hill, M. A., Jennrich, R. I., & Toporek, J. D. (1981). *BMDP statistical software*. Berkeley: University of California Press.

Gottesman, I. I., & Shields, J. (1982). *Schizophrenia: The epigenetic puzzle*. London & New York: Cambridge University Press.

Guze, S. B., Cloninger, C. R., Martin, R. L., & Clayton, P. J. (1983). A follow-up and family study of schizophrenia. *Archives of General Psychiatry, 40*, 1273–1276.

Häffner, H. (1981). Der Krankheitsbegriff in der Psychiatrie. In R. Degkwitz & H. Siedow (Eds.), *Standorte der Psychiatrie: Vol. 20. Zum umstrittenen psychiatrischen krankheitsbegriff* (pp. 16–54). Munich: Urban & Schwarzenberg.

Kendell, R. (1982). The choice of diagnostic criteria for biological research. *Archives of General Psychiatry, 39*, 1334–1343.

Kraepelin, E. (1887). *Psychiatrie* (2nd ed.). Leipzig: Ambr. Abel.

Lewine, R. R. J., Fogg, L., & Meltzer, H. Y. (1983). Assessment of negative and positive symptoms in schizophrenia. *Schizophrenia Bulletin, 9*, 368–376.

MacLean, C. J., Morton, N. E., Elston, R. C., & Yee, S. (1976). Skewness in commingled distributions. *Biometrics, 32*, 695–699.

Nie, N. H., Hull, C. H., Jenkins, J. G., Steinbrenner, K., & Bent, D. H. (1975). *Statistical package for the social sciences* (2nd ed., pp. 434–467). New York: McGraw-Hill.

Pogue-Geile, M. F., & Harrow, M. (in press). Negative and positive symptoms in schizophrenia and depression: A follow-up study. *Schizophrenia Bulletin.*

Sydenham, T. (1979). Observationes medicae (1676). In J. Swan (Ed.), *The entire works of Thomas Sydenham newly made English from the originals* (spec. ed.). Birmingham, AL: Classics of Medicine Library. (Reprinted from original work published in Cave, London, 1742)

3

On the Heterogeneity of Schizophrenia

WILLIAM T. CARPENTER, JR.
University of Maryland

DOUGLAS W. HEINRICHS
University of Maryland

ALTHEA M. I. WAGMAN
University of Maryland

INTRODUCTION

Schizophrenia may be medicine's prime example of a diversity of clinical manifestations within a single diagnostic class. Remarkable differences occur between cases in factors such as age of onset, constellation of psychotic features, course of illness, premorbid personality, prognostic features, presence of deficit symptoms, neurologic dysfunction, response to treatments, insight into illness, and the extent to which the personality is torn asunder. There are at least three general models that could account for such heterogeneity, each with different implications for classification, treatment, and the formulation of research questions.

In the "single disease-multiple site" model, schizophrenia is analogous to syphilis. There is a common etiologic factor affecting different anatomic sites in different cases, thereby accounting for the variability of signs, symptoms, and pathophysiology. Within this framework, the study of factors determining individual variations in vulnerability to the pathogenic agent and ascertaining the mechanisms that determine sites of insult are important. However, the search for a key causative factor and a specific treatment—the "silver bullet"—that corrects or prevents its pathogenic impact is preeminent. This model suggests that an etiologically specific treatment could be developed and applied to all schizophrenic patients.

A second model postulates a single disease with multifactorial etiology. The common pathogenic process is thought to result from the interaction of a number of etiologic factors. The variability between cases is explained in terms of differences in the relative contribution of these factors and their interaction. Although host and environment variability is assumed, as in the first model, this second model encourages efforts to identify multiple etiologic factors and to understand their interdependence. Application of this model results in the development of a number of specific treatment and prevention strategies targeted to different components of the complex etiologic mix. If the multiple disease manifestations result from the perturbations of a final common path, then a unitary treatment approach is plausible.

The preceding models share the premise of a single disease entity, the second being an extension of the first. The third approach, the "multiple disease" model, is quite different. It posits that schizophrenia defines a syndrome rather than a disease entity. The syndrome is associated with any of a number of distinct diseases, each with its own etiology, pathogenesis, and clinical manifestations and prognosis. As each disease entity is ultimately defined, principles of the first two models may guide investigators; however, premature application of a disease-entity model to a heterogeneous syndrome is perilous. This viewpoint encourages a search for variables that allows the delineation of discrete diseases within the larger syndrome. No single treatment approach is expected to be optimal for all schizophrenic-syndrome patients, but a series of therapeutic strategies is anticipated. Finding the appropriate treatment for each patient rather than the blanket application of a standard treatment is critical to the clinical task.

The absence of conclusive evidence favoring one model over another complicates the task of nosology and classification. The first two models assume that schizophrenia is a proper disease class—that, in spite of considerable variability, sufficient core features exist in all bona fide cases to establish a basis for recognizing the presence of schizophrenia and assigning to other extant classes individuals who do not meet definitional requirements. The syndrome model, however, assumes that, until underlying disease entities are identified, classification serves only to define the outer boundaries of the syndrome and would not be expected to reflect within-class homogeneity.

Recent progress in nosology and classification, as represented in the movement from DSM-II (American Psychiatric Association, 1968) to DSM-III (American Psychiatric Association, 1980) is consonant with the first two models, but is less adequate if the syndrome model is valid. Increasing the within-class homogeneity of schizophrenia by defining it as a chronic psychotic illness with a more restricted range of diagnostically relevant symptomatology is valuable; nonetheless, sufficient heterogeneity persists to permit application of the syndrome model within this more narrowed grouping. The primary issue, however, relates to classification of cases excluded from schizophrenia by the more restrictive DSM-III criteria. The syndrome model invites broad boundaries with a subsequent narrowing of class as putative disease entities are defined and assigned new categories. Understandably, problems have arisen as a result of the arbitrary reduction of boundaries of the syndrome by simply reassigning cases to other established classes (in this case the affective disorders) or by creating new classes which are not putative disease entities.

ASTRONOMICAL APPROACHES TO PSYCHIATRIC NOSOLOGY

The underlying assumptions of modern-day approaches to the classification and nosology of psychosis will be illustrated with overdrawn astronomical analogies. At issue is the nosology of the so-called functional psychoses dealing with the broad range of psychotic illness not presently attributable to identifiable etiologies. This population approximates that defined by the criteria for DSM-II schizophrenia as used by the casual diagnostician.

The Antimatter Approach

The antimatter approach reduces the heterogeneity of schizophrenia by annihilating cases from the periphery. The key to this approach is to vigorously assert a set of stringent criteria for schizophrenia and to claim that all cases not meeting said criteria are ipso facto nonschizophrenics. The fact that such cases may fit the definitions provided by Kraepelin (1971) and Bleuler (1911/1950) is beside the point. The fact that such cases may meet other sets of operationalized criteria for schizophrenia merely demonstrates the inadequacies of rival systems. The validity of any approach is assumed to parallel its ability to annihilate cases. Whatever set of stringent criteria is used, the class schizophrenia is reduced in heterogeneity, but the nature of the new-found homogeneity depends upon the nature of the defining criteria (Berner, Katschnig, & Simhandl, 1984). This approach is not concerned with the annihilated cases and provides no basis for the study of psychosis other than the delineation of "very true schizophrenia." Although holding promise for the eradication of schizophrenia, the antimatter approach does not reduce the prevalence of psychotic illness or provide a new nosologic structure.

The Black Hole Approach

This approach answers the question of what to do with annihilated cases of schizophrenia. There has been an increasing tendency for psychiatry in the United States to force cases not tightly held to the core of any given nosologic niche into the vortex of the affective disorders. It takes little imagination to visualize the affective disorders as an enormously powerful space vacuum that find the slightest similarity in emotional display sufficient to draw psychotic cases into its sphere. The strength of this gravitational pull even attracts cases involving mood-incongruent psychotic illness (American Psychiatric Association, 1980). Good-prognosis schizophrenia is another diagnostic entity lost in the process. The fact that good-prognosis schizophrenia can be distinguished from chronic schizophrenia because family pedigree fails to manifest an excess of chronic schizophrenia is taken as suggesting the redefinition of this category into that of an affective disorder (Carpenter & Stephens, 1982). Additional attraction is also found within psychopharmacology. Therapeutic responsivity to drugs typically used in the affective disorders (e.g., lithium) is taken as providing a basis for reassigning schizoaffective and acute schizophrenic cases to the affective disorders despite the fact that these drugs are not disease specific. (Apparently, predicate logic is found not only in schizophrenia, but also in nosologists!) The resulting heterogeneity of the affective disorders will provide the next generation with a formidable challenge, similar in many respects to that brought on by the recent broad and indiscriminant use of the term *schizophrenia*. The black hole analogy may be imperfect, but one of the features it shares with the noncritical expansion of the affective disorders is its inability to emit light.

The Satellite Approach

The satellite approach assumes that the galaxy of psychosis has been defined and that two major stars are known. These are the two psychoses characterized by Kraepelin (1971) as dementia praecox and manic-depressive insanity. There are other bodies that are separate, but not independent, from the two major bodies. These satellites are classified with the assumption that they are consonant with a predefined orbital system, but must await further observation before it can be determined which of the two stars they actually orbit. DSM-III psychoses not classified elsewhere (e.g., schizoaffective psychosis, schizophreniform psychosis) represent satellites of either schizophrenia or the affective psychoses. Here, particularly, the satellites await further exploration to determine to which solar system they belong. Although a fair concession to lack of knowledge, this view tenaciously holds the doubtful assumption that there are only two major psychoses.

The Nova Approach

This approach assumes heuristic value in postulating more than two major stars in the psychosis galaxy and that sufficient information is at hand to hypothesize the location and characteristics of some new stars. From this vantage, one wishes to reduce the heterogeneity of both affective psychoses and schizophrenia rather than to reduce the heterogeneity of one by increasing it in the other. Cases excluded from schizophrenia are singled out for study rather than ignored as nuisance variance. Having defined the two major psychoses, attention turns to positing the approximate location and definitional qualities of third, fourth, fifth, etc. disorders. This approach does not preclude the possibility that some clusters of ambiguous cases may prove to belong to one of the two major classes, but assumes that this is not generally the case. The approach has been eschewed in the development of DSM-III, but is identified by such well known contributions in the literature as Leonhard and the cycloid psychoses (1979), Monroe in the episodic dyscontrol psychoses (1970, 1982), Langfeldt in the differentiation between schizophreniform psychosis and "true" schizophrenia (1937, 1939; Eitenger, Laane, & Langfeldt, 1958), and the Scandinavian view of psychogenic psychoses (Faergerman, 1963; McCabe & Stromgren, 1975; Stephens, Shaffer, & Carpenter, 1982). The approach promises multiple sources of light in an otherwise darkened galaxy. On planet Earth, the nova approach is especially welcomed by diagnosticians in the Third World countries, who have long observed the inadequacies of standard nomenclature for dealing with the array of acute psychotic conditions they have encountered (Kendell, 1984). It is also a welcomed development for the investigator interested in the full range of psychosis, because it offers a new typography rather than the less promising task of weighing the relative merits of proportional shifts of cases between two major psychoses.

Unlike the satellite categories in DSM-III, new classes derived from the nova approach will have considerable intrinsic interest. For example, DSM-III psychotic-symptom criteria are the same for schizophrenia and schizophreniform psychosis, with the distinction based on whether a six-month period of illness has transpired. Schizophreniform psychosis is of little interest to the investigator because it is expected to be a mixture of disease entities, including schizophrenia that has not yet developed, one or another of the affective disorders whose picture is confused early in the course of illness, and perhaps other undefined classes of psychosis. This contrasts with Langfeldt's use of the term *schizophreniform* (1937, 1939; Eitenger *et al.*, 1958), where cross-sectional differences in psychotic manifestation provide a basis for distinguishing two putative disease entities. The same issue is apparent in contrasting DSM-III's brief-reactive psychosis and the Scandinavian psychogenic psychoses (Faergerman, 1963; McCabe & Stromgren, 1975; Stephens *et al.*, 1982). In the former, the presence of an obvious stressor and a duration of reaction in days defines the core of the syndrome. In the latter, however, postulated psychopathologic mechanisms with anticipated clinical features are defined. Psychogenic psychosis is thus a potential nova, whereas the principal asset of the brief-reactive-psychoses class is to avoid premature classification of cases.

REDUCTION OF HETEROGENEITY WITHIN THE SCHIZOPHRENIA SYNDROME

The syndrome model utilizing the nova-type scheme of classification has considerable heuristic appeal for the study of schizophrenia. The challenge is to define subgroups with within-group homogeneity as the first step in identifying more discrete disease entities. For this purpose there are advantages associated with liberalizing the inclusion criteria to assure that the effects of markers, risk factors and clinical features are appropriately manifested in each subdivision.

Experimental Markers

Markers may subdivide a syndrome according to etiology, course, treatment, or other considerations (Zubin, 1979; Zubin & Steinhauer, 1981). Putative biochemical and genetic markers have generated the greatest recent interest, although they have not yet proven decisive in subcategorizing the schizophrenia syndrome. An illustrative example is the finding that decidedly low activity of the monamine oxidase enzyme in platelets was a heritable trait with considerable excess in chronic forms of schizophrenia (Baron, Levitt, Gruen, Kane, & Asnis, 1984; Wyatt *et al.*, 1980). Markers, of course, need not be biochemical. Other promising markers have been explored in EEG and evoked potential (Friedman, Vaughan, & Erlenmeyer-Kimling, 1982; Itil, 1977; Saitoh *et al.*, 1984; Shagass, 1979; Small, Milstein, Sharpley, Klapper, & Small, 1984), brain imaging (Andreasen, Olsen, Dennert, & Smith, 1982; Maser & Keith, 1983; Weinberger, Wagner, & Wyatt, 1983; Weinberger & Wyatt, 1982), autonomic-nervous-system arousal physiology (Dawson & Nuechterlein, 1984; Spohn & Patterson, 1979; Zahn, 1977), an array of information-processing variables (Nuechterlein & Dawson, 1984), cognitive patterns of familial communication (Singer, Wynne, & Toohey, 1978), and eye-tracking (Lipton, Levy, Holzman, & Levin, 1983), among other dimensions. The fact that the payoff has been minimal to date does not negate the promise of this approach, especially when the marker is a stable trait measure. It is inevitable that blind alleys will be explored before experimental procedures can be applied to the task of assigning individual cases to a specific disease class.

Risk Factors

Certain populations are at increased risk for developing schizophrenia. The variables used to identify such populations are referred to as *risk factors*. Such variables are usually assumed to be involved in etiology (e.g., genetic risk) or are correlated with a yet-to-be-determined causal factor (e.g., winter birth). If the various disease entities within the schizophrenia syndrome are etiologically distinct, it is reasonable to investigate the proposition that risk factors can subdivide the population into more homogeneous etiologic entities. A small number of subjects investigated by Kinney and Jacobsen (1978) illustrates this point. The presence of a positive family history for schizophrenia or postnatal CNS trauma was used to signify high risk. The low-risk cohort was observed to have an excess in winter births, suggesting that this risk factor is independent. The investigator testing genetic models would select cases according to family history risk factors, whereas one studying the pathophysiologic consequences of winter birth would seek winter-born cases with a negative family history. Putative risk factors include genetic (Crowe, 1982; Matthysse & Kidd, 1976; Neale & Oltmanns, 1980), gestational and birth complications (McNeil & Kaij, 1978), winter birth (Pulver, Sawyer, & Childs, 1981; Pulver, Stewart, Carpenter, & Childs, 1983), and, perhaps, familial communication deviance (Singer *et al.*, 1978). The relationships among such factors require assessment. Some, no doubt, are positively correlated and represent the same pathologic process. Others may correlate positively because they represent additive causal factors. Those that are inversely related merit special attention as potential markers of discrete subgroups of schizophrenia.

Clinical Features

This is the traditional approach to the problem of heterogeneity, with the best-known effort being the identification of such subtypes of schizophrenia as catatonic, paranoid, and hebephrenic. For example, age of onset differentiates paranoid from nonparanoid schizophrenia (Larson & Nyman, 1970); frequency of schizophrenia in the family history differentiates hebephrenic from catatonic and paranoid subtypes (Fowler, Tsuang, Cadoret, & Monnelly, 1974; Tsuang, Fowler, Cadoret, & Monnelly, 1974; Winokur *et al.*, 1974), and twin studies suggest a high degree of subtype concordance in twin pairs concordant for schizophrenia (Farmer, McGuffin, & Gottesmann, 1984).

Another well-established approach is based on prognostic variables. Good and poor prognostic features and the overlapping concepts of acute and chronic and reactive and process schizophrenia define cohorts with important differences in family history, course of illness, treatment responsiveness, and other considerations (Strauss & Carpenter, 1979).

A more recent trend is to identify a specific psychopathologic attribute found in some, but not all, patients with schizophrenia and to utilize this attribute when subdividing the syndrome. Promising clinical features for this purpose include formal thought disorder, restricted affective processes, and hallucinatory phenomena. To illustrate this approach we will describe the distinction between schizophrenia with and schizophrenia without the deficit syndrome.

DICHOTOMIZING SCHIZOPHRENIA WITH THE DEFICIT SYNDROME

Deficit functioning in schizophrenia has been important in conceptualizing schizophrenia since Kraepelin's initial description of its clinical features (1971). Many efforts at characterizing subdivisions of schizophrenia overlap with the identification of the deficit syndrome. For example, good versus poor premorbid functioning may well overlap with a designation of the deficit syndrome appearing prior to psychosis in one group and not in the other. Chronic and nonchronic subdivisions also overlap to some extent, with an excess of the deficit syndrome associated with the chronic condition. However, it is also possible to have chronic psychosis without the deficit syndrome (e.g., many cases in the paranoid subtype).

Strauss, Carpenter, and Bartko (1974) drew on an aspect of Hughling Jackson's neurologic concepts to call attention to a distinction between positive, or expressive, symptomatology; negative, or deficit, symptomatology; and social impairment. Crow (1980; Crow, Frith, Johnstone, & Owens, 1980) subsequently conceptualized negative symptoms as associated with a type of schizophrenia with irreversible course (Type II). The division of schizophrenia into Types I and II was postulated to be associated with a number of differential features, and some evidence validating this concept has been presented. Andreasen and Olsen (1982) used this positive–negative distinction to define three patient groups: positive, negative, and mixed. Negative patients differed significantly from the other groups in a number of important demographic and clinical variables.

Debates concerning the relevance of negative symptoms, their stability over time, and their response to antipsychotic medication stem from confusion arising from the various ways in which negative symptoms are conceptualized. There is general agreement concerning certain core negative symptoms, such as poverty of content of speech and restricted affect, but even this is subject to debate (Allen, 1984). A principal point of confusion, however, results from failure to distinguish social manifestation of the illness from illness-specific negative symptoms. For example, withdrawal from social relationships may reflect a reaction to positive symptoms (e.g., seclusiveness of the paranoid patient) and environmental circumstances, including stigma, as well as a manifestation of a negative symptom such as diminished social drive.

A second point of confusion arises from the failure to distinguish between negative symptoms as a primary reflection of illness versus negative symptoms that are secondary to the illness. Restricted emotional expression, for example, may be any one of the following: an adaptive response to florid psychotic experience, a drug-induced side effect, an intense dysphoric affect curtailing the full range of experience and expression of other affects; or the result of a long-term impoverished environment. Failure to distinguish primary from secondary negative symptoms prolongs the debate as to whether negative symptoms are responsive to antipsychotic medication. From the above example, one would anticipate that a reduction in psychotic experience produced by antipsychotic drugs could lead to a reduction in that form of restricted affective expression secondary to florid psychosis.

A third problem is due to confounding the longitudinal typology with cross-sectional data. We prefer to conceptualize deficit symptoms as enduring negative symptoms that cannot be explained as secondary phenomena and that continue to be manifest during times of positive symptom reduction or remission, during on and off periods of medication, and between illness and episodes. Frequently, psychopathologic traits underlying the deficit syndrome are evident prior to initial positive-symptom episodes.

Utilizing the definition that deficit symptoms are negative symptoms that are primary and enduring illness qualities, we have attempted to distinguish schizophrenic patients with and without this syndrome. Definitions of negative symptoms, deficit symptoms, and the deficit syndrome are detailed elsewhere, as are the methods used in our study (Carpenter, 1984). In the study, patients were classified as deficit-syndrome patients if they manifested primary, enduring negative symptoms. This exercise also identified patients without such symptoms. All patients met criteria for Research Diagnostic Criteria (RDC) schizophrenia or schizoaffective, mainly schizophrenic, disorder. We identified 15 deficit-syndrome patients and matched them with 15 nondeficit-syndrome patients according to age, sex, and race. Subsequent comparisons between these two cohorts support the following propositions:

1. Negative symptoms are found in nondeficit patients, but correlation of symptom manifestations over repeated assessment periods is negligible. In contrast, negative symptom ratings in deficit patients are significantly positively correlated over time.
2. Positive psychotic symptoms are independent of the deficit characterization rather than inversely related to it. Psychosis scores were similar in the two cohorts.
3. Longitudinal clinical judgment is supported by significantly higher cross-sectional ratings of blunted affect on the Brief Psychiatric Rating Scale (BPRS) in the deficit cohort.
4. The finding that the two cohorts were similar on IQ, age of onset, years of education, and duration of illness suggested that the deficit concept is not synonomous with poor premorbid adjustment or chronicity.

5. Extensive similarity between cohorts on a battery of neuropsychological tests disconfirms the hypothesis that the deficit syndrome represents a generalized and progressive dementia.

6. Discrete test results from the neuropsychological battery revealing significant differences, with the deficit cohort having inferior performance (e.g., differences on tactile discrimination and Wisconsin Card Sort), suggest that the deficit syndrome is additionally characterized by impairment of frontal and parietal association cortex functioning.

Findings of the study suggest that it is feasible to define two importantly distinct clinical subgroups within schizophrenia whose similarity on certain key variables (e.g., psychosis scores, education level) permits interpretation of differences to be related to the psychopathologic trait of interest. Subgrouping on the basis of the deficit syndrome is critical in testing treatments designed to reduce deterioration in schizophrenia, and the deficit subgroup may be the crucial subgroup for examining etiologic hypotheses of long-standing psychopathology.

CONCLUSIONS

Assumptions made about the heterogeneity of schizophrenia have profound importance in directing future research, setting expectations for future therapies, and shaping classification and nosology. There are important advantages to a syndromal model for schizophrenia, and for assuming more than two major classes of functional psychoses. Within the syndromal paradigm, a range of variables may be potentially useful in establishing more homogeneous subgroups as a step toward identifying discrete disease entities. The implications of a preliminary study using the presence or absence of the deficit syndrome as such a variable are discussed.

REFERENCES

Allen, H. A. (1984). Positive and negative symptoms and the therapeutic organization of speech. *British Journal of Psychiatry, 144*, 611–617.

American Psychiatric Association. (1968). *Diagnostic and statistical manual of mental disorders* (2nd ed.). Washington, DC: APA.

American Psychiatric Association. (1980). *Diagnostic and statistical manual of mental disorders* (3rd ed.). Washington, DC: APA.

Andreasen, N. C., & Olsen, S. (1982). Negative versus positive schizophrenia. *Archives of General Psychiatry, 39*, 789–794.

Andreasen, N. C., Olsen, S. A., Dennert, J. W., & Smith, M. R. (1982). Ventricular enlargement in schizophrenia: Relationship to positive and negative symptoms. *American Journal of Psychiatry, 139*, 297–301.

Baron, M., Levitt, M., Gruen, R., Kane, J., & Asnis, L. (1984). Platelet monoamine oxidase activity and genetic vulnerability to schizophrenia. *American Journal of Psychiatry, 141*, 836–842.

Berner, P., Katschnig, H., & Simhandl, C. (1984). Diagnosis of schizophrenia. *Integrative Psychiatry, 2*, 3–9.

Bleuler, E. (1950). *Dementia praecox or the group of schizophrenias* (J. Zinkin, Trans.). New York: International Universities Press. (Original work published 1911)

Carpenter, W. T. (1984). *Deficit and non-deficit forms of schizophrenia.* Presented at the second bi-annual winter Workshop on Schizophrenia, Davos, Switzerland.

Carpenter, W. T., & Stephens, J. H. (1982). Prognosis as the critical variable in classification of the functional psychoses. *Journal of Nervous and Mental Disease, 170*, 688–691.

Crow, T. J. (1980). Molecular pathology of schizophrenia: More than one disease process? *British Medical Journal, 280*, 66–86.

Crow, T. J., Frith, C. D., Johnston, E. C., & Owens, D. (1980). Schizophrenia and cerebral atrophy. *Lancet, 2*, 1129–1130.

Crowe, R. R. (1982). Recent genetic research in schizophrenia. In F. Henn & H. Nasrallah (Eds.), *Schizophrenia as a brain disease* (pp. 40–60). London & New York: Oxford University Press.

Dawson, M. E., & Nuechterlein, K. H. (1984). Psychophysiological dysfunctions in the developmental course of schizophrenic disorders. *Schizophrenia Bulletin, 10*, 204–232.

Eitenger, L., Laane, C. L., & Langfeldt, G. (1958). The prognostic value of the clinical picture and the therapeutic value of physical treatment in schizophrenia and the schizophreniform states. *Acta Psychiatrica Scandinavica, 33*, 33–53.

Faergerman, P. M. (1963). *Psychogenic psychoses.* London: Butterworth.

Farmer, A. E., McGuffin, P., & Gottesman, I. I. (1984). Searching for the split in schizophrenia: A twin study perspective. *Psychiatry Research, 13*, 109–118.

Fowler, R. C., Tsuang, M. T., Cadoret, R. J., & Monnelly, E. (1974). A clinical and family comparison of paranoid and nonparanoid schizophrenia. *British Journal of Psychiatry, 124*, 346–351.

Friedman, D., Vaughan, H. G., & Erlenmeyer-Kimling, L. (1982). Cognitive brain potentials in children at risk for schizophrenia: Preliminary findings. *Schizophrenia Bulletin, 8*, 514–531.

Itil, T. M. (1977). Qualitative and quantitative EEG findings in schizophrenia. *Schizophrenia Bulletin, 3*, 61–79.

Kendell, R. E. (1984). Reflections on psychiatric classification for the new architects of DSM-IV and ICD-10. *Integrative Psychiatry, 2*, 43–47.

Kinney, D. K., & Jacobsen, B. (1978). Environmental factors in schizophrenia: New adoption study evidence. In L. C. Wynne, R. L. Cromwell, & S. Matthysse (Eds.), *The nature of schizophrenia: New approaches to research and treatment* (pp. 38–51). New York: Wiley.

Kraepelin, E. (1971). *Dementia praecox and paraphrenia.* (R. M. Barclay, Trans.). Huntington, NY: Krieger Publishing.

Langfeldt, G. (1937). *The prognosis in schizophrenia and the factors influencing the course of the disease.* Copenhagen: Munksgaard.

Langfeldt, G. (1939). *The schizophrenic states.* Copenhagen: Munksgaard.

Larson, C. A., & Nyman, G. E. (1970). Age of onset in schizophrenia. *Human Heredity, 20*, 241–247.

Leonhard, K. (1979). *The classification of the endogenous psychoses* (5th ed.). New York: Irvington Publishers.

Lipton, R. B., Levy, D. L., Holzman, P. S., & Levin, S. (1983). Eye movement dysfunctions in psychiatric patients: A review. *Schizophrenia Bulletin, 9*, 13–32.

Maser, J. D., & Keith, S. J. (1983). NIMH activities: CT scans and schizophrenia—Report on a workshop. *Schizophrenia Bulletin*, *9*, 265–283.

Matthysse, S. W., & Kidd, K. K. (1976). Estimating the genetic contribution to schizophrenia. *American Journal of Psychiatry*, *133*, 185–191.

McCabe, M. S., & Stromgren, E. (1975). Reactive psychoses: A family study. *Archives of General Psychiatry*, *32*, 447–454.

McNeil, T. F., & Kaij, L. (1978). Obstetric factors in the development of schizophrenia: Complications in the birth of preschizophrenics and in reproduction by schizophrenic parents. In L. C. Wynne, R. L. Cromwell, & S. Matthysse (Eds.), *The nature of schizophrenia: New approaches to research and treatment* (pp. 401–429). New York: Wiley.

Monroe, R. R. (1970). *Episodic behavioral disorders*. Cambridge, MA: Harvard University Press.

Monroe, R. R. (1982). DSM-III-style diagnoses of the episodic disorders. *Journal of Nervous and Mental Disease*, *170*, 664–669.

Neale, J. M., & Oltmanns, T. F. (1980). *Schizophrenia*. New York: Wiley.

Nuechterlein, K. H., & Dawson, M. E. (1984). Information processing and attentional functioning in the developmental course of schizophrenic disorders. *Schizophrenia Bulletin*, *10*, 160–203.

Pulver, A. E., Sawyer, J. W., & Childs, B. (1981). The association between season of birth and the risk for schizophrenia. *American Journal of Epidemiology*, *114*, 735–749.

Pulver, A. E., Stewart, W., Carpenter, W. T., & Childs, B. (1983). Risk factors in schizophrenia: Season of birth in Maryland, USA. *British Journal of Psychiatry*, *143*, 389–396.

Saitoh, O., Niwa, S., Hiramatsu, K., Kameyama, T., Rymar, K., & Itoh, K. (1984). Abnormalities in late positive components of event-related potentials may reflect a genetic predispositon to schizophrenia. *Biological Psychiatry*, *19*, 293–303.

Shagass, C. (1979). Possible contributions of evoked potentials to the vulnerability hypothesis. *Psychopharmacology Bulletin*, *15*, 34–35.

Singer, M., Wynne, L., & Toohey, M. (1978). Communication disorders and the families of schizophrenics. In L. Wynne, R. L. Cromwell, & S. Matthysse, (Eds.), *The nature of schizophrenia: New approaches to research and treatment* (pp. 499–511). New York: Wiley.

Small, J. G., Milstein, V., Sharpley, P. H., Klapper, M., & Small, I. F. (1984). Electroencephalographic findings in relation to diagnostic constructs in psychiatry. *Biological Psychiatry*, *19*, 471–487.

Spohn, H. E., & Patterson, T. (1979). Recent studies of psychophysiology in schizophrenia. *Schizophrenia Bulletin*, *5*, 581–611.

Stephens, J. H., Shaffer, J. W., & Carpenter, W. T. (1982). Reactive psychosis. *Journal of Nervous and Mental Disease*, *170*, 657–663.

Strauss, J. S., & Carpenter, W. T. (1979). The Prognosis of schizophrenia. In L. Bellak (Ed.), *Disorders of the schizophrenic syndrome* (pp. 472–491). New York: Basic Books.

Strauss, J. S., Carpenter, W. T., & Bartko, J. J. (1974). Towards an understanding of the symptom picture considered characteristic of schizophrenia: Its description, precursors and outcome. *Schizophrenia Bulletin*, *2*, 61–69.

Tsuang, M. T., Fowler, R. C., Cadoret, R. J., & Monnelly, E. (1974). Schizophrenia among first-degree relatives of paranoid and non-paranoid schizophrenics. *Comparative Psychiatry*, *15*, 295–302.

Weinberger, D. R., Wagner, R. L., & Wyatt, R. J. (1983). Neuropathological studies of schizophrenia: A selective review. *Schizophrenia Bulletin*, *9*, 193–212.

Weinberger, D. R., & Wyatt, R. J. (1982). Brain morphology in schizophrenic in vivo studies. In F. A. Henn & H. Nasrallah (Eds.), *Schizophrenia as a brain disease* (pp. 148–175). London & New York: Oxford University Press.

Winokur, G., Morrison, J., Clancy, J. *et al.* (1974). The Iowa 500: The clinical and genetic distinction of hebephrenic and paranoid schizophrenia. *Journal of Nervous and Mental Disease, 159*, 12–19.

Wyatt, R. J., Potkin, S. G., Bridge, T. P. *et al.* (1980). Monoamine oxidase in schizophrenia: An overview. *Schizophrenia Bulletin, 6*, 199–207.

Zahn, T. P. (1977). Autonomic nervous system characteristics possibly related to a genetic predisposition to schizophrenia. *Schizophrenia Bulletin, 3*, 49–60.

Zubin, J. (1979). Markers of vulnerability to mental disorders. *Psychopharmacology Bulletin, 15*, 47–49.

Zubin, J., & Steinhauer, S. R. (1981). How to break the logjam in schizophrenia. *Journal of Nervous and Mental Disease, 169*, 477–492.

General Discussion

Dr. Irvin Gottesman:* One of the themes that ran through all three papers was whether or not the differences that are observed among individuals who are called "schizophrenic" represent qualitative distinctions or merely quantitative differences along some unifying dimension. I think that when you press Crow, for example, he won't say that the differences between Type I and Type II are qualitative differences; and he himself has observed individuals moving over time from one type to the other type, even though it is more frequent to go from Type I to Type II.

So I would raise with you the general question as to whether or not we are dealing here with a Baskin-Robbins or Howard Johnson theory of schizophrenia, that is, we have 31 flavors, but everyone clearly recognizes that they are all ice cream. Is the difference between chocolate and strawberry a qualitative difference, or is it a quantitative difference?

One of the ways that the term "heterogeneity" was *not* used so far is specifically with regard to those disorders that imitate schizophrenia, and which we call phenocopies. Information has been compiled from Davison and Bagley (1969), Gottesman and Shields (1982), and Propping (1983). I like that term because it reminds you that they are not the "real McCoy." Table 1 lists possible central nervous system or somatic phenocopies of after-the-fact schizophrenia-like psychoses. In the literature you will find one or more cases who have a clinical diagnosis of schizophrenia but who, on further examination—sometimes at autopsy—turned out to have one of these other disorders.

We need to have the starting material of probands in family studies of schizophrenia cleaned of these kinds of possibilities; otherwise they just perpetuate the confusion about the extent of etiological heterogeneity.

Table 2 lists some pharmacological phenocopies which are, regrettably, too common, maybe more so in New York, Chicago, Philadelphia, St. Louis, and Los Angeles. On admission after acute exposure to some of these substances, some of which may have been prescribed by a physician, you will find individuals who are acting, at least cross-sectionally, in a manner that gets them a diagnosis of schizophrenia.

* St. Louis, Missouri.

Table 1. Possible CNS/Somatic Phenocopies of SC-like Psychoses

Epilepsy (temporal lobe)	Pernicious anemia
Brain tumors	Pellagra
Narcolepsy	Lupus erythematosus
Brain trauma	Acute rheumatism
Congenital CNS malformation	Chorea minor
Encephalitis	Cushing's disease
Cerebral embolism after heart surgery	Hyperthyroidism
Cerebral ischemia	Hepatic encephalopathy
Progressive paralysis	Uremia
Hypoglycemia	Aqueduct stenosis

Lastly, Table 3 presents some "genocopies" of schizophrenia-like psychoses in that these individuals have a different genetic disease from schizophrenia. On first examination or without full knowledge that these individuals really had one of these other disorders, they still, cross-sectionally, received the diagnosis of schizophrenia. These are other examples of the kind of heterogeneity that we don't have to live with once we are made aware of the possibilities. The good news is that no one investigator has to face very many of these confusers to the diagnosis of schizophrenia, because each of them tends to be rather rare. Take Huntington's disease, for example. It makes sense to ask whether or not the mother or the father had Huntington's before you give someone a diagnosis of schizophrenia.

James Shields and I used the psychiatric twin register that began at the Maudsley Hospital in 1948. We collected from 16,000 consecutive admissions all the individuals who were twins and then selected all those twins who had a diagnosis of schizophrenia or possible schizophrenia. We then submitted the case histories to our panel of blindfolded clinicians. Note that Dr. Welner

Table 2. Possible Pharmacological Phenocopies of SC-like Psychoses

Amphetamine	Phencyclidine
Methamphetamine	Alcohol
Ephedrine	Disulfiram
LSD	Phenelzine
Cocaine	Mandrax
Atropine	Bromide
Dopa	Thallium
Carbidopa	Carbon Monoxide
Biperiden	Glucocorticoids
Amantadine	Isoniazid
Cimetidine	Digitalis
Cannabis	

Table 3. Possible "Genocopies" of SC-like Psychoses

Turner (45, XO) or Noonan syndrome
XXY karyotype and XXX
Erythropoietic protoporphyria
Niemann–Pick's disease, late type
Gaucher's disease, adult type
Fabry disease
"Amaurotic idiocy," juvenile type
Congenital adrenal hyperplasia
Homocystinuria
Wilson's disease
Huntington's disease

was the judge in the Danish adoption studies. We asked him to do his thing with our case histories from our Maudsley twins, and we asked him to wear two hats: First the "soft spectrum" hat and then to take that off and use the hat he was reared with, his "environmental hat" of Scandinavian psychiatry and the traditions of Strömgren and Langfelt and Essen-Möller. You can see from Table 4 a tremendous difference in the yield from the case histories.

There were 120 case histories. Many of the individuals, of course, were perfectly normal clinically, even though they were the co-twins of our schizophrenics. So from the pile of 120 case histories, Joseph Welner picked out 81 as schizophrenic or schizophrenic spectrum, but when we asked him to revert to his original training, the yield reduced to 42. Now, I am not saying that one number is better than another. I am presenting this as the kind of clinical heterogeneity that is legitimate for us to investigate as part of the schizophrenia problem.

From the United Kingdom hospital charts—our starting point—we had 70 cases. From our six-judge blindfolded consensus, which we did in the regular consensus fashion, the judges did not know about the co-twin and did not know whether they were dealing with identical or fraternal

Table 4. Yields of Schizophrenic Cases from Operational Criteria versus Diagnostician Judgments: Part 1

Diagnostician-based Judgments			
J. Welner (Danish adoption study schizophrenia "soft spectrum")	81	CATEGO S, P, or O	52
		J. Welner ("classical" Danish)	42
United Kingdom hospital chart	70	E. Essen-Möller ("classical" Swedish)	34
Six-judge consensus	69		
E. Slater ("neo-Kraepelinian")	62	CATEGO S only	17

Note: After I. I. Gottesman and J. Shields, 1976.

twins. They gave us 69 cases. Slater, who described himself as a neo-Kraepelinian, still was quite close to the consensus and not very far off from what yield we obtained when we asked John Wing to rate our cases and then feed them into the CATEGO program that he used for the PSE. We did not use the PSE interview with our twins, so he had to abstract the symptoms from our cases. That procedure yielded a nice healthy number of 52.

If we impose the strictest criteria from the PSE frame of reference, our sample almost disappears. So you can destroy your sample if you are being too puristic when imposing structured criteria.

Now I want to show you the new wrinkle on this, and that is where we shift from the clinical point of view to the operational checklist point of view; we get results, for the most part, that are quite comparable to what we obtained from seasoned clinicians (see Table 5). But in a sense, we revealed the difficulties of working with too strict a list of criteria. If we imposed Taylor and Abrams criteria, we looked like we did when we imposed CATEGO category S only. We almost lost our sample, and we would have been hard pressed. In other words, instead of waiting just 16 years before we started our work, we would *only* have had to have waited 32 years in order to get a decent sample size. We had the same problem with Carpenter and Strauss when we used a six-symptom cut-off that was much better when we used five. If we impose strict Schneiderian first-rank symptoms, you can detect the kind of overlapping Venn diagrams that are generated by this kind of information. We are hard pressed. We only had 17 cases, rather than the nice number that we got with the RDC. That will make all of you who use the RDC happy. We were very happy.

Surprising to us was that, using the criteria for Feighner probable, which included Feighner definite, we obtained 53 cases. The reason we think, in hindsight, that we were so fortunate there—we didn't think we would get that much of a yield—was because we were using longitudinal

Table 5. Yields of Schizophrenic Cases from Operational Criteria versus Diagnostician Judgments: Part 2

Current Operational Criteria			
RDC broad	54	Flexible 5 cut-off	33
Feighner probable	53	First-rank symptoms	17
RDC narrow	49	Flexible 6 cut-off	16
Tsuang & Winokur Pa + Heb	49[a]	Taylor and Abrams	16
Feighner definite	46		

[a] Minimum estimate, as does not count balance of "given" cases who are undifferentiated.

Note. From P. McGuffin, A. E. Farmer, I. I. Gottesman, R. M. Murray, and A. M. Reveley (1984) observations of our subjects who had been called schizophrenics. So we were not dealing with the cross-sectional approach that you clinicians have to face on the front line. We were very lucky in that we had, at the time we did this, a minimum of 6 years follow-up information on each of our cases and on some of them we now have about 50 years follow-up since their first diagnosis and admission for schizophrenia.

You can impose the concept of heterogeneity when you restrict yourself to talking about the course of the illness. Even though Manfred Bleuler observed variation in the courses of schizophrenia in his Swiss sample over a period of about 20 years, he still concluded that this did not reflect etiological heterogeneity. I have been talking to him for some years about this general problem, trying to get him to tell me what his father meant when his father used the phrase, "the group of schizophrenias." he says that people misinterpreted his father in thinking that he meant that there was qualitative heterogeneity with regard to the etiology of schizophrenia. His father used the term "the group of schizophrenias" as a challenge to future generations to see whether or not there was indeed qualitative heterogeneity, or only a kind of quantitative heterogeneity along a dimension of severity. That is the way he interprets his own data and the way he interprets his father's point of view.

Another kind of heterogeneity I wish to note is in regard to the modes of transmission of schizophrenia. If you put together all of the various suggestions in the literature and try to make room, in a diplomatic fashion, then you can come up with the kind of a combined model that builds in both etiological heterogeneity and clinical heterogeneity, as shown in Figure 1. It leaves room for some cases that are primarily environmental. It doesn't give them a lot of room. Some of the phenocopies that I mentioned earlier, say, induced by phencyclidine or LSD, would be placed in such a category. The largest proportion of cases are multifactorially caused with a large dose

Figure 1. Schematic overview of the genetic constitutions of schizophrenics on a model combining the distinct heterogeneity theory, the monogenic theory, and the multifactorial polygenic theory. (After I. E. Gottesman and J. Shields, 1982, *Schizophrenia: The epigenetic puzzle*. London & New York: Cambridge University Press.)

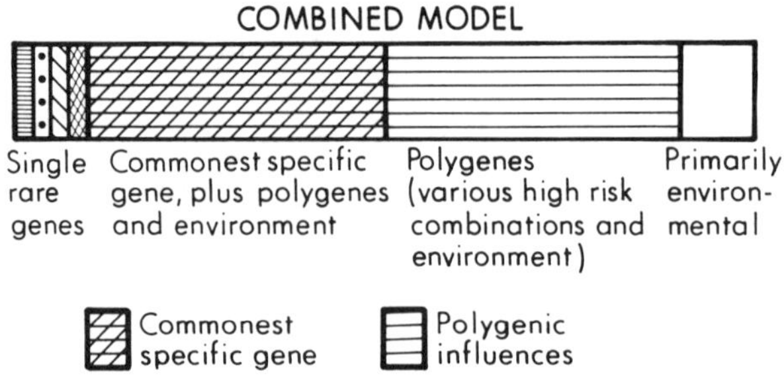

of something genetic, but it is not the something genetic that we associate with the simpler, Mendelizing disorders. We make room for those on the far left-hand side. This is just a suggestion. Don't take the proportions literally.

I was happy to have Dr. Kety point out that Schneider was indeed arbitrary in defining the first-rank symptoms that constitute what he saw as genuine schizophrenia. Most people haven't had the opportunity to read Schneider, even though his work is available in English. His is a remarkably superficial approach to a very important area, even though he is one of the most heavily cited individuals when it comes to talking about schizophrenia in the modern era.

I don't agree with Dr. Kety that Bleuler and Kraepelin had a friendly relationship with each other. They actually had a sibling rivalry kind of relationship, and Kraepelin thought that Bleuler had really gone overboard in his admiration for Sigmund Freud.

I would ask Dr. Cloninger to comment on how generalizable he thinks his five- or six-item symptom scale might be. Would, for example, he be willing to let Dr. Dohrenwend or Dr. Lee Robbins use that as a screening inventory in the field, and would he comment on what looks like something illogical: How can he expect us to believe that a 5-item scale could have a psychometric kind of reliability? And for Dr. Carpenter, I think I have already put my questions to him earlier and asserted, as I think he did, that Crow doesn't think there is a firm barrier between Type I and Type II schizophrenia. When it comes to talking about other ways of cutting up this pie, when I see all the research that is accumulating on season of birth, I want to ask whether you are not recommending an astrological or a zodiacal dimension; how much can you find out about somebody knowing their zodiac sign in regard to their risk for schizophrenia.

Dr. C. Robert Cloninger:* I think it is an important question to address, just how the schizophrenic-symptom scale should currently be used. In general, of course, for just reliability of measurement, it would be better from a psychometric standpoint to have a long, unwieldy scale that would take so much time that no one would ever want to use it. From a more practical point of view, I think what we have found is that these symptoms are highly correlated, and that they are highly discriminating and stable within this large population.

Now, let me point out that, actually, what we are doing is requiring multiple symptoms out of a fairly small set, whereas if you compare that to DSM-III, you only need one out of a certain set. So I think requiring a multiplicity of symptoms is probably a more robust test, especially given what appears to be the factor structure of the syndrome, which is very

* St. Louis, Missouri.

tightly linked. I think the scale is something that is simple to apply and appears to have remarkable prognostic as well as diagnostic utility; it not only can yield increasing information as to whether or not someone is schizophrenic, but can also tell us something about stability and certainty of diagnosis. I would encourage people to try it out in multiple populations. It is only by tests of other populations that we are really going to see how generalizable it will be.

I could say that it would be possible for us to double the length of the scale by adding other symptoms that were eliminated since they were highly correlated with the core. I mean, in the discriminate analysis, you are trying to pick the smallest, most efficient subset, and there are other variables that could be eliminated, such as delusions of reference and so forth, that are also closely related to this but not quite as specific. For example, delusions of reference are excluded, even though they are highly correlated with the core syndrome of auditory hallucinations, delusions of persecution, and delusions of control, because they are more contaminated with the depressive syndrome. That is, they are more highly correlated with the depressive syndrome.

Dr. Jean Endicott:* My understanding is that this set of items was derived from primarily an outpatient sample—

Dr. Cloninger: Half and half.

Dr. Endicott: Half and half. Because I was struck by the fact that you did cross-validate on a half sample within, but I was wondering if you had newly admitted inpatients with a lot of acute psychotics, psychotic affectives, and whether or not it would hold up, and have you applied it to a newly admitted inpatient sample?

Dr. Cloninger: No, we haven't done that yet and we should. However, our samples already include substantial numbers of acute psychotics. These include manic psychoses, depressive psychoses, and other acute undiagnosed psychoses. We found our scale differentiated schizophrenics from these other psychotics as well as from nonpsychotics. Because our sample included such psychotic patients who eventually required hospitalization, I think our results can be generalized to both in-patient and out-patient samples, and would encourage applications in a wide variety of clinical settings.

Dr. Endicott: Okay. My point is that it might hold up very well in primarily out-patient samples, but given the nature of the symptoms—

Dr. Sam Greenhouse†: I have two comments on Dr. Kety's paper. The first relates to an apparent logical gap, which he usually is not guilty of, and, therefore, needs some clarification. In his preliminary remarks, he implied the rejection of a new procedure, such as operational kinds of

* New York, New York.

† Washington, D.C.

classification schemes as opposed to the Bleuler—Kraepelin scheme, simply because they differed.

Now, it seems to me when one proposes a new measuring instrument to replace an older, well established instrument, the only reasonable inference we can make is when both rulers give the same results. When they differ, it is not clear to me that you can immediately reject the new procedure.

The second comment, and more important, relates to the slide. If I remember correctly, the interviews of the relatives, the adoptees, were not done in the blind and, therefore, it seems to me it would have been a much more persuasive way of showing replicability if instead of having an outside group just look at the written interviews, they actually conducted new interviews of all the relatives of the adopted children.

With regard to Dr. Cloninger's comments, I would suggest that his high correlations among the six clusters, at least among the top three, would indicate that you could further reduce to two and even perhaps one and still be able to accomplish the same kinds of diagnostic classifications as achieved with the three. I also wonder whether the discriminate analysis was based upon a linear assumption only or whether interactions among his symptoms were also included.

Dr. Gottesman: Dr. Kety, do you want to comment on the first?

Dr. Seymour Kety:* Regarding my description of the cordial relationships between Bleuler and Kraepelin to which Dr. Gottesman took exception, that was based on Bleuler's generous references to Kraepelin as the originator of the syndrome and on my recollection of a conversation with Manfred Bleuler, who told me that as a youth he had the opportunity to listen to his father and Kraepelin discussing schizophrenia during Kraepelin's annual visits to Bleuler's home. It is quite clear that Kraepelin disagreed with Bleuler's interpretations of the symptoms of schizophrenia in terms of Freud's "complexes." But the first half of Bleuler's monograph is a phenomenological description of schizophrenia, which is remarkably similar to the dementia praecox of Kraepelin, which he acknowledged.†

In response to Dr. Greenhouse's pertinent comments, I should indicate that in the case of an empirical collection of symptoms into a particular syndrome like schizophrenia, there is a standard against which attempts at revision should be compared and that is the original syndrome. Anyone is free to describe a new syndrome, test its reliability, sensitivity, specificity,

* Bethesda, Maryland.

† Lothar Kalinowsky was kind enough, after hearing this discussion, to send me his translation of a paragraph from Kraepelin's *Lebenserinnerungen* [(p. 77), in H. Hippius, G. Peters, & D. Ploog (Eds.), 1983, Berlin & New York: Springer-Verlag]: "It was a particular pleasure for me when Bleuler visited with us for some time. He had just intensely studied the question of deterioration. In lively exchanges of opinion at the bedside of patients, we could come to the conclusion that our experiences on most points were in mutual agreement."

and popularity and promulgate it under a new and appropriate name. If the syndrome is to be called schizophrenia, however, its validity depends upon how faithfully it reproduces the original concept of schizophrenia in addition to being more parsimonious, economical, and operational. In the case of the "new ruler" (to apply Dr. Greenhouse's term to DSM-III schizophrenia), it has yielded results, to which I referred in the adoption studies, that are quite consistent with and probably sharper than results with a global diagnosis that attempted to take full advantage of Kraepelin's description of dementia praecox. The deviations of DSM-III schizophrenia from Kraepelin and Bleuler are in omission rather than commission, and it is quite possible that it defines a more homogeneous but large subgroup of the original syndrome. Ongoing studies on course and outcome, response to treatment, distribution in families, and biological characteristics should help to determine whether that is so and how the criteria may be changed to improve the homogeneity of the subgroup it describes.

In the Copenhagen adoption study, the interviewer did not know to which group the relative he was interviewing belonged and noted any clues to that relationship that the subject inadvertently gave him during the interview. Our later analysis indicated that the clues did not influence his observations appreciably or affect the results. More important than the fact that the two studies used the same interviews was the fact that they used the same sample. We are presently engaged in a similar study using interviews on an entirely different sample: adoptees and relatives in the rest of Denmark, outside of Copenhagan.

Dr. Irwin Feinberg:* I would like to point out that Bleuler's definition of the disease required the presence of certain fundamental symptoms occurring in the absence of primary impairment of memory, perception, and other aspects of cognition ("the intact simply functions"). The latter was a very important part of his definition. I think that when we return a little further to understanding the illness as he described it, we will find that the kinds of cognitive abnormalities that are now being alleged to occur as deficits in schizophrenia are not real. Instead, they reflect the problems of testing schizophrenics—problems of cooperation, problems of motivation—and perhaps with respect to the findings of Dr. Carpenter, the statistical problems of multiple tests of significance.

Dr. William T. Carpenter, Jr.†: I agree with the comments about memory function. Crow claims his evidence counters Bleuler's view of intact memory and clear sensorium in schizophrenia, but his test relies on mental-status data that may not represent impairment in memory processes. Concerning our data, we do not report that a memory problem distinguishes deficit from

* San Francisco, California.
† Baltimore, Maryland.

nondeficit. The two cohorts had similar results on the few tasks reflecting memory.

Dr. Gottesman raised another question concerning Crow's concept. Crow does not allow for movement from Type II to Type I, yet it is evident that some patients with negative symptoms remit. Differentiating negative symptoms from deficit symptoms as we suggest may resolve this problem in Crow's hypothesis, for I believe it is the deficit syndrome rather than negative symptoms that characterize Type II schizophrenia. Our nondeficit patients often have negative symptoms. The deficit-syndrome patients are not likely to have full remission of negative symptoms.

Dr. Gottesman also asked about the zodiac, but since he did not explain his preference for the zodiac over "earth signs" or the "planetary ruler," I assume his curiosity is about the season-of-birth data. Excess winter births in schizophrenic persons have been replicated over and over, north and south of the equator, in temperate and intemperate climates. The finding has not yet yielded to explanation as artifact, and it may be associated with (or mark) a risk factor of note. Some already claim it supports a viral hypothesis or that it is linked to birth complications, but there is not yet a basis for interpretation of this finding.

4

Paul Hoch Award Address

Schizophrenia at the Crossroads: A Blueprint for the 1980s

JOSEPH ZUBIN, STUART R. STEINHAUER, RICHARD DAY, AND DANIEL P. VAN KAMMEN
Veterans Administration Medical Center, Pittsburgh, Pennsylvania and University of Pittsburgh School of Medicine

INTRODUCTION

It is a great honor to be doubly blessed by the Hoch Award. In my presidential address to this association in 1951 (a third of a century ago) at the birth of biometrics, I laid out the blueprint for the biometric approach to psychopathology. Seventeen years later in 1968, you honored me with the Paul Hoch Award and I then presented some of the achievements during those 17 years—our adolescent period. Now, today, 16 years later, as you honor me a second time, the adult period has been reached—age 33. If you see fit to give me a third award, it would be in the year 2000, but you better not do so, because then I suppose I would get to keep it for good!

At the inception of our Biometrics Research Unit in 1956, we were practically alone, except for a few scattered centers in St. Louis and Iowa, and the Biometrics Branch at NIMH headed by Morton Kramer. Since then, the biometric movement has spread so rapidly that we have had to run ahead fast in order not to get trampled by the crowd. We are especially pleased to note that some of our efforts, such as the vulnerability model and the work in information processing, especially the research in attention, has spread to many U.S. centers, and even to European countries, where the reception has been even more encouraging.

In contemplating whether to give another accounting covering the last 16 years of the biometric effort, I began to realize that we are still far from fulfilling the 1951 blueprint. For this reason, I decided not to talk of the past but of the future. Since moving to Pittsburgh to establish a new Biometrics

Unit, I decided that I would cut loose from the constraints of the past and invited Drs. van Kammen, Steinhauer, and Day, members of the team that is now establishing a new multidisciplinary approach to schizophrenia research at the Highland Drive Veterans Administration Medical Center in Pittsburgh, to join me in the preparation of this presentation.[1] I would like at this point to pay my respects to those who launched and supported the work of the old Biometrics Research Unit in New York and the new unit in Pittsburgh. In New York, the late Paul Hoch, then Commissioner of Mental Hygiene, launched the unit, and my debt to him is immeasurable. With the passage of time, his foresight in launching the Biometrics Research Unit is astounding and I believe it has exceeded even his expectations. Dr. Benjamin Passa- most helpful in the expansion of the unit. The heads of the sections and their collaborators who carried out the mandate of the unit over the last 30 years, and who now administer independent programs, were, in alphabetical order:

1. Anthropology—Muriel Hammer
2. Biostatistics—Joseph Fleiss
3. Diagnosis—Barry Gurland and Larry Sharpe
4. Family Research and Drug Addiction—Denise Kandel
5. Evaluation Research—Robert L. Spitzer and Jean Endicott
6. Learning Theory and Behavior Modification—Kurt Salzinger, Suzanne Salzinger, Stephanie Portnoy, and Richard Feldman
7. Psychometrics and Clinical Measurement—Eugene I. Burdock and Anne S. Hardesty
8. Psychophysiology—Samuel Sutton, Gad Hakerem, Patricia Tueting, and Mitchell Kietzman
9. Sociology—Ruth Bennett and David Wilder
10. Vulnerability Project—Bonnie Spring

Drs. E. I. Burdock and Anne Hardesty left the Biometrics Research Unit to establish a Biometrics Laboratory at New York University and Bonnie Spring transferred her vulnerability project to Harvard University.[2] These researchers verified for me the words of the sages: "Much have I learned from my teachers, even more from my colleagues, but from my pupils more than from any of them."

1. In addition to the schizophrenia research programs at the Highland Drive VA, there is another center of schizophrenia research at Western Psychiatric Institute and Clinic, including Gerard Hogarty's program involving expressed emotion, family therapy (with Carol Anderson) and attention parameters (with Diane Wagener), as well as the schizophrenia module headed by S. Charles Schulz, which covers research dealing with movement disorders, neuroleptic resistant patients, and various biological parameters.

2. Now at Texas Tech University.

I owe a great deal to Dr. Thomas Detre, Director of Western Psychiatric Institute and Clinic, for inviting me to Pittsburgh; to Dr. David Kupfer, our new chairman of the Department of Psychiatry; and to Mr. Carl Cossu, Director, Dr. Peter Stajduhar, Chief of Staff, Dr. Gerhard Werner, Coordinator, Clinical Education, and Dr. Gerald Goldstein, formerly Research Coordinator, at the Veterans Administration Medical Center, Pittsburgh, Pennsylvania. The Western Psychiatric Institute and Clinic staff have been most helpful, especially Drs. Evelyn Bromet, Nancy Day, Shirley Hill, and J. R. Jennings. In a sense, the award is really being given to these collaborators, both past and present, for without them the work would have been impossible.

Our Biometrics Research Program is continuing at the Highland Drive Veterans Administration Medical Center in Pittsburgh. Although our major thrust during the past several years has been in the domain of psychophysiological research in schizophrenia, we have recently extended the program to the investigation of psychosocial factors and their impact on recidivism.

THE BIOMETRIC PERSPECTIVE

Each of the collaborators in the preparation of this blueprint has his or her own particular point of view and should in no way be held responsible for the inevitable distortion that may result in any attempt to lay them on the procrustean biometric bed I have provided. When their turn comes for the award they will call the tune and I will be glad to oblige.

Let me spell out the major biometric questions that face the student of schizophrenia today. This is no small task, because asking the right question is perhaps the most important thing we can do. As John Tukey (1962) has said (called to my attention by Connie Duncan-Johnson, in press): "Far better an approximate answer to the *right* question, which is often vague, than an exact answer to the *wrong* question, which can always be made precise" (pp. 13–14).

A review of the questions that I raised in 1951 indicates that they are still with us now. Unlike old soldiers they do not even fade. The primary questions are still

1. How can we further improve classification?
2. How can we fathom etiology?
3. How can we improve treatment?
4. How can we evaluate it?

Some of these questions have been around so long that they have become chronic. However, several new, revolutionary developments in the biometrics of psychopathology have occurred since 1968. Prognosis of schizophrenia seems to have changed for the better; the classification problem has been revolutionized; a search for biological, neurophysiological, and behavioral indicators of vulnerability to schizophrenia—markers as they have come to be called—has begun; biochemical and psychosocial treatment regimens have undergone clinical trials for their evaluation. Space does not permit me to review them all. Following Medawar's injunction, we shall limit ourselves to the soluble.

In order to indicate what to expect in this presentation, I want to make a confession. After a lifetime of working in schizophrenia and living through the various revolutions that the concept has undergone, I feel that I have become a heretic with regard to some of the current views of the psychiatric establishment, and because confession is supposed to be good for the soul, I want to list my heresies:

1. Schizophrenia is far more benign in outcome than what we have been led to believe.
2. It is an episodic disorder and not the persistent chronic condition that DSM-III makes it out to be—the only persistent quality it has is vulnerability on the part of the patient to the development of one or more episodes.
3. Chronicity is not an essential part of its natural history but reflects either the persistence of premorbid personality or iatrogenic, ecogenic, or nosocomial artifacts. This also holds true of the negative symptoms that go along with chronicity.
4. It is a unitary rather than a multiple disorder, but may arise in a variety of ways.

It must be remembered that the heresies of today often become the dogmas of tomorrow, which in turn give way to the heresies of the day after tomorrow. Luckily, there are no more burnings at the stake!

What Are the Reasons for Optimism about the Outcome of Schizophrenia?

There is ample reason to be more optimistic today, but the dire nature of schizophrenia, during the episode, dampens our enthusiasm. It is difficult to demonstrate the change for the better in this country, because of the absence of lifetime follow-up studies, but data from such studies in Europe (Bleuler, 1972/1978; Ciompi, 1980b; Huber, Gross, Schüttler, & Linz, 1980; Watt, Katz, & Shepherd, 1983) give overwhelming evidence for a better outcome than is generally believed. Several follow-back studies of shorter duration in so-called chronic or long-term cohorts in this country

Table 1. Frequency of Hospitalization among First Admissions during the Total Follow-up Period

Frequency measure	*n*	%
Never released	6	8.8
Released and rehospitalized and never released again	9	13.2
Rehospitalized more than once followed by release	32	47.1
Released and never rehospitalized	21	30.9
Total	68	100.0

show surprisingly somewhat similar results, as reported by Courtney Harding in this volume. It is clear from these studies that schizophrenia, far from being a persistent, chronic, deteriorating state, is actually an episodic illness. As shown in Table 1, the proportion of the first admissions in Bleuler's study having only one episode with remission was 30.9% and the proportion having an episodic course with final remission was 47.1%. Thus fully 78% were episodic.

Although rehospitalization is conventionally regarded as an exacerbation of an ongoing illness, the vulnerability hypothesis postulates that many rehospitalizations are often related to the onset of a new episode following a period of recovery and freedom from symptomatology.

Although there are quite a number of other studies that demonstrate the episodic nature of schizophrenia, they were not all as well controlled as the studies done by Bleuler, who made a personal follow-up of each of his probands. We shall, therefore, limit our consideration to only those studies that give evidence of careful follow-up and only to first admissions, because they give a clearer picture of outcome.

The five year follow-up of the World Health Organization (WHO) patients in a still-incomplete study (personal communication, N. Sartorius) reports the preliminary findings that the proportion of total follow-up time during which the patients were in psychotic episodes ranged from a high of 66.9% to a low of 18.8% in Ibadan. Ibadan and Agra were the two centers in which the highest proportion of patients were found to have had a single psychotic episode, followed by a remission without further relapses, over the 5-year period. An average of 21% of the patients in the developed countries were continuously ill throughout the 5-year period compared to only 12% in the developing countries. Thus, there seems to be a tendency for more episodic courses in patients in developing countries.

Another study confirming the episodic nature of schizophrenia is the Buckingshampshire County Study (Watt *et al.*, 1983). This was a 5-year follow-up of all the schizophrenics admitted from the catchment area of this county of approximately 500,000 individuals feeding into a single mental hospital. This study is more epidemiologically representative of the course

Table 2. Clinical Course of Schizophrenic First Admissions during 5-year Follow-Up (1975–1980)

Clinical course	Males		Females		Total	
	N	%	*N*	%	*N*	%
One episode only–no impairment	4	15.4	7	31.8	11	23.0
More than one episode with no or minimal impairment	9	34.6	8	36.4	17	35.4
Impairment after first episode with subsequent exacerbations and no return to normality	1	3.8	3	13.6	4	8.3
Impairment increasing with each of several episodes and no return to normality	12	46.2	4	18.2	16	33.3
Total	26	100	22	100	48	100

of schizophrenic illness. Table 2 shows the course of illness for the first admissions.

Considering the total column only, 23% had only one episode and 35% had more than one episode with a final remission, yielding a total of 58% with an episodic course. It is interesting to note that the females had a much better episodic course than the males, with 31.8% having only one episode and 36.4% having more than one episode with final remission, for a total of 68.2% with an episodic course.

The superior outcome for the females is even more striking as shown in Figure 1, which shows the percentage of first-admission schizophrenics discharged and not readmitted during the last few decades.

Although the proportion of males vascillated around 35%, the corresponding proportion for females increased during the last four decades from

Figure 1. Percentage of first-admission schizophrenics discharged and not readmitted during the subsequent 5 years. Striped = males; white = females; black = total. (Adapted from Watt, Katz, and Shepherd, 1983, Fig. 3, p. 668.)

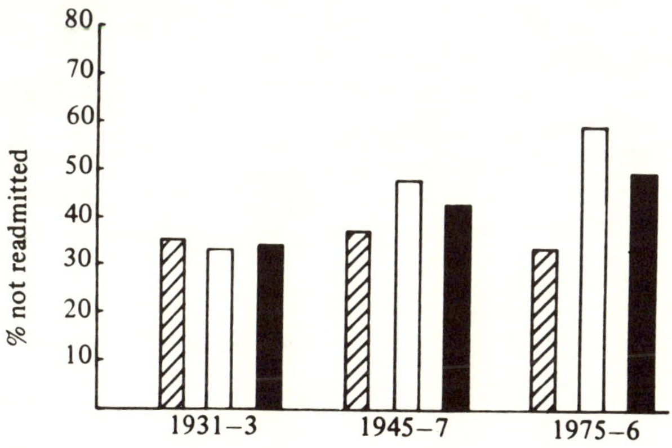

33% to 60%. This superior outcome for females should be investigated more thoroughly, because the sources of recidivism may be revealed in such an analysis.

Further evidence of the episodic course of schizophrenia even in patients whose duration of illness extended for 15 or more years after the initial episode is given in the study of Shmaonova, Lieberman, Lobova, and Kramelashvill (1983). Some 30% had only one episode, 25% two episodes, 16% three episodes, and the rest had from 4 to 11 episodes in decreasing frequencies. It is not clear whether these data represent exacerbations of an ongoing episode, "attacks," or new episodes.

The Revolution in Descriptive Psychopathology

This revolution had many causes. Its early beginnings can be traced to Adolf Meyer and, later, to Nolan D. C. Lewis (D. Zubin & Zubin, 1977), who recruited me to help in the revision of the Mental Status Examination Handbook in 1944 (Lewis, 1944). This work was interrupted by military service, but on my return from the war first Eugene Burdock and then Anne Hardesty and Gad Hakerem helped to launch an attack on improving the psychiatric interview, in the form of a Ward Behavior Interview (Burdock, 1960). They in turn initiated Robert L. Spitzer and, later, Jean Endicott into the preparation of items for structured clinical interviews, in which effort Joseph Fleiss and Jacob Cohen also participated. At the same time, with the help of Morton Kramer, the now-classic US–UK Project was organized. This project demonstrated the usefulness of systematic interviewing and its potential for clarifying diagnoses both here and abroad. This was accomplished by Barry Gurland with the collaboration of Lawrence Sharpe and Joseph Fleiss and a team of devoted assistants in the U.S., and by John Cooper, Robert Kendell, and John Copeland and their associates in the U.K. This study, together with the WHO Pilot Study of Schizophrenia and the pioneering work of the St. Louis school under Eli Robbins, laid the foundation for the revolution in diagnosis, which culminated under the direction of Spitzer and Endicott in a series of interview instruments and, finally, in DSM-III and the Research Diagnostic Criteria.

The reception of the Schedule for Affective Disorders and Schizophrenia (SADS) and DSM-III by the profession indicates that a great need has been filled. A few issues have been raised regarding this revolution. The first is the question of the definition of schizophrenia. It is high time we realized that rigorous, mathematically tight definitions do not hold for nature, only for abstract mathematics. If we tried to introduce such rigor into psychopathology we would end up with rigor mortis. If it were necessary that a category be defined rigidly, such widely useful concepts as "species" would go by the board. As Julian Huxley (1940) has pointed out:

> There is no single criterion of species. Morphological difference; failure to interbreed; infertility of offspring; ecological, geographical, or genetical distinctness—all those must be taken into account, but none of them singly is decisive. Failure to interbreed or to produce fertile offspring is the nearest approach to a positive criterion. It is, however, meaningless in apogamous forms, and as a negative criterion it is not applicable, many obviously distinct species, especially of plants, yielding fertile offspring, often with free Mendelian recombination in crossing. A combination of criteria is needed, together with some sort of flair. (p. 11)

It should be borne in mind that certain dangers may lurk in the standardization of interviewing and diagnosis. In the course of their training, researchers and clinicians have to develop certain required skills, such as interviewing, apparatus handling, research design and statistics. Unfortunately, in the course of this onerous training, they often let their imagination lag. ". . . skill without imagination is craftmanship and gives us many useful objects such as wickerwork picnic baskets. . . ," says Tom Stoppard (1973), but it is not creative. There is a great need for reviving the imagination of our researchers. For example, the skill in interviewing and diagnosis has reached a point where some now consider it possible to determine the diagnosis by following blindly the skills learned in the training process. This routine interviewing, good as it is for meeting daily clinical needs, is not sufficient for research and diagnosis and may stultify our knowledge as of 1984. We need to reintroduce the curiosity and creativity that developed the current available skills in the first place, in order to permit innovations to occur. Standardized craftsmanship leads to sterility, as has been the case with intelligence testing. Only with the development of the information-processing approach and the rise of cognitive psychology have the shackles of standardized tests been removed as an obstacle blocking further research in intelligence. Looking at the patient, listening to his or her style, developing empathic relationships instead of merely noting the answers to the items on the interview, become prerequisites for the improvement of interviewing techniques and diagnosis. For diagnosis is, in fact, a mini-experiment in which a series of hypotheses are examined for their tenability until the most tenable hypothesis regarding the diagnosis is reached.

But why, despite the improvement in our techniques, is it still so difficult to determine the presence of a schizophrenic syndrome? Despite the advances made in descriptive psychopathology, genetics, biochemistry, and biophysics, we have not yet found the etiology of any of the mental disorders and must still depend on behavioral syndromes. But the behavior of the patient is determined not only by his current mental disorder but also by his underlying premorbid personality, and it is this mixture that is presented at the time of admission. If we could dissect the behavior due to the mental disorder from the behavior due to premorbid personality and to the interaction of the two, we could recognize the focal disorder in isolation from its surround and probably find this factor characteristic of all similarly afflicted patients. What we perceive, however, is not the effect of the focal disorder alone, but the effect of the illness, which reflects the premorbid personality, and the focal disorder, and their interaction. This is why no two schizophrenics are alike—their focal disorder may be the same but their illness is different. The relation between premorbid personality and psychopathology is still moot and involves such thorny issues as the distinction between "trait" and "state."

The Search for Etiology

Another new direction that has developed during the last 16 years is the investigation of markers for the various scientific etiological models that have been suggested for schizophrenia (J. Zubin & Steinhauer, 1981). These include the biologically based genetic, internal environment, neurophysiological, and neuroanatomical models on the one hand, and the environmentally based ecological, developmental, and learning models on the other hand.

In view of the multiplicity of models, an interdisciplinary supermodel had to be developed to encompass them as submodels for an understanding of etiology. This gave rise to the vulnerability model (J. Zubin & Spring, 1977), as depicted in Figure 2.

Briefly stated, the vulnerability model assumes that schizophrenia is essentially episodic, developing in a vulnerable individual when subjected to exogenous or endogenous stressors. When the episode terminates the patients return to their premorbid level of adjustment. For the good premorbid patients, we consider the ending of the episode and the return of the patient to his or her premorbid niche, a recovery, or at least a remission. For the poor premorbids, it is difficult to know whether the episode has ended, because a return to the premorbid level still does not enable them to function and they are often mistakenly considered as persisting in their episode. However, not all the vulnerable who undergo stressors necessarily develop episodes. The moderating variables of premorbid personality, social networks, and ecological niches, if favorable, may cushion the impact of the stressor and the episode is aborted (J. Zubin, Magaziner, & Steinhauer, 1983).

One of the obstacles to accepting the vulnerability model is the problem presented by the so-called chronic or long-term patients. Is chronicity an essential part of the natural development of an episode, a side effect, or is it an artifact? It is generally agreed today by what might be called the psychiatric establishment that schizophrenia is a chronic disorder or even a disease that persists throughout the life of the individual bearing that diagnosis, that it is essentially genetically transmitted, and that complete recovery is rather rare, because residual symptoms of the disorder develop

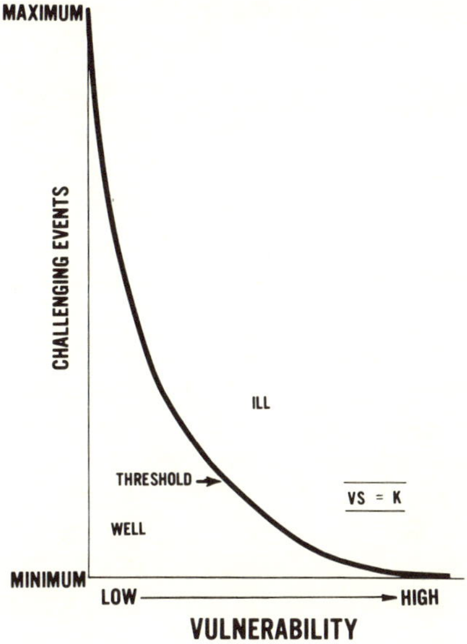

Figure 2. Relation between vulnerability and challenging life events. The equation for this hypothetical curve is $VS = K$, where V is the degree of vulnerability, S is the degree of stress induced by the challenging event, and K is a constant. (Adapted from Zubin and Steinhauer, 1981, Fig. 2, p. 481.)

that characterize the person throughout life and prevent a return to society to the fullest degree.

The thesis presented here challenges the established view and provides the tentative evidence for a newly emerging view of this disorder, which might be summarized as follows: Although the established view maintains that the person diagnosed as schizophrenic is essentially sick but may have intermittent periods of wellness, the new view maintains that this person is essentially well but may have one or more intemittent episodes of illness.

This view challenges chronicity as a natural part of the disorder. It maintains that the persistent feature of this disorder is not its continued existence, but the presence of a vulnerability that may or may not develop into an episode. It considers genetics to be neither a sufficient nor a necessary etiological agent, nor the only possible etiological agent. Many of the residual symptoms masquerading as chronicity may be artifacts produced by the reaction of the individual himself, the peer group, and society as a whole to the acute episode that had developed. It may also reflect the return to the poor premorbid personality at the end of the episode, or the toxic niche to which the patient returns.

In view of the fact that chronicity is generally regarded as an expected stage in the course of schizophrenia, it is well to examine the evidence for and against the proposition that chronicity is indigenous to schizophrenia. Against this proposition are the following arguments:[3]

3. The arguments pro and con chronicity follow the paradigm presented by Ciompi (1980a).

Arguments against Chronicity as an Indigenous Component of Schizophrenia

1. *Not universal:* Not all schizophrenics develop chronic states. Bleuler found no more than 10% continuously hospitalized after first admission in his follow-up study.

2. *Prevalence is exaggerated:* The apparent prevalence of chronicity is due to the accumulation of a small proportion of chronics, but even of these, in Bleuler's follow-up, 30% remain in the hospital for lack of any other home.

3. *General trend in outcome is remission rather than chronicity:* Long-term follow-up studies (Bleuler, Ciompi, Huber) indicate that the general trend is toward improvement rather than deterioration. Sporadic recovery can occur even after a lifetime of chronicity.

4. *Environment rather than heredity is associated with chronicity:* Long-term outcome is often independent of family history of schizophrenia—environment rather than heredity may influence the appearance of chronicity. Such moderating variables as social networks, ecological niches, and premorbid personality, if favorable, may mitigate the impact of stressors but, if unfavorable, may exacerbate the impact leading to chronicity.

5. *Chronicity is associated with psychosocial factors:*

a. Life events play a triggering role in recidivism and in maintenance of chronic episodes.

b. Labeling impact prevents readjustment, especially occupationally.

c. Highly critical families play a role in the prolongation and resumption of schizophrenia episodes.

6. *Negative symptoms do improve with neuroleptic treatment and do respond to amphetamines* (Boronow & van Kammen, 1982).

Arguments in Favor of Indigenous Nature of Chronicity

1. *Irreversibility of negative symptoms*:

a. It has been claimed that the presence of irreversible negative symptoms characterizies chronic schizophrenia, but negative symptoms may be associated with chronicity because they may have been premorbidly present, and when the episode ends, the patients return to their premorbid level including their negative symptoms. As evidence for this possibility, 70% of Bleuler's probands had deviant premorbid personalities including negative symptoms, and about 58% of these poor premorbids were regarded as attaining a moderately severe or severe end state (chronic) (Zubin *et al.*, 1983). Furthermore, deviant behavior can develop due to institutionalization and isolation and may be mistakenly regarded as a natural consequence of schizophrenia. For example, negative symptoms are also seen in long-term prisoners, neglected residents of old age homes, nursing homes, etc.

b. It is often difficult to distinguish chronic schizophrenics from other chronic patients in the back wards of institutions, but these symptoms often disappear under social stimulation (Paul, 1977; Wing, 1970).

2. *Biochemical or organic basis*: No generally accepted evidence is available for any specific somatic, biochemical, or other organic basis for chronic schizophrenia. Chemical intervention, though effective in the acute phase against positive symptoms, is not generally effective in the chronic phase against negative symptoms; the latter may be more amenable to psychosocial intervention.

3. *Ubiquity of chronicity*: It has been claimed that chronicity is ubiquitous and that it transcends differences in environments. However, cross-cultural studies indicate that developing countries have better outcomes and hence less chronicity than developed countries (World Health Organization, 1974, 1978).

Thus, it may be concluded that the proposition that chronicity is *not* an indigenous part of the course of schizophrenia (except in a small proportion of cases) is quite tenable in view of currently available evidence (Ciompi, 1980b; Cutting, 1983; J. Zubin, in press; J. Zubin, Kietzman, & Steinhauer, in press).

The Future Perspective

DIAGNOSIS

Although it is not always easy to discern the trend of the future, some trends cast their shadows before them. With regard to descriptive psychopathology, it is quite clear that diagnosis has made tremendous strides. In contract with the 1920s and 1930s, when it was primarily an academic exercise without any significance for treatment or outcome, it has now become one of the most important single activities of the clinician. The wholesale acceptance of diagnosis by the law and by agencies dealing with third-party payments is sometimes a frightening spectacle. Witness, for example, the problem in P.K.U. where a certain titre of phenylalanine (in some states) makes it incumbent upon the clinician to intervene; or the shift from the criminal court to the clinic in cases in which embezzlement to support compulsive gambling changes a crime into an illness. There no doubt will be attempts to curb the law from running ahead of science or even keeping up with it. The law and third-party payments need to be handicapped at least a decade behind science in order to permit the tentative findings of science to be verified.

Another problem in descriptive psychopathology is the need to objectify the individual symptoms that form the basis of our syndromic diagnoses. Just as we have developed research criteria for diagnoses, we desperately need research criteria for the definition of anxiety, depersonalization, thought disorder, and so forth.

It will become necessary to separate diagnosis (an everyday clinical service) from classification (a scientific endeavor free from marketplace considerations and local social–cultural implications). There is a need for an Academy of Scholars to study the problem of taxonomy in psychopathology. Perhaps it would be necessary to first establish an academy for the taxonomy of human behavior, to lay a foundation for the classification of normative behavior before entering the arena of deviant behavior.

Another trend of the future is the development of approaches to the study of the validity of diagnosis as opposed to its reliability. We have gone as far as we can go with the latter, and further polishing of reliability independently of validity would turn us into craftsmen rather than scientists. There are signs that construct-validity approaches are beginning to develop that may provide a DSM of the future with objective indicators for at least some of the diagnostic categories. Elsewhere, I have laid out a blueprint for the study of vulnerability consisting of (1) discovery of markers to identify the vulnerable, (2) development of techniques for investigating the life-event triggers necessary to elicit the vulnerability, and (3) determination of moderating variables that prevent an episode from developing even when a life-event trigger strikes a vulnerable individual (J. Zubin *et al.*, 1983; J. Zubin & Steinhauer, 1981).

MARKERS

In future tests of the vulnerability hypothesis it will become necessary to find means of identifying the vulnerable, regardless of whether they do or do not exhibit their vulnerability in the form of an episode. These indicators of vulnerability generally have gone under the name of vulnerability markers. These refer to specific types of performance or characteristics that identify individuals who either had schizophrenic episodes in the past, are having one presently, or have a higher risk of developing an episode in the future.

The ideal marker is one that occurs only in schizophrenics and not in normal controls or in nonschizophrenic mental patients. At present, there are no such ideal markers. What we currently mean by a marker is a characteristic or behavior that discriminates (occurs significantly more frequently) schizophrenic from normal controls or nonschizophrenic mental patients. To simplify our discussion we shall tentatively refer only to the discrimination between schizophrenics and normal controls, and not deal with the discrimination between schizophrenics and nonschizophrenic mental patients.

Because of the heterogeneity of schizophrenia, it is not likely that pathognomonic markers will be found. More often these markers will also be found, albeit less frequently, in normals and in nonschizophrenic mental patients. Consequently, we may have to depend upon patterns across several markers to identify individuals vulnerable to schizophrenia. In analyzing the nature of the marker, that is, whether it is a vulnerability marker or episode marker, we have to determine the pattern it presents across the three time periods of pre-episode, episode, and postepisode, and whether or not it exists significantly more frequently or less frequently in first-degree relatives.

Table 3 shows the various types of markers in accordance with their pre-episode, episode, postepisode status and their familial frequency in siblings or other first-degree relatives. Because the starting point is usually a patient in the hospital with an episode, it is difficult to determine, without suitable follow-up or follow-back, whether the marker under investigation is an episode marker or a vulnerability marker.

Vulnerability Markers. A vulnerability marker should be present in the pre-episode, episode, and postepisode periods, and it also should be present in greater frequency than chance in unaffected first-degree relatives. We distinguish two types of vulnerability markers: (1) familial, which characterizes first-degree relatives with a frequency exceeding chance expectancy, and (2) nonfamilial, which does not exceed chance. Thus, marker *A* satisfies all the requirements for a vulnerability marker. *AA* is present during all the three specified periods but is not characteristic of first-degree relatives; hence it is probably nonfamilial. *D* is a vulnerability marker that disappears after the episode ends but nevertheless is found in first-degree relatives. Apparently the episode extinguishes the marker. Once a marker is established it can be applied to screen the general population for the presence of vulnerable individuals.

Episode Markers. The starting point in the search for episode markers is the individuals who are presently having an episode. *B* is such an episode marker because it waxes and wanes with the episode but does not characterize unaffected first-degree relatives. Once the marker is found, it may be applied to patients to determine whether the episode is still present, or to the general population to identify those who are undergoing an undetected episode.

Residual Markers. E and *G* are markers that make their appearance during the episode, but persist after the episode. It is still to be determined whether they are indigenous to the disorder or result from iatrogenic, nosocomial, or ecogenic factors.

Prodromal and Early Signs of Incipient Episodes. There are also certain prodromal characteristics that usually appear when an episode is imminent.

Table 3. Types of Markers by Pre-episode, Episode, and Postepisode Status, and Presence in First-degree Relatives

Marker	Pre-episode	Postepisode	First-degree relatives	Type of marker	
A	+	+	+	+	Vulnerability
AA	+	+	+	–*	Vulnerability
B	–	+	–	–	Episode
BB	–	+	–	+	?
C	+	–	+	+	Vulnerability
CC	+	–	+	–	Vulnerability (nonfamilial)
D	+	–	–	+	Vulnerability, normalized by episode
DD	+	–	–	–	Vulnerability (nonfamilial), normalized by episode
E	–	+	+	–	Residual effect of episode
EE	–	+	+	+	?
F	+	+	–	+	Vulnerability, normalized by episode
FF	+	+	–	–	Vulnerability (nonfamilial), normalized by episode
G	–	–	+	–	Residual effect of episode
GG	–	–	+	+	?
H	–	–	–	–	Nondifferential for schizophrenia
HH	–	–	–	+	Invulnerability

+ = Marker significantly more frequent in schizophrenics and/or first-degree relatives than in normal controls during the designated period
–* = Marker significantly less frequent in schizophrenics and/or first-degree relatives than in normal controls during the period
– = Marker not differential during the period
? = Doubt whether the pattern across the periods occurs in nature

These harbingers are not invariably followed by an episode and, therefore, are not regarded as markers but as predictors of a possibly approaching episode.

Invulnerability Markers. The *HH* marker, which is present in excess only in unaffected first-degree relatives of schizophrenics but not in the probands themselves, presents an interesting possibility. Perhaps an *HH* marker is an indicator of *invulnerability*, a characteristic that is antithetical to schizophrenia even as Meduna thought epilepsy was. Thus, although the first-degree relatives may share other vulnerability markers with their probands, the presence of the *HH* marker counteracts the vulnerability indicated by the other marker and eliminates the vulnerability of the individual. Similarly, the *AA* marker, which is absent in first-degree relatives in a proportion significantly below that in the general population but is present in the probands in pre-episode, episode, and postepisode intervals, may identify the individuals who are resistant to being vulnerable to schizophrenia. Had this marker been absent in the probands, they too may have not been vulnerable, even though they may have had other vulnerability markers. A search for such markers would indeed be a worthwhile endeavor.

BIOLOGICAL PERSPECTIVE

Among the many aspects that the biological approach provides, we have selected two as our chief guides in thinking during the coming years about biological aspects of schizophrenia: (1) the multiple biological roots of the disorder and (2) the role of the changing homeostasis of the internal environment of the patient.

We shall make the following assumptions:

1. Even though schizophrenia may be a phenomenologically unitary disorder, the etiology of schizophrenia is heterogeneous and/or multifactorial as was described previously in the seven scientific models.
2. The homeostatic disturbances observed in the incipient stage of the disorder can serve as an early indication of the imminence of an episode, as an exacerbation of an ongoing episode, or even as an early indication of the therapeutic response to treatment.

Heterogeneous Etiology

There seems to be increasing evidence that not all schizophrenia is genetically based. The recent evidence of brain atrophy in some schizophrenic patients, as reported by the Maudsley group, indicates that CT scan abnormalities occur more frequently in patients without schizophrenic relatives (Reveley, Reveley, Clifford, & Murray, 1982). Although normal lateral ventricle size is largely genetically controlled, the schizophrenic probands in pairs of discordant identical twins have the larger ventricles (Reveley, 1975). If some environmental event can cause this discrepancy in ventricular size, then a viral etiology becomes a tenable hypothesis for nonfamilial schizophrenia. The most recent data on seasonality of schizophrenic births support this notion (Watson, 1984). It is very intriguing that certain viruses have a preference for specific neurotransmitter systems such as dopamine, norepinephrine, or serotonin (Lycke & Roos, 1970; Shaskan, 1983). Lycke and Roos (1970) proposed that dopamine receptors could regulate viral entrance into a cell. Shaskan (1983) hypothesized that MAO may act as a virus receptor. Low-platelet MAO activity has been proposed as a vulnerability marker for schizophrenia and found to be associated with long-term hospitalization, neuroleptic treatment, and, ironically, with good premorbid functioning and extraversion. It also seems to correlate with severity of psychosis ($r = .62$, $N = 21$, $p < .003$).

Goldberg (this volume) addressed the differences between sporadic and genetic schizophrenia in great detail. It will be important in future studies of platelet MAO activity and in cognate studies to separate the patients with genetic loading from those without. Platelet MAO activity may turn out to be a moderating variable modifying the illness once it sets in (van Kammen *et al.*, 1981).

Brain atrophy such as enlarged ventricle size and cortical atrophy has been shown to be present in a substantial number of schizophrenic patients. This brain atrophy, which may be caused by brain damage, raises the possibility of pre- or perinatal trauma or anoxia or viral infection. Recently, Schulsinger *et al.* (1984) reported that obstetric complications in schizophrenic mothers led to wider ventricles in those of their children who became schizophrenic. This finding supports the concept that the CT scan abnormalities are associated with neuronal injury. Schulsinger *et al.* also proposed that perinatal trauma or anoxia may be necessary to bring out psychosis in patients with schizotypal personalities. Because 10% of schizophrenics have a familial history of the disorder and there is an excess of winter births among schizophrenic patients, prenatal infection may be an etiological agent. However, the absence of epidemics or higher rates of schizophrenia in the children of mental hospital staff militates against this possibility.

Brain atrophy in schizophrenic patients is associated with decreased CSF dopamine turnover (van Kammen *et al.*, 1981). Other findings include cognitive impairment and negative symptoms in patients with brain atrophy. This suggests that a subgroup of schizophrenic patients can now be identified by biological means.

Episodic Instability in Internal Environment as an Early Warning Sign Preceding Psychotic Behavior

The leading biological hypothesis of schizophrenia of the decade is the dopamine hypothesis. In reality, this appears to be a hypothesis of *psychotic* decompensation. Because psychotic decompensation is a dynamic process that develops over time, biological markers of impending relapse could perhaps be found. Close scrutiny of the pharmacological evidence for the dopamine hypothesis implicates the norepinephrine (NE) system as well (van Kammen & Antelman, 1984). Both neurotransmitter systems interact with each other and are involved with the autonomic nervous system. Autonomic arousal seems to increase prior to relapse. Rather than a trait marker, increased CSF NE may be a state-dependent early warning sign of psychotic decompensation (van Kammen & Antelman, 1984). However, the state of the internal environment may not be synononomous here with clinical status, and changes in the former precede changes in the latter (van Kammen *et al.*, 1982).

Other evidence supporting the possibility of identifying biochemical early warning signs comes from the amphetamine challenge test (van Kammen *et al.*, 1982). The concept of instability or episodic dysregulation in the interval environment preceding psychosis is consistent with the stress diathesis or vulnerability model of schizophrenia. Environmental stress can sensitize the internal environment or make it stress-tolerant. The amphetamine challenge test exposes the sensitivity to stress in the patients. In 50 patients treated with neuroleptics, the responses to the test identified beforehand those who would relapse following withdrawal from neuroleptics, an identification that could not be made clinically.

The two concepts of etiological heterogeneity and episodic instability do not contradict each other; they support and complement each other. They also promise a better methodological testing of, for instance, the dopamine hypothesis, by taking different etiologies and state dependency into account. These concepts do not identify a specific dopamine disorder, but provide for the possibility of several dopamine-related disturbances—be they supersensitivity of dopamine receptors, overactive regulator protein, different dopamine receptors, impaired dopamine release or utilization, impaired peptidergic, serotonergic, gabaergic or noradrenergic activity. Conversely, the same etiologies could be involved with different disorders including sporadic schizophrenia, affective disorders, and impulse disorders. These concepts also suggest that we should not expect to find a specific diagnostic marker applicable to all schizophrenic patients. So far that seems to hold true.

In summary, we see the next decade as breaking new ground in the following areas:

1. Defining the state-dependent dopamine and norepinephrine disturbances that precede an episode.
2. Identifying relapse-prone and neuroleptic-responsive patients, which will allow us to treat patients pharmacologically only as needed, something that Marvin Herz has also proposed (Herz, 1982).
3. Identifying patients who should be treated with lithium, propranolol, clonidine, or other nonneuroleptic agents.
4. Understanding the PET, brain-blood flow, and CT-scan findings in relationship to specific subgroups of patients and clinical states.

5. Separating and identifying different genetic and sporadic forms of schizophrenia.

6. Development of antipsychotic drugs without risk of extra-pyramidal side-effects or tardive dyskinesia (D-receptor antagonists).

PSYCHOPHYSIOLOGICAL PERSPECTIVE

One of the more exciting approaches to research in schizophrenia during the past decade has been the application of information-processing theory to psychopathology. In reviewing such activities, it is clear that much of the neurophysiological and other psychophysiological data are closely related to some purely behavioral techniques, such as reaction time, dichotic listening, and span of apprehension.

Significantly different performance for schizophrenics compared to normals have been reported so frequently and consistently that we tend to attribute any poorer performance on the patients' part to a "generalized performance deficit," rather than to a specific deviation characteristic of schizophrenia only.

Triggered by the incisive criticisms of Chapman and Chapman's (1973) more careful research, investigators have employed designs that attempt to control for such generalized deficits. For example, we had originally demonstrated that in a reaction-time task, schizophrenics not only performed more slowly than normals, but also had an unusually prolonged response to cross-modal stimuli, that is, stimuli that differed in sensory modality from the immediately preceding stimulus (Sutton, Hakerem, Zubin, & Portnoy, 1961; Waldbaum, Sutton, & Kerr, 1975). A recent dissertation by Manuzza (1982) of the Department of Psychophysiology laboratories at New York State Psychiatric Institute has reevaluated crossmodal retardation in schizophrenics from the perspective of the Chapmans' argument, and has demonstrated that the crossmodality retardation in schizophrenia is neither artifactual nor due to generalized deficit. Where does one go to next with such data? The logical step seems to be a determination of whether the findings are only meaningful across groups of subjects, or whether they can be applied to patients individually.

There are several important reasons for emphasizing a search for discriminating measures that can be used to characterize individuals rather than groups. One of the primary reasons is to establish new criteria for diagnostic subgroups. The iterative technique, advocated by Sutton (1973), suggests that the finding of identifiable differences that discriminate subgroups of schizophrenic patients on the basis of an experimental variable can be used as the stepping-off point for reexamining the confluence of symptomatology in such patients. Thus, the laboratory differences may provide a guide for directing the clinician to search more carefully for features that identify different types of patients.

Differences on experimental variables within the patient group may ultimately be used as a clinical tool to predict the type of therapeutic regimen that is most effective for each patient. An extension of this approach is to observe the reaction of patients to different pharmacotherapies, using a favorable reaction to assist in establishing diagnosis. This is an approach that currently seems to have gained greater headway in classification of depressive illnesses. A comparable type of discrimination that has been studied somewhat more among schizophrenics is the use of pharmacologic challenges that exacerbate symptoms among those who are apparently still within their episodes (Angrist & van Kammen, 1984; van Kammen *et al.*, 1982).

An example of the beginning of an evolution from characterization of overall group differences to individual characterization is the study of event-related potentials in schizophrenics. I take considerable pride in my participation in the "discovery"[4] by Dr. Samuel Sutton of the P300 component in our laboratories in 1964 (Sutton, Braren, Zubin, & John, 1965; Sutton, Tueting, Zubin, & John, 1967). P300 refers to a scalp-positive wave that occurs with a latency of approximately 300 msec, and is most closely related to the informational significance associated with an event, rather than primarily the physical characteristics of the event (Donchin, 1979; Sutton *et al.*, 1967). As detailed elsewhere (Steinhauer & Zubin, 1982), P300 was found while we were looking for evoked potential correlates of the effect of certainty and uncertainty in the cross-modality reaction time phenomena. Only the response of normal subjects had been recorded 17 years ago, and we still did not know whether P300 had any relevance for the study of schizophrenia. Not until 1972 did Roth and Cannon (1972) and then Levit in our own laboratories report that greatly diminished P300 amplitudes occur among schizophrenics (Levit, Sutton, & Zubin, 1973). Since that time, decreased P300 amplitude in schizophrenia has been one of the most robustly reported phenomena, replicated in laboratories all over the world, notably in the work of Shagass in Philadelphia and Roth, Pfefferbaum and Kopell in Palo Alto, among others. A more comprehensive survey of this literature is provided by J. Zubin *et al.* (in press). In a preliminary analysis, P300 has been reported by Friedman, working with the high-risk sample of

4. The discovery of P300, the cross-modality effect in reaction time, the findings of the US–UK Project, the development of semistructured interviewing, DSM-III, and RDC, and the development of the "immediacy hypothesis" were the high-water marks of our biometric endeavors.

Erlenmeyer-Kimling (Friedman, Vanghan, & Erlenmeyer-Kimling, 1982), to be significantly attenuated in the high-risk offspring of schizophrenics.

In our current studies in Pittsburgh, we have been examining P300 during a modified counting task. Not only do we find that P300 amplitudes are reduced, we also find a difference in the pattern of responses across experimental conditions, which suggests that many of the patients are utilizing information primarily from immediately preceding trials only (a phenomenon reflective of Salzinger's immediacy hypothesis), rather than responding to more complex aspects of sequential probabilities, which normal subjects seem to do quite naturally (Steinhauer & Zubin, 1982). Having observed these effects in the grouped data, we looked more closely at the responses of individual subjects, and realized that the pattern across conditions could be specified for individual subjects. There is increased confidence in the use of these patterns because parallel findings are observed in the pupillary dilation response and, to some degree, in cardiac changes, which are recorded simultaneously with the event-related potential. Thus, we may begin to classify patients on the basis of either amplitude alone, or patterning of this amplitude across experimental conditions. We can now indicate, even for smaller amplitude responses, whether the patient shows a pattern like that of normals or one of several identifiable different patterns not found in normals. As a result, we may consider using the laboratory findings for fractionating the schizophrenia group into subtypes.

The point of this brief discussion of the psychophysiological perspective has been not only to illustrate that it has been possible to change an emphasis from group differences to individual differences, but also to indicate the future of the information-processing approach in the study of schizophrenia. As it appears now, our objective is to utilize techniques that tell us something about the manner in which processing activities differ in schizophrenics—the what, where, when, and how that we have described in other papers (Kietzman, Spring, & Zubin, 1980; Zubin, in press). We need to understand what is different about the use of information among (at least a subgroup of) schizophrenics, and whether the type of deviation in processing activity occurs consistently in different situations. It does little good to continue to find a difference in overall response level between normals and schizophrenics in our electrophysiological, positron emission, biochemical, and behavioral measures, unless we use the knowledge to lead to new approaches to classification, treatment, and etiology.

Given the recent trend away from global research, which looked only for evidence that some construct such as arousal or attention was different in schizophrenia, to the more specifically guided experiments that seek to delineate stages of processing activity, there seems every reason to be optimistic about what the near future will reveal about the bases of schizophrenia. An exemplary model in the experimental psychopathology domain is the meta-like analysis of the skin-conductance orienting response undertaken by researchers from six different laboratories in Great Britain, West Germany, and the United States in attempting to bring order to previously divergent findings (Bernstein *et al.*, 1982).

PSYCHOSOCIAL PERSPECTIVE

The term *psychosocial factors* presently covers a diverse spectrum of studies, including research on the personality factors antedating the onset of schizophrenic psychoses and studies of the effects of stress and the familial environment on the course and outcome of the illness, as well as the work that focuses on how socioeconomic and cultural factors are related to the frequency and phenomenology of schizophrenic disorders. It covers a significant part of the research being done by psychologists, social psychiatrists, epidemiologists, sociologists, and anthropologists. We wish to take note of some of the more exciting work being carried on in this field and direct our attention toward what we consider to be some of the most interesting areas of future inquiry.

Many of the earlier hypotheses, such as those having to do with social-class position and the effects of poverty, have not proved to be as helpful as may have been initially expected. Yet, there remain significant findings in this area that we need to address. For example, there is much evidence to indicate that schizophrenic patients have a better course and outcome in the less developed and non-Western countries (World Health Organization, 1978). This has been documented in several studies by very reputable transcultural investigators (e.g., Lambo in Nigeria, Rin and Lin in Taiwan, Murphy in Mauritius, WHO in India, Waxler in Sri Lanka), and we are still lacking an adequate explanation for these international differences (Day, 1982).

In the past, the international work has focused on the development of a common language designed to facilitate communication across different cultural and theoretical traditions. A necessary part of this movement has been an emphasis on the aspects of schizophrenic disorders that are universal across cultures and time. Given the situation in the late 1950s when we were designing the US-UK Project (Cooper *et al.*, 1972), such a bias was understandable. Yet, a careful reading of the literature that has emerged from all of these large-scale international studies indicates that the cross-cultural variations in the schizophrenic syndrome are just as obvious and striking as are the commonalities. It is also our impression that a renewed interest is developing in the careful study of the degree and types of variation found in schizophrenia cross-culturally. Interestingly enough, much of the impetus for this type of work seems to be a product of the new generation of psychiatrists emerging in the developing countries. Many of these investigators are saying that our established classification systems fail to adequately describe what they see in their own clinical practice. In summary, it is our feeling that a renewed interest in and sensitivity to the influence of sociocultural factors on the genesis, phenomenology, course, and outcome of schizophrenic disorders will be one of the really exciting areas of theoretical and empirical work in the immediate future.

Closer to home, psychosocial research over the past 10 years has shown a growing emphasis on the application of biometric methods to the study of the social environment and its implications for the basic vulnerability to episodes of schizophrenia. Perhaps the most exciting work that has taken place in the past 10 years has occurred in the arena of the family. The research on the expressed emotion (EE) of family members and its relationship to schizophrenic relapse immediately comes to mind. Research in this area began in Great Britain and has now spread to the United States (see Kuipers, 1979), as well as to a number of non-English-speaking and non-Western countries. Hogarty (this volume) and Goldstein (this volume) describe some of the work going on in Pittsburgh and Los Angeles, respectively. The EE data reported so far have been striking, and we think that it is safe to assume that the work done in this area is going to have a substantial and permanent impact on the way we think about and treat the schizophrenias (Falloon *et al.*, 1982; Leff *et al.*, 1982). In addition to EE measures, research into communication deviance (CD) in the families of schizophrenic patients has also made significant progress in recent years. Of particular interest are the data suggesting that EE and CD may be independent measures that interact together to determine the probability of a negative outcome in specific cases (Doane *et al.*, 1981; Goldstein, 1983). It may well be that communication deviance in the family is associated more with the *etiology* of the condition, that is, a vulnerability marker, whereas expressed-emotion variables affect the short-term course of the illness, that is, may only serve as triggers. In the area of acute stressors such as life events, there has been an ongoing interest in their roles as triggers for specific episodes of the disorder (Day, 1981; Dohrenwend, 1981). We have seen the early drafts of some new international research, carried out by the World Health Organization, that support the involvement of life events in the onset of a majority of acute schizophrenic episodes.

All of this work is just a beginning, and it will be a long time before data are available that will permit the construction of a fully elaborated theory of the effects of psychosocial variables on the schizophrenias. We do believe, however, that such a theory is possible and represents a worthwhile goal for our future research. In this connection, it is valuable to give some thought to the areas that are most in need of study and would make the greatest contribution to the elaboration of our current knowledge.

It should be recalled that the greatest proportion of the work we have just discussed has involved schizophrenic patients and their families. It is also clear that the vast majority of so-called chronic or long-term schizophrenic patients do not live in family settings. We need to branch out and take advantage of the new concepts we have developed in order to increase the breadth and depth of our generalizations. In brief, the chronic long-term patient living outside of the family requires renewed attention in light of the data that have been collected over the past 10 years.

A second area where much work still remains to be done concerns the buffering factors that act to mitigate the effects of toxic factors such as expressed emotion and life events. The buffering factor about which we have the greatest knowledge is, of course, neuroleptic medications. Still, a large percentage of patients relapse while actively taking their medications and it is vital that we discover the role played by other exacerbating or buffering factors such as the patient's social network, ecological niche, and premorbid personality. Here we should emphasize the implications of social support and social network systems for the continuing health of patients with a schizophrenic vulnerability. There is a great need to expand our current knowlege to include systems that operate outside the immediate family milieu such as the extended nonkinfolk system and systems involving the peripheral members of the network (Hammer, 1983; Hammer, Makiesky-Barrow, & Gutwirth, 1978). If we consider the entire social network in which the proximate social network is imbedded, we can better understand the entire social matrix in which the individual lives—the microcosm that represents the portion of the macrocosm. It is this matrix that determines health and well being, illness, and even mortality.

In our study of recidivism in schizophrenia at the Highland Drive Veterans Administration Medical Center in Pittsburgh, we have been impressed by the large number of outpatients that never fully achieve a proper remission from illness. Instead, they remain actively psychotic while living in the community. How much of this chronic symptomatology can be explained by the fact that these people leave to hospital only to return to toxic community settings where they exist within alienating, lonely, and, sometimes, downright frightening social circumstances? We believe that we can prove that more than just a negligible proportion of this chronic symtomatology is socially induced.

This raises a final point. Let us recall that schizophrenia, as we know it, involves a central or acute syndrome, as well as long-term states of impaired functioning. The studies we have reviewed in this report have focused almost exclusively on the problems of florid relapse and the appearance of positive symptomatology. Our work in the Veterans Administration system has made us acutely aware of the absence of new and exciting inroads into the problems of so-called chronic deficit states or long-term episodes. Important theoretical and practical advances are yet to be made in this area. The most recent data from long-term European follow-up studies indicate that, contrary to general opinion, the majority of the schizophrenics need not have a disastrous outcome. We firmly believe that when we take the time to do the requisite research, we are going to find out that the greatest part of the "iceberg" of disability is actually a socially induced artifact and not an inherent part of the illness process itself. If we are correct in this, we may also speculate that it is in this area, the study of chronic states of disability and impairment, that psychosocial researchers have the greatest potential contribution to make. It is our position that schizophrenia, in the vast majority of cases, is an episodic condition and need not result in the chronic deficit states that we have come to both expect and to accept as a self-fulfilling prophecy.

SUMMARY

It is clear that the greatest advance in the 1970s has been in descriptive psychopathology and, to prevent this success from becoming a failure in the 1980s, we must encourage innovative imagination to overcome the drift toward rigid application of standardized procedures.

Concerning the improved outlook in outcome of schizophrenia, the evidence from long term follow-up studies in Europe indicates that a significant proportion of schizophrenics have only one episode, from which they recover, and that an even larger proportion show an episodic course of several episodes with final remission. Only a small proportion remain chronically ill, but they are the ones who accumulate in our facilities and give schizophrenia its undeserved reputation for chronicity. The evidence has also shown that there is considerable doubt whether much of the chronicity that overwhelms our daily practicioners and engenders pessimism is indigenous to schizophrenia. There is reason to believe that it may be an artifact engendered by iatrogenic, ecogenic, and nosocomial factors.

As for vulnerability markers, several potential candidates have been found with frequencies greater than chance expectancy both in probands and in their unaffected first-degree relatives.

1. Crossover index in reaction time (Shakow)
2. Smooth pursuit eye movement index (Holzman)
3. Continuous performance task (Kornetsky, Mirsky *et al.*)
4. Span of apprehension (Asarnow)
5. Dichotic listening with distraction (Spring)
6. Platelet MAO

We have yet to determine whether these markers are vulnerability markers, episode markers, or residual markers.

Although the specificity of each of these markers for schizophrenia is still to be established, the possibility exists that patterns across these markers may serve to identify subgroups of schizophrenia and thus to reduce the apparent heterogeneity of global schizophrenia.

The availability of such markers and the proposed behavioral and chemical challenges for eliciting episode markers, as well as the possibility of early warning signs of the imminence of an episode, indicate that the future bodes well for supplementing the current clinical diagnoses and treatment with objective indicators that may succeed in reducing the heterogeneity of our nosological categories and reduce the excessive use of neuroleptics and other treatment modalities. These, together with the development of more knowledge about the role of the psychosocial factors in the development of episodes or in their triggering, ought to provide more efficient methods for therapeutic and preventive intervention.

ACKNOWLEDGMENTS

The authors wish to thank Ms. Wendy Ferzacca for valuable assistance in the preparation of the manuscript. This work was supported by the Medical Research Service and the Health Services Research and Development Service of the Veterans Administration, and by NIMH grant MH30915.

REFERENCES

Angrist, B., & van Kammen, D. P. (1984). C.N.S. Stimulants as tools in the study of schizophrenia. *Trends in Neuroscience*, *7*, 388–390.

Bernstein, A. S., Frith, C. D., Gruzelier, J. H., Patterson, T., Straube, E., Venables, P. H., & Zahn, T. P. (1982). An analysis of the skin conductance orienting response in samples of American, British, and German schizophrenics. *Biological Psychology*, *14*, 155–211.

Bleuler, M. (1978). *The schizophrenic disorders: Long-term patient and family studies*. New Haven, CT: Yale University Press [*Die Schizophrenen Geistesstorungen im Lichte Langjahriger Kranken*. Stuttgart: Thieme, 1972].

Boronow, J. D., & van Kammen, D. P. (1982). *Amphetamine lowers negative schizophrenic symptoms*. Presented at the American Psychiatric Association meeting—New Research Section, May.

Burdock, E. I. (1960). A ward behavior rating scale for mental hospital patients. *Journal of Clinical Psychology*, *16*, 246–247.

Chapman, L. J., & Chapman, J. P. (1973). Problems in the measurement of cognitive deficit. *Psychological Bulletin*, *79*, 380–385.

Ciompi, L. (1980a). Ist die chronische Schizophrenie ein Artefakt?—Argumente und gegenargumente [Is chronic schizophrenia an artifact?—Arguments and counter arguments]. *Fortschritte der Neurologie und Psychiatrie*, *48*, 237–248.

Ciompi, L. (1980b). The natural history of schizophrenia in the long term. *British Journal of Psychiatry, 136*, 413–420.

Cooper, J. E., Kendell, R. E., Gurland, B. J., Sharpe, L., Copeland, J. R. M., & Simon, R. (1972). *Psychiatric diagnosis in New York and London* (Maudsley Monograph Series No. 20) New York: Oxford University Press.

Cutting, J. (Sect. Ed.). (1983). Schizophrenic deterioration. *British Journal of Psychiatry, 143*, 77–84.

Day, R. (1981). Life events and schizophrenia: The triggering hypothesis. *Acta Psychiatrica Scandinavica, 64*, 97–122.

Day, R. (1982). Research in the course and outcome of schizophrenia in traditional cultures. In M. J. Goldstein (Ed.), *Preventive intervention in schizophrenia: Are we ready*? National Institute of Mental Health, DHHS Publication No (ADM) 82–1111, pp. 197–219.

Doane, J., West, K. L., Goldstein, M. J., Rodnick, E. H., & Jones, J. E. (1981). Parental communication deviance and affective style. *Archives of General Psychiatry, 38*, 679–685.

Dohrenwend, B. P. (1981). Recent stressful life events and episodes of schizophrenia. *Schizophrenia Bulletin, 7*, 12–23.

Donchin, E. (1979). Event-related potentials: A tool in the study of human information processing. In H. Begleiter (Ed.), *Evoked brain potentials and behavior* (pp. 13–88). New York: Plenum Press.

Duncan-Johnson, C. C. (in press). P300 applications to research on schizophrenia. *Electroencephalography and Clinical Neurophysiology*.

Falloon, I. R. H., Boyd, L., McGill, C. W. *et al.* (1982). Family management in the prevention of exacerbations of schizophrenia. *New England Journal of Medicine, 306*, 1437–1440.

Friedman, D., Vaughan, H. G., Jr., & Erlenmeyer-Kimling, L. (1982). Cognitive brain potentials in children at risk for schizophrenia: Preliminary findings and methodological considerations. *Schizophrenia Bulletin, 8*, 514–531.

Goldstein, M. J. (1983). Family interaction: Patterns predictive of the onset and course of schizophrenics. In H. Stierlin, L. C. Wynne, & M. Wirsching (Eds.), *Psychosocial intervention in schizophrenia* (pp. 5–19). Berlin & New York: Springer-Verlag.

Hammer, M. (1983). Care and extended social networks in relation to health and illness. *Social Science and Medicine, 7*, 405–411.

Hammer, M.,Makiesky-Barrow, S., & Gutwirth, L. (1978). Social networks and schizophrenia. *Schizophrenia Bulletin, 4*, 552–545.

Herz, M. I. (1982). Intermittent medication for stable schizophrenic outpatients: An alternative to maintenance medication. *American Journal of Psychiatry, 138*(7), 918–922.

Huber, G., Gross, G., Schüttler, R., & Linz, M. (1980). Longitudinal studies of schizophrenic patients. *Schizophrenia Bulletin, 6*, 592–605.

Huxley, J. S. (1940). Introductory: Towards the new systematics. In J. S. Huxley (Ed.), *The new systematics*. London & New York: Oxford University Press (Clarendon).

Kietzman, M. L., Spring, B., & Zubin, J. (1980). Perception, cognition, and attention. In H. I. Kaplan, A. M. Freedman, & B. J. Sadock (Eds.), *Comprehensive textbook of psychiatry/III* (pp. 334–371). Baltimore: Williams & Wilkins.

Kuipers, L. (1979). Expressed emotion: A review. *British Journal of Social and Clinical Psychology, 18*(18), 237–243.

Leff, J., Kuipers, L., Berkowitz, R., *et al.* (1982). A controlled trial of social intervention in the families of schizophrenic patients. *British Journal of Psychiatry, 141*(141), 121–134.

Levit, R. A., Sutton, S., & Zubin, J. (1973). Evoked potential correlates of information processing in psychiatric patients. *Psychological Medicine, 3*, 487–494.

Lewis, N. D. C. (1944). *Outlines for psychiatric examinations*. New York: New York State Department of Mental Hygiene.

Lycke, E., & Roos, B. E. (1970). The monoamine metabolism in viral encephalitis of the Mouse. I. Virological and biochemical results. *Brain Research, 23*, 235–246.

Manuzza, S. (1982). *The modality shift effect in schizophrenia - fact or artifact?* Doctoral dissertation, City University of New York.

Paul, G. L. (1977). *Psychosocial treatment of chronic mental patients: Milieu versus social-learning programs.* Cambridge, MA: Harvard University Press.

Reveley, M. A. (1975). Genetics of platelet MAO activity in discordant schizophrenic and normal twins. *British Journal of Psychiatry, 142*, 560–565.

Reveley, M. A., Reveley, A. M., Clifford, C. A., & Murray, R. M. (1982). Cerebral ventricular size in twins discordant for schizophrenia. *Lancet*, March 6, 1982, 540–541.

Roth, W. T., & Cannon, E. H. (1972). Some features of the auditory evoked response in schizophrenics. *Archives of General Psychiatry, 27*, 466–471.

Schulsinger, F., Parnas, J., Peterson, E. T., Schulsinger, H., Teasdale, T. W., Mednick, S. A., Moller, L. & Sivlerton, L. (1984). Cerebral ventricular size in offspring of schizophrenic mothers: A preliminary study. *Archives of General Psychiatry, 41*, 602–606.

Shaskan, E. G. (1983). Is there functional significance for dopamine antagonist binding sites on lymphoid cells? *Advances in Biological Psychiatry, 12*, 123–141.

Shmaonova, L. M., Lieberman, Yu.I., Lobova, E. K., & Kramelashvili, V. V. (1983). Frequency of acute schizophrenic episodes. *Psychiatric Journal of the University of Ottawa, 139*, (7), 5–16.

Steinhauer, S., & Zubin, J. (1982). Vulnerability to schizophrenia: Information processing in the pupil and event-related potential. In E. Usdin & I. Hanin (Eds.), *Biological markers in psychiatry and neurology* (pp. 371–385). Oxford: Pergamon Press.

Stoppard, T. (1973). Artist descending a staircase. In *Albert Bridge and other plays* (p. 83). New York: Grove Press.

Sutton, S. (1973). Fact and artifact in the psychology of schizophrenia. In M. Hammer, K. Salzinger, & S. Sutton (Eds.), *Psychopathology: Contributions from the social, behavioral and biological sciences* (pp. 197–213). New York: Wiley.

Sutton, S., Braren, M., Zubin, J., & John, E. R. (1965). Evoked-potential correlates of stimulus uncertainty. *Science, 150*, 1187–1188.

Sutton, S., Hakerem, G., Zubin, J., & Portnoy, M. (1961). The effect of shift of sensory modality on serial reaction time: A comparison of schizophrenics and normals. *American Journal of Psychology, 74*, 224–232.

Sutton, S., Tueting, P., Zubin, J., & John, E. R. (1967). Information delivery and the sensory evoked potential. *Science, 155*, 1436–1439.

Tukey, J. W. (1962). The future of data analysis. *Annals of Mathematical Statistics, 33*, 1–67.

van Kammen, D. P., Bunney, W. E., Jr., Docherty, J. P., *et al.* (1982). d-Amphetamine-induced heterogeneous changes in psychotic behavior in schizophrenia. *American Journal of Psychiatry, 139*, 991–997.

van Kammen, D. P., & Antelman, S. M. (1984). Minireview: Impaired noradrenergic transmission in schizophrenia. *Life Sciences, 34*, 1403–1413.

van Kammen, D. P., Malas, K. L., Sternberg, D. E., Murphy, D. L., Lerner, P., Lake, C. R., Dalton, L. A., & Bunney, W. E., Jr. (1981). Platelet monoamine oxidase (MAO) and clinical variables in schizophrenia: Interrelationships with spinal fluid norepinephrine (NE) and dopamine-beta-hydroxylase (DBH). *Psychopharmacology Bulletin, 17*(3), 207–209.

Waldbaum, J. K., Sutton, S., & Kerr, J. (1975). Shift of sensory modality and reaction time in schizophrenia. In M. L. Kietzman, S. Sutton, & J. Zubin (Eds.), *Experimental approaches to psychopathology* (pp. 167–176). New York: Academic Press.

Watson, C. G. (1984). Schizophrenic birth seasonality in relation to the incidence of infectious diseases and temperature extremes. *Archives of General Psychiatry, 41*, 85–90.

Watt, D. C., Katz, K., & Shepherd, M. (1983). The natural history of schizophrenia: A 5-

year prospective follow-up of a representative sample of schizophrenics by means of a standardized clinical and social assessment. *Psychological Medicine*, *13*, 663–670.

Wing, J. K. (1970). *Institutionalism and schizophrenia*. London & New York: Cambridge University Press.

World Health Organization (1974). *International pilot study of schizophrenia*. Geneva: Wiley.

World Health Organization (1978). *Schizophrenia: An international follow-up study*. London: Wiley.

Zubin, J. (in press). Implications of the vulnerability model for DSM-IV. In T. Millon & G. Klerman (Eds.), *Contemporary directions in psychopathology: Toward the DSM–IV*. New York: Guilford.

Zubin, J., Kietzman, M. L., & Steinhauer, S. R. (in press). General clinical psychology in relation to psychiatry. In *Handbook of psychiatry* (Vol. 5). London & New York: Cambridge University Press.

Zubin, J., Magaziner, J., & Steinhauer, S. R. (1983). The metamorphosis of schizophrenia: From chronicity to vulnerability. *Psychological Medicine*, *13*.

Zubin, J., & Spring, B. (1977). Vulnerability: A new view of schizophrenia. *Journal of Abnormal Psychology*, *86*, 103–126.

Zubin, J., & Steinhauer, S. R. (1981). How to break the logjam in schizophrenia: A look beyond genetics. *Journal of Nervous and Mental Disease*, *169*, 447–492.

Zubin, D., & Zubin, J. (1977). From speculation to empiricism in the study of mental disorder: Research at the New York State Psychiatric Institute in the first half of the twentieth century. *Annals of the New York Academy of Sciences*, *291*, 104–135.

SECTION TWO

BIOLOGICAL BASES

5

Regional Cerebral Blood Flow in Schizophrenia

RAQUEL E. GUR
University of Pennsylvania

THE XENON-133 TECHNIQUE

The introduction by Kety *et al.* (1948) and Kety and Schmidt (1945) of the nitrous oxide method for measurement of cerebral blood flow (CBF) in man provided the basis for later developments in the study of regional cerebral blood flow (rCBF) and metabolism. The xenon-133 inhalation method, first described by Mallett and Veall (1963, 1965), is a noninvasive procedure that enables repeated measurements in the same subject. A two-compartmental exponential model was proposed (Obrist, Thompson, Wang, & Wilkinson, 1975) in which a faster clearing compartment, presumably gray matter, is separated from a slower clearing compartment, considered to be white matter and extracerebral tissue. The procedure entails inhalation of trace amounts of isotope (5–7 mCi/liter) mixed with air through a face mask for one minute. The uptake and clearance of isotope from the brain is monitored by collimated sodium iodide crystal detectors placed over the scalp. Endtidal air is used to estimate isotope concentration and $p\mathrm{CO}_2$ of arterial blood. The CBF is computed from the clearance rates as described by Obrist *et al.* (1975). A number of CBF indices have been described and applied in the study of normals and pathological populations (Obrist *et al.*, 1975; Risberg, Ali, Wilson, Wills, & Halsey, 1975) and their stability and sensitivity has been evaluated (Obrist & Wilkinson, 1985).

The studies conducted in our laboratory, which will be presented in this chapter, used the initial slope (IS), defined as the tangent at time zero of an equivalent bolus injection (Obrist & Wilkinson, 1979), as the CBF index. IS is sensitive to blood flow in the fast-clearing gray matter compartment.

RESTING rCBF IN SCHIZOPHRENIA

Initial studies on whole-brain CBF showed no consistent differences between schizophrenics and normals (Della Porta *et al.*, 1964; Gordan, Estess, Adams, Bowman, & Simon, 1955; Hoyer & Oesterreich, 1975; Kety *et al.*, 1948; Wilson, Schieve, & Scheinberg, 1952). The application of the intracarotid injection technique enabled measurements of rCBF in one hemisphere at a time. Using this method in a sample of 9 chronic elderly schizophrenic females, Ingvar and Franzen (1974a, 1974b) found decreased frontal flows in the left hemisphere. However, a sample of 11 young schizophrenics showed hyperfrontality.

The introduction of the xenon-133 inhalation method permitted studies of bilateral rCBF in schizophrenics. Mathew *et al.* (1981) reported lower right hemisphere flows in 6 unmedicated chronic schizophrenics, compared to 6 matched controls. In a subsequent study (Mathew, Duncan, Weinman, & Barr, 1982) of 23 unmedicated schizophrenics and 18 controls, general decreased flows were reported for the schizophrenics. Global reduction in resting flows were also found by Ariel *et al.* (1983), who compared 29 medicated schizophrenics to 22 controls. The interpretation of these studies is hindered, however, by lack of control for $p\text{CO}_2$ (Mathew *et al.*, 1982) and demographic variables (Ariel *et al.*, 1983), such as sex and education.

Sex differences in rCBF have been documented (Gur *et al.*, 1982). Although there have been no systematic studies correlating rCBF specifically with education, this factor certainly contributes to dietary habit and general health, which may influence the integrity of the cerebrovascular system.

No resting rCBF differences were obtained by Gur *et al.* (1983) in a study of 15 medicated schizophrenics and 25 controls, matched for age, sex, education, and socioeconomic background.

In a subsequent study (Gur *et al.*, 1985) of 19 unmedicated schizophrenics and 19 matched controls, resting flow differences were observed. Specifically, whereas normal controls had symmetric flows, unmedicated schizophrenics had higher left than right hemispheric flows. This finding is consistent with behavioral data suggesting left hemispheric overactivation in schizophrenics (Gur, 1978; Schweitzer, Becker, & Welsh, 1978).

Sheppard *et al.* (1983) obtained consistent results in a sample of unmedicated schizophrenics and matched controls. CBF was measured by positron emission tomography with oxygen-15-labeled water.

ACTIVATED rCBF IN NORMALS

Since neural activity produces increased energy metabolism and metabolic activity is, in turn, highly coupled with CBF (Reivich, 1974), the physiologic measures could be used in experimental research where human subjects are engaged in specific tasks. This will enable rigorously controlled investigation of brain regions that participate in these behavioral functions. Supporting the feasibility of such investigations, increased rCBF was demonstrated with the xenon-133 technique for simple sensory stimulation as well as during the execution of motor movements (e.g., Lassen, Roland, Larsen, Melamed, & Soh, 1977; Halsey, Blauenstein, Wilson, Wills, & Greenspoon, 1977). Visual stimulation produced increase in rCBF in the area of primary and association visual cortex, and auditory stimulation increased rCBF in the auditory cortex. Rhythmical movement of the eyes produced bilateral increase in rCBF in areas corresponding to the "frontal eye fields" (Lassen *et al.*, 1977). Rhythmical movement of the hand (Olesen, 1971), fingers, lips, and toes activated the respective contralateral motor areas.

The sensitivity of the physiologic techniques to blood flow changes produced by sensory stimulation suggests that they can also be used to map more complex cognitive functions. This was initially examined by Ingvar and Risberg (1967), using the intracarotid xenon-133 technique. Increased rCBF was found during cognitive activity compared to resting baseline. Risberg and Ingvar (1973) measured rCBF in the dominant hemisphere in a group of chronic alcoholics. A visually presented reasoning task and an auditory digit-span-backward task were administered. Increased rCBF, compared to resting, was observed in the occipital, temporo-occipital, parietal, and frontal regions for the former task, and anterior frontal, prerolandic, and posterior temporal regions showed rCBF increase for the latter task.

With the same technique, Carmon, Lavy, Gordon, and Portnoy (1975) found greater increase in the left hemispheres that were studied during a verbal memory task compared to when listening to music. By contrast, greater increase occurred for right hemispheres studied while listening to music, compared to the same verbal task.

With the xenon-133 inhalation technique, which permits bilateral determination of rCBF, Risberg, Halsey, *et al.* (1975) compared hemispheric rCBF during rest to laterality of flow during performance of a verbal analogies task and a spatial (Street's incomplete figures) task. The subjects were right-handed volunteers who were rewarded for good performance. The rewarded subjects showed greater left-hemispheric increase for the verbal task and greater right-hemispheric increase for the spatial task. A group of subjects who were not rewarded for performance showed much weaker effects.

Gur and Reivich (1980) administered the same tasks to a group of 36 right-handed males. The main finding was that, while the verbal task produced highly significant lateralized increases in rCBF in the expected left hemisphere, the spatial task produced greater right hemispheric increase in 17 of the 36 subjects and reverse asymmetry in 17 subjects (the remaining 2 subjects showed the same laterality of rCBF as during rest). This suggests that the Gestalt completion task could be solved either by right-hemispheric or by left-hemispheric strategies, whereas the verbal task was more "hard-wired" to the left hemisphere. However, the evidence that right-hemispheric lesions produce greater impairment on the Gestalt completion test suggests that right hemispheric strategies are superior. In support of this possibility, the subjects who showed greater right-hemispheric increase for the spatial task performed better than subjects who showed greater left hemispheric increase.

In a subsequent study with 62 young normals (Gur *et al.*, 1982), the Gestalt completion test was substituted by a spatial line orientation task developed by Benton, Varney, and Hamsher (1975). The task is highly sensitive to right-hemispheric lesions and similar tasks were shown to produce left visual field superiority in tachistoscopic studies. As before, each subject underwent 3 flows, in a counterbalanced order; resting, performing a verbal task, and performing a spatial task. This time, both the verbal and the spatial task produced significant lateralized increase in rCBF. Furthermore, the effects were influenced by handedness and sex, factors reputed to affect the direction and degree of hemispheric specialization (see Figure 1).

The findings with rCBF were replicated in a positron emission tomography (PET) study (Gur *et al.*, 1983). The verbal and spatial tasks produced

Figure 1. Initial slope (IS) index of blood flow to the left (——) and right (– – –) hemispheres for the total sample and for right- and left-handed females (○) and right-and left-handed males (□) during performance of resting (R), verbal (V), and spatial tasks (S). (From Gur *et al.* 1982.)

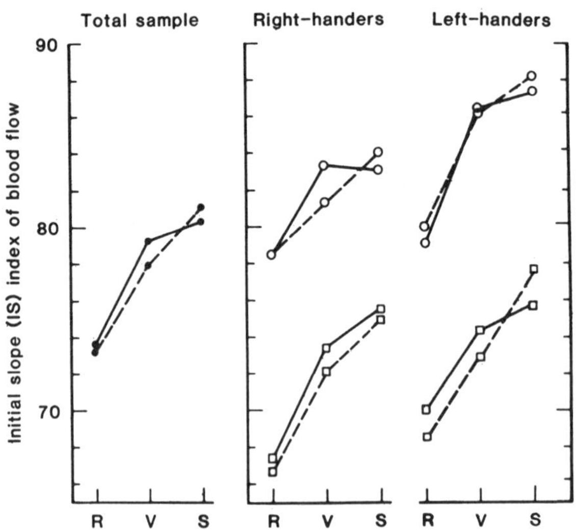

the expected increased metabolism in the left and right hemispheres, respectively. This effect was significant in the superior temporal and inferior parietal regions ("Wernicke's area"). In addition, there were significant task effects on laterality of metabolism in the frontal eye fields.

ACTIVATED rCBF IN SCHIZOPHRENIA

Ingvar and Franzen (1974a, 1974b) administered Raven's Progressive Matrices test to the sample of 11 young schizophrenics, and a nonstandard picture-naming task to the elderely patients. They reported normal increases in gray-matter flow in the measured left hemisphere, for the young patients. However, there was not a normal control group in this study.

With the exception of Ingvar and Franzen's investigation, rCBF was measured in schizophrenics only in the resting state. Such studies have limited potential for revealing regional brain abnormalities that may underly the psychological disturbances associated with schizophrenia. More pertinent information can be obtained by studying the differences between schizophrenics and normals in regional brain activity during engagement in psychological tasks requiring functions that are presumably disturbed in schizophrenia.

Because our earlier work suggested left-hemispheric dysfunction and overactivation in schizophrenia (Gur, 1977, 1978, 1979), we applied the paradigm (described in the preceding section of this paper) that produced reliable lateralized hemispheric rCBF increase in normals.

In our first study of medicated schizophrenics (R. Gur *et al.*, 1983) 15 inpatients (7 males and 8 females) participated. Diagnosis was made on the basis of DSM-III criteria. Patients were screened for medical and neurological disease, as well as for history of alcoholism, drug abuse, or electroconvulsive treatment. They were compared to 25 controls (11 males and 14 females), who matched the patients in age (schizophrenic mean age 28.5, controls age 29.5), sex, education, and socioeconomic background. All subjects were right-handed. Each subject participated in 3 rCBF measurements, as described in the preceding section.

As mentioned previously, there were no differences between schizophrenics and controls in resting flows. The normal pattern of higher anterior relative to posterior flows (Risberg, 1980) was found in both groups ($p < .001$). During cognitive activity, controls had greater left-hemispheric increase for the verbal task, and greater right-hemispheric increase for the spatial task. The pattern of rCBF changes was identical to the earlier normal sample (Gur *et al.*, 1982). Schizophrenics, however, had no asymmetry in rCBF for the verbal task, and greater left-hemispheric increase for the spatial task (see Figure 2).

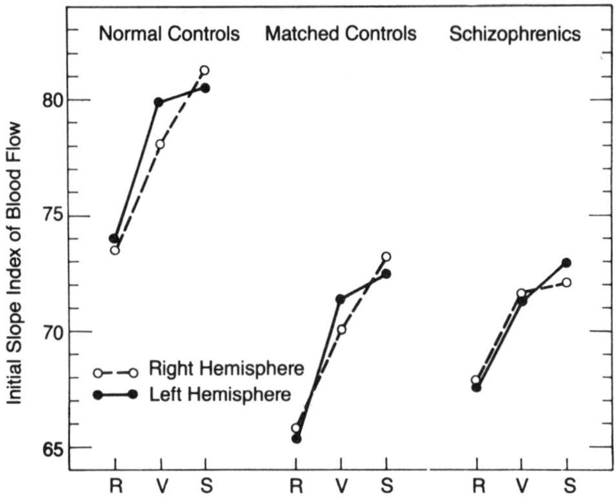

Figure 2. Regional cerebral blood flow in two hemispheres of schizophrenics and matched controls when resting (R), solving verbal analogies (V), and performing spatial task (S). Normal control values are from Figure 1 for comparison with latest matched sample. (From Gur *et al.*, 1983.)

There was an interaction of sex with diagnosis and task ($p < .02$). Schizophrenic females, unlike any other group, had highest flows during the verbal task rather than the spatial task. Severity of illness, length of illness, level of medication, or performance did not account for these effects.

The pattern of overall flow changes during cognitive activity observed in schizophrenic females is unusual. Greater rCBF increase for the spatial than for the verbal task has been a consistent finding in our study with normals. The pattern of hemispheric flow changes also deviates from normals. Specifically, the left hemisphere in schizophrenics fails to activate more than the right hemisphere, for the verbal task. However, there is greater left-hemispheric increase rather than right-hemispheric increase, for the spatial task. This may permit more precise characterization of hemispheric abnormalities in schizophrenics in light of the hypothesis of left-hemispheric dysfunction and overaction in schizophrenia (Gur, 1978). The dysfunction may be due to the relative failure of the left hemisphere to become active for verbal tasks. Instead, the left hemisphere overactivates to the "inappropriate" spatial task.

Our second study (Gur *et al.*, 1985) included 19 unmedicated schizophrenics and 19 matched controls, who were selected in the same way as the subjects in the first study. The sample included 11 males and 8 females in each group. The research procedures were identical to those described above.

Resting flows, as mentioned earlier, were higher in the left hemisphere for schizophrenics ($p < .05$). As before, anterior flows were higher than posterior flows ($p < .001$). During cognitive activity, two abnormalities emerged as statistically significant. Schizophrenics showed higher flows for the verbal than spatial task. This was observed in anterior regions for males, and for both anterior and posterior regions for females. Left-hemispheric overactivation for the spatial task was evident both for males and females.

Evaluation of the effect of medication showed differences between acute medicated and unmedicated schizophrenics in resting flows. Medicated schizophrenics had more symmetric flows, whereas unmedicated schizophrenics had higher left-hemispheric flows, more so in precentral regions.

To assess the relation between clinical status and rCBF, the sample of medicated and unmedicated patients was divided, on the basis of the Brief Psychiatric Rating Scale (BPRS) median score, into low- and high-severity groups. High-severity patients had higher resting left-hemispheric flows. During cognitive activation they showed less increase in rCBF than the low-severity group. These preliminary findings suggest that these two major variables—medication status and degree of psychopathology—should be further evaluated. This can be done by repeated studies in the same patients before and following treatment. It will also permit addressing the issue of trait-state as it relates to rCBF and neuropsychological functioning.

The findings of left-hemisphere increased flows, even for the spatial task, supporting the hypothesis of left-hemispheric overactivation, also raises the question of right-hemispheric functioning in schizophrenia. The right hemisphere, in addition to its role in spatial functioning, has been linked to attention and arousal.

Thus far, studies of psychological factors influencing regional brain physiology have focused on the effects of cognitive tasks. However, these techniques may also be suitable for the study of conation and affect. Attention is a central conative function whose anatomic substrates have recently been studied in a systematic fashion. Single-cell recordings demonstrated the existence in the inferior parietal region of neurons that are selectively activated by visual fixation and pursuit of motivationally relevant objects. The connectivity of area PG in the monkey brain, which is in the caudal part of the inferior parietal lobe, has been studied extensively by Mesulam and colleagues using the horseradish peroxidase technique.

Based on this connectivity, Mesulam (1981) has suggested that attention to sensory targets may depend on the coordinated activity of a neural network that includes the inferior parietal lobule, the cingulate cortex, and the frontal eye fields. In humans, there is a distinct hemispheric asymmetry in that unilateral sensory neglect occurs much more frequently following right-hemispheric lesions.

To test the hypothesized asymmetry in the attentional network, PET scans of subjects who were given sensory stimuli in the left and right visual fields in order to examine metabolic asymmetries in primary sensory cortices, were evaluated. Contralateral effects of stimulation were demonstrated in these subjects for the primary sensory cortices (Greenberg *et al.*, 1981). However, the experimental design has also permitted an examination of the effects of an attentional task. To assure central fixation, the subjects were given an attentional task in which a light-emitting diode was placed in central fixation. The light source dimmed occasionally, and the subjects were told to pay attention to this light source, and indicate when dimmings occurred. The PET scans of these stimulated subjects were compared to scans obtained from control subjects who were studied while their eyes were blindfolded and their ears plugged. These control subjects were not given an attentional task. The results showed greater right-hemispheric metabolism in stimulated subjects compared to controls specifically for the inferior parietal region (IP), with no significant lateralization effects in control regions.

The attentional network was examined in further detail in a subsequent study, using a scanner with better resolution. The results were replicated for the IP, with subjects attending to stimuli showing significantly higher right-hemispheric laterality of metabolism compared to controls. In addition, the same effects were obtained for the "frontal eye fields," the prefrontal cortex, and the calcarine cortex, but not in the cingulate gyrus or any of the control regions (Reivich, Gur, & Alavi, 1983). Diffuse increase in r CBF for a variety of attentional tasks was also reported by Roland and colleagues (Roland, 1982; Roland *et al.*, 1982). The increases occurred most consistently in the parietal cortex, and appeared most pronounced in right-hemispheric regions. The frontal eye fields also showed consistent activation.

The possibility of right hemispheric dysfunction in the attentional network in schizophrenia can be evaluated by measurement of rCBF during attentional tasks.

CONCLUSIONS

Developments in neuroimaging now enable the study of brain–behavior relations in psychiatric patients. Schizophrenics, who manifest significant behavioral abnormalities, are of particular interest. The xenon-133 inhalation technique provides a method for evaluation of brain activity during psychological stimulation. Our data so far suggest abnormalities in the pattern of rCBF in schizophrenics: left-hemispheric overactivation is a consistent finding. It is yet to be determined whether specific differences, related to nature and degree of psychopathology, will emerge. As we advance our knowledge of the normal brain and achieve better mastery of multiple techniques, a better integration of methods will follow. It is likely that this approach will contribute to the understanding of brain–behavior relations in schizophrenia.

ACKNOWLEDGMENT

This work was supported by NIMH grant MH 30456.

REFERENCES

Ariel, R. N., Golden, C. J., Berg, R. A., Quaife, M. A., Dirksen, J. W., Forsell, T., Wilson, J., & Graber, B. (1983). Regional cerebral blood flow in schizophrenia with the Xenon ^{133}Xe method. *Archives of General Psychiatry, 40*, 258–263.

Benton, A. L., Varney, N. R., & Hamsher, K. (1975). *Judgment of line orientation.* Iowa City: University of Iowa Hospitals.

Carmon, A., Lavy, S., Gordon, H., & Portnoy, Z. (1975). Hemispheric differences in rCBF during verbal and nonverbal tasks. In *Brain work* (pp. 414–423). Copenhagen: Munksgaard.

Della Porta, P., Maiolo, A. T., Negri, V. U., *et al.* (1964). Cerebral blood flow and metabolism in therapeutic insulin coma. *Metabolism, Clinical and Experimental, 13*, 131–140.

Gordan, G. S., Esters, F. M., Adams, J. E., *et al.* (1955). Cerebral oxygen uptake in chronic schizophrenic reaction. *Archives of Neurology and Psychiatry, 73*, 544–545.

Greenberg, J. H., Reivich, M., Alavi, A., Hand, P., Rosenquist, A., Rintelman, W., Tusa, R., Stein, A., Christmas, D., Fowler, J., MacGregor, B., & Wolf, A. (1981). Metabolic mapping of functional activity in man with 18F-fluorodeoxyglucose technique. *Science, 212*, 678–680.

Gur, R. C., Gur, R. E., Obrist, W. D., Hungerbuhler, J. P., Younkin, D., Skolnick, B. E., & Reivich, M. (1982). Sex and handedness differences in cerebral blood flow during rest and cognitive activity. *Science, 217*, 659–661.

Gur, R. C., Gur, R. E., Rosen, A. D., *et al.* (1983). A cognitive-motor network demonstrated by positron emission tomography. *Neuropsychologia, 21*, 601–606.

Gur, R. E. (1977). Motoric laterality imbalance in schizophrenia: A possible concomitant of left hemisphere dysfunction. *Archives of General Psychiatry, 34*, 33–37.

Gur, R. E. (1978). Left hemisphere dysfunction and left hemisphere overactivation in schizophrenia. *Journal of Abnormal Psychology, 87*, 226–238.

Gur, R. E. (1979). Cognitive concomitants of hemispheric dysfunction in schizophrenia. *Archives of General Psychiatry, 36*, 269–274.

Gur, R. E., Gur, R. C., Skolnick, B. E., Caroff, S., Obrist, W. D., Resnick, S., & Reivich, M. (1985). Brain function in psychiatric disorders. III. Regional cerebral blood flow in unmedicated schizophrenics. *Archives of General Psychiatry, 42*, 329–334.

Gur, R. E., Skolnick, B. E., Gur, R. C., Caroff, S., Obrist, W. D., Younkin, D., & Reivich, M. (1983). Brain function in psychiatric disorders. I. Regional cerebral blood flow in medicated schizophrenics. *Archives of General Psychiatry, 40*, 1250–1254.

Halsey, J. H., Blauenstein, U. W., Wilson, E. M., Wills, E. L., & Greenspoon, E. (1977). The differing rCBF responses to left and right hand movement, with comparison of several flow indices. *Acta Neurologica Scandinavica, 56* (Suppl.), 264–265.

Hoyer, S., & Oesterreich, K. (1975). Blood flow and oxydative metabolism of the brain in patients with schizophrenia. *Psychiatria Clinica*, *8*, 304–313.

Ingvar, D. H., & Franzen, G. (1974a). Abnormalities of cerebral blood flow distribution in patients with chronic schizophrenia. *Acta Psychiatrica Scandinavica*, *50*, 425–462.

Ingvar, D. H., & Franzen, G. (1974b). Distribution of cerebral activity in chronic schizophrenia. *Lancet*, *2*, 1484–1486.

Ingvar, D. H. & Risberg, J. (1967). Increase in regional cerebral blood flow during mental effort in normals and in patients with focal brain disorders. *Experimental Brain Research*, *3*. 195–211.

Kety, S. S., & Schmidt, C. F. (1945). The determination of cerebral blood flow in man by the use of nitrous oxide in low concentrations. *American Journal of Physiology*, *143*, 53.

Kety, S. S., Woodford, R. B., Harmel, M. H., *et al.* (1948). Cerebral blood flow and metabolism in schizophrenia. *American Journal of Psychiatry*, *104*, 765–770.

Lassen, N. A., Roland, P. E. Larsen, B., Melamed, E., & Soh, K. (1977). Mapping of human cerebral functions: A study of the regional cerebral blood flow pattern during rest, its reproducibility and the activations seen during basic sensory and motor functions. *Acta Neurologica Scandinavica*, *56* (Suppl.), 262–263.

Mallett, B. L., & Veall, N. (1965). The measurement of regional cerebral clearance rates in man using Xenon-133 inhalation and extracranial recording. *Clinical Science*, *29*, 179–191.

Mathew, R. J., Duncan, G. C., Weinman, M. L., & Barr, D. L. (1982). Regional cerebral blood flow in schizophrenia. *Archives of General Psychiatry*, *39*, 1121–1124.

Mathew, R. J., Meyer, J. S., Francis, D. J., Schooler, J. C., Weinman, M., & Mortel, K. F. (1981). Regional cerebral blood flow in schizophrenia: A preliminary report. *American Journal of Psychiatry*, *138*, 112–113.

Mesulam, M. M. (1981). A cortical network for directed attention with unilateral neglect. *Annals of Neurology*, *10*, 309–325.

Obrist, W. D., Thompson, H. K., Wang, H. S., & Wilkinson, W. E. (1975). Regional cerebral blood flow estimated by 133-Xe inhalation. *Stroke*, *6*, 245–256.

Obrist, W. D., & Wilkinson, W. E. (1979). The non-invasive Xe-133 method: Evaluation of CBF indices. In A. Bes & G. Geraud (Eds.), *Cerebral circulation* (pp. 119–124). Amsterdam: Elsevier/North-Holland.

Obrist, W. D., & Wilkinson, W. E. (1984). Stability and sensitivity of CBF indices in the noninvasive ^{133}Xe method. In A. Hartmann & S. Hoyer (Eds.), *Measurement of cerebral blood flow and cerebral metabolism in man* (pp. 30–36). Berlin & New York: Springer-Verlag.

Olesen, J. (1971). Contralateral focal increase of cerebral blood flow in man during arm work. *Brain*, *94*, 635–646.

Reivich, M. (1974). Blood flow metabolism couple in brain. In F. Plum (Ed.), *Brain dysfunction in metabolic disorders* (p. 888). New York: Raven Press.

Reivich, M., Gur, R. C., & Alavi, A. (1983). Positron emission tomographic studies of sensory stimuli, cognitive processes and anxiety. *Human Neurobiology*, *2*, 25–33.

Risberg, J. (1980). Regional cerebral blood flow measurements by Xe-inhalation: Methodology and applications in neuropsychology and psychiatry. *Brain and Language*, *9*, 9–34.

Risberg, J., Ali, Z., Wilson, E. M., Wills, E. L., & Halsey, J. H. (1975). Regional cerebral blood flow by the 133 xenon inhalation. *Stroke*, *6*, 142–148.

Risberg, J., Halsey, J. H., Wills, E. L., & Wilson, E. M. (1975). Hemispheric specialization in normal man studied by bilateral measurement of the regional cerebral blood flow. *Brain*, *98*, 511–524.

Risberg, J., & Ingvar, D. H. (1973). Patterns of activation in grey matter of the dominant hemisphere during memorizing and reasoning. *Brain*, *96*, 737–756.

Roland, P. E. (1982). Cortical regulation of selective attention in man. A regional cerebral blood flow study. *Journal of Neurophysiology*, *48*, 1059–1078.

Roland, P. E., Meyer, E., Shibasaki, T., *et al.* (1982). Regional cerebral blood flow changes in cortex and basal ganglia during voluntary movements in normal human volunteers. *Journal of Neurophysiology*, *48*, 467–480.

Schweitzer, L., Becker, E., & Welsh, H. (1978). Abnormalities of cerebral lateralization in schizophrenic patients. *Archives of General Psychiatry*, *35*, 982–985.

Sheppard, G., Gruzelier, J. H., Manchanda, R., Hirsch, S. R., Wise, R., Frackowiak, R., & Jones, T. (1983). ^{15}O positron emission tomographic scanning in predominantly never-treated acute schizophrenic patients. *Lancet*, *31*, 1448–1452.

Wilson, W. P., Schieve, J. F., & Scheinberg, P. (1952). Effect of series of electric shock treatments on cerebral blood flow and metabolism. *Archives of Neurology and Psychiatry*, *68*, 651–654.

COMMENTARY

Dr. Malcolm Bowers:* If there are a couple of questions for Dr. Gur, she is willing to consider them at this time.

Dr. Athan Karras†: Your patients, if I remember correctly, are off medication for one week, and it is possible that there is a rebound effect from being off medication for such a short time that might account for the differential effects between the hemispheres. Your overactivation could simply be, at this time, a rebound phenomenon, and you may need patients who are off their medication for a longer period of time. You see rebound phenomena in a variety of physiological and biochemical phenomenon.

Dr. Gur: That's correct. Eleven of the 19 patients were not on medication at all. Some of them have never been treated and this was their first psychiatric admission. They had no trace of phenothiazine or any drug in their drug screen. Eight of the patients had detectible levels of neuroleptics and were washed out for a week. I agree with you that this is a concern, but there were no differences when we looked at the 11 and the 8 separately. It might be that their admission most of the time was precipitated by stopping medications, and by the time they came in, there were only barely detectible levels, and then we kept them off for a week. If it would have been possible, it would have been better to keep them off for a longer time, but there were other clinical considerations that had to take place, and since there were no differences between the 8 and the 11, I am not sure that the results can be explained on this basis.

* New Haven, Connecticut.

† New York, New York.

Dr. Irwin Feinberg:* I just wanted to ask what the standard error of your measurements was, because you were talking about significant differences where the difference was about three percent, the difference between, say 65 and 67 cc/100 grams/minute. Is that right?

Dr. Gur: We are dealing with a within-subject design where the same subjects participate in three flows. If we had three populations of patients, the first getting only baseline, the second getting only verbal, the third getting only spatial, then the standard errors are a factor.

But, because the design is a within-subject design the standard error is not a factor. Furthermore, the differences were small but consistent, yielding significant results.

Dr. Gerry Bruder†: I just wanted to comment on what I think are some very interesting sex differences in the slide we have in front of us. What it seems to show me is that for the spatial task, the greater right flow than left flow seems to be predominantly for male normals. If you look at the normal data, the greater right flow than left flow is predominantly for males, whereas for females, both hemispheres seem to light up in the spatial task. That goes along with our behavioral data in the auditory modality, and other visual data that suggest that the advantage for the right hemisphere for spatial tasks is predominantly for males. Also, I think it is interesting that, in terms of differentiating between schizophrenics and normals regarding the blood-flow data, it seems to be that for males, the task that would do the best job would probably be the spatial task. The difference, the hyperflow on the left, is for the males predominantly in the spatial task, whereas for the females it seems the verbal test might be better for differentiating in terms of the flow, with greater flow in the left hemisphere.

Dr. Gur: That's correct. We are in the process now of applying similar auditory modality tasks doing regional cerebral blood flow. This will help assess if the auditory modality is similar to what we will expect from the results obtained for visual modality and based on the neuropsychological literature. I suspect that we will come up with similar results to use if we apply the same procedure.

Dr. Henry Nasrallah‡: I have a quick question about the subtyping of your patients. You mentioned paranoid and undifferentiated. What method of subtyping did you use, and did you find any difference between the paranoids and nonparanoids?

Dr. Gur: We have not seen differences. It doesn't mean that the differences are not there. The sample is small, and this may be partly why we don't see differences. Once we have larger samples we will be able to

* San Francisco, California.

† New York, New York.

‡ Iowa City, Iowa.

examine the paranoid–nonparanoid dimension, and also other differences. When we look at the BPRS or other rating scales, and do item-by-item analysis, there are those items that go along with the general findings and those that do not. So it appears that the first step is to look item by item and look at those that differentiate between the two populations. I did not present data on probe by probe, and there are differences in probe by probe as far as the correlation with BPRS. However, the sample is small, and I think that before drawing any conclusion, I look at it more as a pilot, which suggests that there are differences.

6

Clinical–Neuropathological Correlations in Schizophrenia: Theoretical Implications

DANIEL R. WEINBERGER
National Institute of Mental Health, Saint Elizabeths' Hospital, Washington, D.C.

In its frustration to find a solution to the unsolved riddle of schizophrenia, psychiatry research has tended to search for peripheral signs of CNS disease. An example of this approach might be finding dopamine or one of its metabolites to be elevated in blood and then making the assumption that "brain" dopamine is high. A major limitation with this approach is its naive tendency to view the brain as a "black box," as if it were physiologically and chemically homogeneous. An alternative approach, searching inside the black box, is infinitely more complex and bewildering. If one undertakes a search in the brain for evidence of CNS disease, it is essential to set theoretical priorities about where to look. Because we have neither the time nor the resources to look everywhere, we must narrow the choice of sites to those of high theoretical probability. It is logical to assume that certain functional neuroanatomical systems are particularly relevant to psychiatric symptoms. Evidence of pathology in such systems is more likely to be pathophysiologically meaningful. In contrast, even if we observed pathology in, for example, the spinal cord, we would have difficulty accepting such findings as pathophysiologically relevant to psychiatric symptoms.

In the case of schizophrenia, the question of where to look for evidence of brain pathology is a controversial one. The common wisdom would suggest that we look in the limbic system. Several lines of circumstantial evidence implicate this brain region. First of all, many of the so-called biogenic amine and peptide-rich tracks that have been a focus of psychiatric research for the last several decades are concentrated in the limbic system. The dopamine hypothesis of schizophrenia implicates limbic structures such as nucleus accumbens, hypothalamus, amygdala, etc. (Meltzer & Stahl, 1976). Another line of evidence involves what might be called "symptomatic schizophrenia," or schizophrenia-like illnesses associated neurological disorders such as trauma, tumor, infections, and seizure disorders. In surveys of such cases, it has been emphasized that schizophrenia-like psychoses are more often related to pathology in limbic and diencephalic regions than in other parts of the brain (Davison & Bagley, 1969). Finally, people who have seizure discharges from limbic sites experience a number of psychic phenomena that qualitatively are not that dissimilar from those reported by patients with schizophrenia (Blumer, 1975; Chapman, 1966). Such experiences also have been induced by stimulating implanted limbic electrodes in human subjects (Gloor, Olivier, Quesney, Anderman, & Horowitz, 1982; Halgren, Walter, Cherlow, & Crandall, 1978). These experiences include complex auditory and visual hallucinations, complex illusions, strong fears, feelings of embarrassment, depersonalization, derealization, varieties of forced thinking which the subject may be unable to resist, as well as ineffable sensations and feelings.

COMPUTED TOMOGRAPHY EVIDENCE OF LIMBIC PATHOLOGY

There is intriguing, though not conclusive, evidence that limbic-diencephalic pathology is associated with schizophrenia per se. Some of this evidence has surfaced from computed tomography (CT) studies. Over the past seven years, numerous CT studies have appeared in the psychiatric literature. These studies are reviewed in detail elsewhere (Weinberger, Wagner, & Wyatt, 1983). From these reports, two fairly consistent findings have emerged, both of which may implicate a loss of brain mass in periventricular limbic and diencephalic brain regions. The findings are enlargement of lateral and third ventricles. Because ventricular enlargement can be seen in patients even at the onset of their schizophrenic illness, it is clearly not the result of chronic psychiatric treatment, either institutional, somatic, or psychotherapeutic (Weinberger, DeLisi, Perman, Targum, & Wyatt, 1982; Nyback, Wiesel, Berggren, & Hindmarsh, 1982; Schultz *et al.*, 1983). At least 25 controlled CT quantitative studies exist, the vast majority of which have observed that schizophrenic patients have larger lateral ventricles than do similarly aged normal individuals (see Figure 1). Third-ventricle enlargement, though less frequently studied, has been at least as consistently found (see Figure 2).

Several issues must be addressed before the CT findings can be considered as possible evidence of limbic–diencephalic pathology and clues to the pathogenesis of schizophrenia. The meaning of these CT observations is far from certain. Even the location of the underlying pathology is in doubt. Although a neuropathological process involving limbic–diencephalic structures and resulting in a reduction of periventricular tissue mass would be associated with ventricular enlargement on CT, such CT changes might also

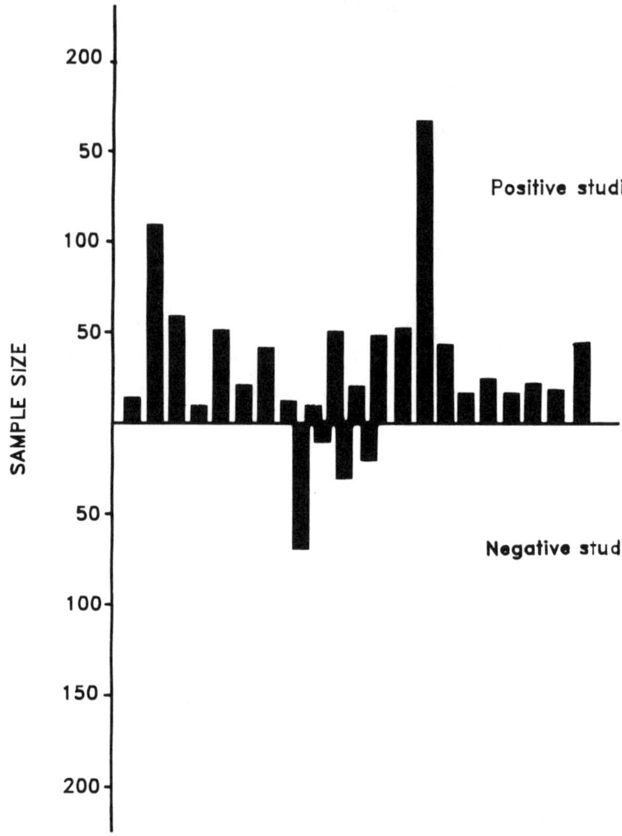

Figure 1. Summary of results of controlled CT studies of lateral ventricular enlargement. References cited elsewhere (Weinberger, 1984; Weinberger, Wagner, & Wyatt, 1983).

reflect distant, nonlimbic (e.g. cortical, white matter, etc.) pathology. This is because ventricular dilatation in the absence of a disorder of CSF flow is a nonspecific, nonlocalizing sign of reduced brain mass. Therefore, such findings are not confirmation of structural neuropathology in the limbic system and diencephalon, as common wisdom has suggested we should find in this illness.

The apparent nonspecificity of the CT findings in schizophrenia has bewildered a number of observers of this literature. Perhaps the meaning of such CT observations is misunderstood. All they tell us is that something has happened to the brain that was not supposed to have happened to it. This is consistent with the fact that there are more reasons that ventricles can become large than there are ways they can look large on a CT scan.

The question of specificity has to be addressed to the underlying pathological process. It is only by understanding the nature and the cause of the pathological process, when and where it occurs, and perhaps what other factors interact with it that one can speak to the issue of specificity. An analogous situation is seen with multiple sclerosis and Alzheimer's disease, both of which may have identical appearances on CT, yet clearly different underlying pathologies.

Another unresolved issue is the question of reversibility. This may seem like a strange question, because one tends to assume that findings suggestive of brain atrophy would be, by definition, irreversible. Yet cases of apparent reversible atrophy on CT scan have been described in association with significant weight loss (Heinz, Martinez, & Haenggeli, 1977), acute alcohol encephalopathy (Carlen, Wortzman, Holgate, Wilkinson, & Rankin, 1978), steroid administration (Rodeck & Campbell, 1979) and Cushing's disease (Heinz *et al.*, 1977). Such cases illustrate that everything that looks like atrophy on a CT scan is not true atrophy in the histopathological sense of the word. Nevertheless, the cases of so-called pseudoatrophy appear to be different from what has been described in schizophrenia. Whereas the most frequent finding in schizophrenia is enlargement of the ventricular system, the typical findings in pseudoatrophy cases have been dilatation of

Figure 2. Summary of results of controlled CT studies of third ventricular size. References cited elsewhere (Weinberger, 1984; Weinberger, Wagner, & Wyatt, 1983).

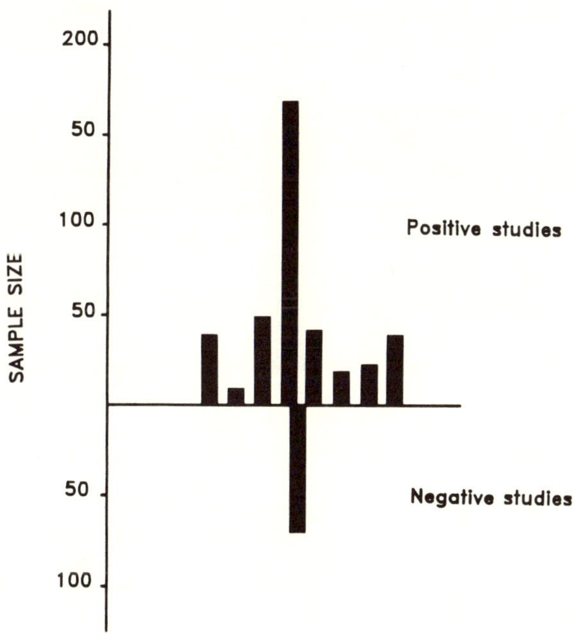

cortical fissures and sulci with ventricular changes being less common. As mentioned above, treatment does not appear to be an important factor in the development of the CT findings. The changes have been observed in patients, at least to some degree, at the onset of their illness, before they have been under psychiatric treatment.

If we assume that the CT findings relate to a pathological process that might be relevant to schizophrenia, and is not reversible or an artifact of treatment, then they should have some clinical implications. Furthermore, not only should the putative neuropathological changes have clinical implications, but cases with marked neuropathology should have more of these clinical manifestations. It is also reasonable to expect that the clinical manifestations bear some relationship or similarity to other symptoms that are associated with a loss of brain mass. If, for example, we found that the CT findings correlated with body weight or with nonspecific serum enzymes, it would suggest a less compelling link to the pathogenesis of the illness. Table 1 lists statistically significant correlations of clinical phenomena with large ventricles on CT. The correlations reported are consistent with the two assumptions described above. These clinical pathological correlations provide the strongest evidence to date of a link between large ventricles and the pathogenesis of schizophrenia.

It goes without saying that pathology observable at the gross level of CT should be observable under the microscope. Although a CT scan image is several steps removed from the actual brain, the CT data provide some clues about the nature of what microscopic pathology might exist. First, as stated above, whatever the pathological process is, it seems to be associated with a reduction in brain mass. In other words, the process is degenerative or dysplastic. Second, the process appears to predate the development of diagnostic symptomatology in late adolescence. This conclusion comes from studies of first-episode schizophreniform patients, some of whom have large ventricles. Because it is unlikely that an adult could develop acute enlargement of the ventricular system without also having neurological symptoms, the chances are that the enlargement had been there for a long time. A third inference that can be drawn from the CT data is that the pathology appears to be nonprogressive. This inference comes from the failure of most studies

Table 1. Clinical Correlations of Large Ventricles in Schizophrenia

1. "Negative" (defect) symptoms (Johnstone *et al.*, 1978)
2. Cognitive impairment (Weinberger & Wyatt, 1982)
3. Minor ("soft") neurological signs (Weinberger & Wyatt, 1982)
4. Disordered smooth-pursuit eye movements (Weinberger & Wyatt, 1982)
5. Frequent extrapyramidal reactions to neuroleptics (Luchins, Jackman, & Meltzer, 1983)
6. Poor premorbid social adjustment (Weinberger, Cannon-Spoor, Potkin, & Wyatt, 1980)
7. Poor response to treatment (Weinberger, Cannon-Spoor *et al.*, 1980)

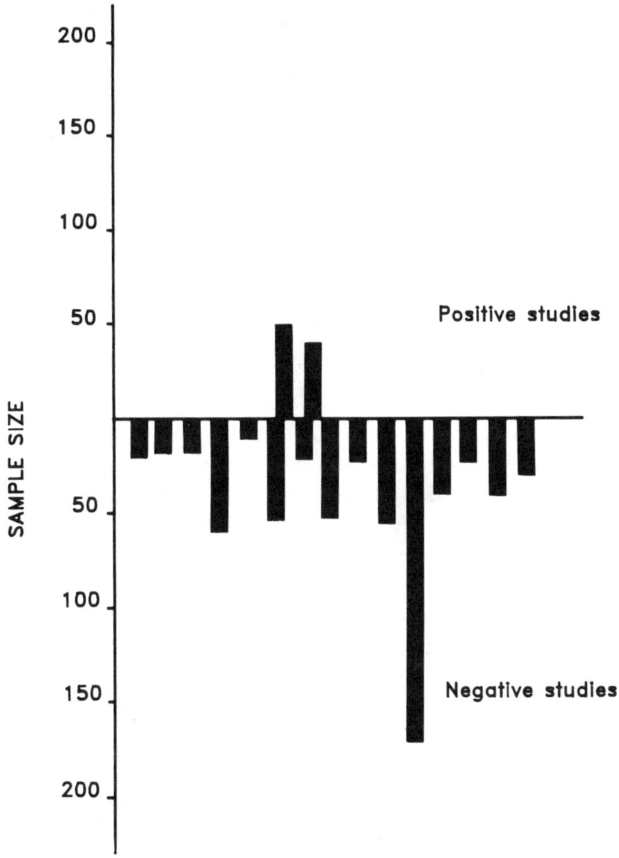

Figure 3. Summary of results of CT studies that examined the statistical correlation between ventricular size (lateral or third ventricles) and length of schizophrenic illness. References cited elsewhere (Weinberger, 1984; Weinberger, Wagner, & Wyatt, 1983).

to find a significant relationship between ventricular size and length of illness (see Figure 3). In summary, the CT scan data suggest that this pathological process is degenerative or dysplastic, that it is a static condition, and that it appears, at least in many individuals, to predate the diagnostic symptomatology.

POSTMORTEM NEUROPATHOLOGY STUDIES AND LIMBIC PATHOLOGY

Despite the disappointing history of early postmortem neuropathology studies in schizophrenia, new studies, utilizing modern diagnostic criteria and innovative procedures, have appeared in the past decade. Unlike studies from the first half of this century, which tended to focus on cerebral cortex, recent investigators have emphasized limbic–diencephalic regions because of their greater theoretical relevance. Table 2 summarizes controlled studies that have emerged in the last 10 years. An X indicates a site of pathological change that significantly differentiates patients with schizophrenia from controls. An O indicates no differences found. Rather than search for a qualitatively pathognomonic "lesion" as earlier researchers had done, these studies have applied techniques (e.g, morphometric analyses, glial stains) to identify primarily nonspecific degenerative changes. This approach is more theoretically consistent with the CT results. These studies are described in greater detail elsewhere (Weinberger *et al.*, 1983). Table 2 illustrates that most of the findings have been in the limbic system and diencephalon, although few studies have looked at the same regions. In addition, it seems that there is no region of the limbic system or diencephalon that has been consistently observed across studies to show degenerative changes in schizophrenia. As stated, most of these studies have been quantitative; for example, Nieto and Escobar (1972) and Stevens (1982) found more evidence of fibrillary gliosis among schizophrenic patients than among psychiatric controls. The study by Bogerts, Mertz and Schonfeldt-Bausch (in press) involved volumetric measurement of selected limbic nuclei. In any particular study, however, there is no consistent pattern of pathological change seen in all or even the majority of schizophrenic patients. What is reported, both across studies and within studies, is quantitatively significant yet patchy, nonspecific changes of various limbic-diencephalic nuclei. It is noteworthy that, as predicted by the CT studies, most of the changes described at postmortem examination have been old and long-standing, not acute. Such postmortem findings probably would have been associated with large ventricles on CT scan.

As with the CT data, there are a number of problems in attempting to interpret these postmortem studies. First, we know very little about the clinical implications of static, subtle pathology of the limbic system and diencephalon. Second, it is difficult to attribute a relatively consistent behavioral syndrome (i.e., schizophrenia) to such patchy involvement of various deep, poorly defined (anatomically, neurochemically, and functionally) limbic–diencephalic regions. Depth-electrode studies from animals and man suggest complex structure-function relationships for limbic sites. There appears to be no nucleus in the limbic system that has a monopoly on a given behavior. In other words, in animals a particular behavior (e.g., orienting response, aggressive behavior) can be elicited by stimulating one of several regions (Isaacson, 1982). Similar findings have been reported in man. For example, similar psychic experiences have been described after stimulation of amygdala, temporal cortex, and hippocampus (Gloor *et al.*,

Table 2. Structural Neuropathology in Schizophrenia: Recent Postmortem Evidence

	Hypothalamus	Amygdala	Hippocampus	Medial pallidum	Thalamus	Substantia innominata	Cerebellum	Other
Nieto and Escobar (1972)	X				X	X		X
Weinberger, Kleinman, Luchins, Bigelow, and Wyatt (1980)							X	
Averbach (1981)						X		
Dom, De Saedeleer, Bogerts, and Hopf (1981)				X	O			X
Stevens (1982)	X	X		X		X	X	X
Bogerts, Hantsch, and Herzer, 1983; Bogerts, Mertz, and Schonfeldt-Bausch (in press)	O	X	X	X	O			X
Kovelman and Scheibel (1984)			X					

1982; Halgren *et al.*, 1978). The complex nature of these structure–function relationships is further exemplified by their variability. The same nucleus, stimulated on different days, will not necessarily result in the same experience (Halgren *et al.* 1978). On some days, stimulation may produce no effect whatsoever.

One probable reason for such confusing findings is the exceedingly complex neuroanatomical connections of this part of the brain. A vast converging network of sensory, autonomic, and nonspecific cortical and subcortical afferents are integrated in each nucleus, which then projects diffusely through an equally complex diverging system of efferents. A relatively simple example of this anatomical complexity is the bed nucleus of the stria terminalis, a small forebrain nucleus that in man probably consists of less than 10,000 neurons. The function of this nucleus is unknown. Figure 4 shows the surprisingly vast connectivities of the small bed nucleus. This figure illustrates that far-reaching bed-nucleus output is under the influence of varied and probably variable input. Nothing less could be expected of a brain region involved in emotional behavior. It is tempting to speculate that the function of this nucleus could be affected by pathology in any of several regions and that, conversely, pathology in bed nucleus might affect function in a number of other regions. The effects, however, are unlikely to be specific or pathognomonic. This assumption follows from the character of the nonspecific inputs and outputs. Depending on variations in the quality and/or volume of inputs, the clinical implications of bed-nucleus pathology might vary even from day to day. Perhaps this example using the bed nucleus is a clue to how patchy limbic pathology could predispose to abnormal behavior.

The preceding theoretical discussion may provide a rationale for accepting subtle limbic pathology as being clinically relevant. It is certainly

Figure 4. Anatomical connections of bed nucleus of the stria terminalis. (From Isaacson, 1982; Nauta and Domesick, 1982.)

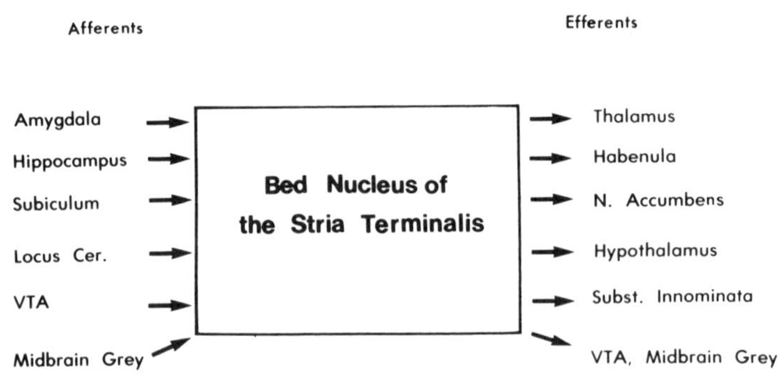

Table 3. Schizophrenia: Defect Symptoms

Improverished thinking
Blunted, flat Affect
Intellectual impairment
Social isolation and withdrawal
Marked impairment in role performance
Impaired personal hygiene and grooming
Loss of initiative, motivation
Hoarding and foraging behaviors
Marked deficit in insight

not clear, however, that such pathology can produce the clinical syndrome of schizophrenia. In fact, if we critically reconsider the basis for the "common wisdom" linking schizophrenia to limbic pathology, namely cases of "symptomatic schizophrenia," we encounter additional problems. Although cases of "symptomatic schizophrenia" may have schizophrenic-like hallucinations and delusions, they also have certain important differences from schizophrenia. For the most part, they have preserved affect, they have preserved insight, the psychosis is ego alien, and their cognition is not impaired or disturbed the way it is in schizophrenia (Davison & Bagley, 1969). These characteristic differences represent the so-called defect symptoms of schizophrenia, those symptoms that separate schizophrenia from other chronic illnesses associated with hallucinations and delusions. Examples of defect symptoms are listed in Table 3. The infrequency of these symptoms in patients with "symptomatic schizophrenia" secondary to limbic pathology (i.e., tumors, etc.) suggests that another functional neuroanatomical system is involved in schizophrenia.

DORSOLATERAL PREFRONTAL CORTEX IN SCHIZOPHRENIA

There is ample reason to believe that this additional neuroanatomical locus involves prefrontal association cortex. Prefrontal cortex, perhaps the most complexly organized and connected part of the human brain, is also one of the last parts of the brain to myelinate (Fuster, 1980). This is particularly true for the so-called dorsolateral or convexity cortex as compared with the orbitomedial prefrontal cortex. Patients with frontal cortical lesions, especially those involving dorsolateral cortex, have clinical features similar to the schizophrenic defect state. These include abnormalities of attention, distractibility, poor concentration, impaired goal-directed behavior, emotional blunting, concreteness, diminished will, overall restriction in thinking, behavior dominated by here-and-now needs, decreased IQ, impared abstraction–sequencing, overall reduction in spontaneous movement, lack of initiative, restlessness, aimlessness, poor social judgment, lack of insight, and decreased concern for personal hygiene (Fuster, 1980; Stuss & Benson, 1984).

In addition to the symptomatological overlap between schizophrenia and frontal cortex damage, some of the clinical findings associated with schizophrenia suggest frontal cortical dysfunction. Most of the so-called minor soft neurological signs long regarded as common in patients with schizophrenia implicate dysfunction in frontal cortex and have been called frontal release signs (Weinberger & Wyatt, 1982). The cognitive deficits and impaired performance on neuropsychological tests frequently reported in schizophrenia are most consistent with frontal dysfunction (Weinberger & Wyatt, 1982). Disordered smooth-pursuit eye movements, though consistent with dysfunction in any of several locations along the pathways for saccadic eye movements, could result from dorsolateral cortical dysfunction involving prefrontal eye fields (Mialet & Pichot, 1981). Recent EEG findings with spectral analysis and topographical mapping display suggest that there is more slowing of underlying rhythms in the dorosolateral frontal than in other cortical regions (Morihisa, Duffy, & Wyatt, 1983).

Although these clinical findings in schizophrenia suggest frontal cortical dysfunction, they are far from conclusive. More convincing evidence has emerged from innovations in functional brain-imaging technology, particularly regional cerebral blood flow (rCBF) and Positron Emission Tomography (PET). These techniques have made it possible to study regional neuronal metabolism in living subjects. The few PET studies of cortical glucose metabolism and oxygen consumption have been thus far inconsistent. Although some patients with frontal hypometabolism have been described (Buchsbaum *et al.*, 1982), other studies have not observed differences between patients and controls (Kling *et al.*, 1984; Sheppard *et al.*, 1983). One explanation for this is that these studies have involved the resting state, a state that is difficult to define and standardize from individual to individual. The "resting state" of a patient with schizophrenia is hardly comparable to that of a normal individual. The differences may bear less of a relationship to pathophysiology than to anxiety or other aspects of the test experience. Another problem with available PET studies is that of prolonged temporal resolution. Approximately 40 minutes of brain activity has to be averaged into one image.

More interesting results have emerged from studies of regional cerebral blood flow using xenon-133 as a radioactive tracer. Because cortical blood flow is tightly coupled to neuronal metabolism (Rosenblum, 1965), monitoring regional blood flow is tantamount under most circumstances to monitoring neuronal metabolism. Ingvar and Franzen (1974), using a xenon-133 intracarotid injection method, reported reduced dorsolateral frontal cortical blood flow in schizophrenia, during both resting and stimulation (sensory and cognitive)(Franzen & Ingvar, 1975). Despite their dramatic observations, the findings have been difficult to interpret because of methodological limitations. The abnormal patients were primarily elderly, controls were younger and alcoholic, and all patients were receiving neuroleptic drugs and were heavily premedicated with phenobarbital.

Recent rCBF investigations have provided conflicting results. Using a noninvasive inhalation technique, Mathew, Duncan, Weinman, and Barr (1982) reported no frontal flow decrease, but reduced overall mean brain flow in schizophrenic patients. The patients, however, were studied only at rest and blood flow was not corrected for blood carbon dioxide tension ($p\mathrm{CO}_2$), a major blood flow covariate. Ariel *et al.* (1983) did report reduced dorsolateral frontal flow, especially on the left, but their study was poorly controlled, not $p\mathrm{CO}_2$ corrected, and also only evaluated the "resting state." Gur *et al.* (1983) studied cortical rCBF during cognitive tasks aimed at differentially activating left and right hemispheres. Although they found subtle differences between neuroleptic-treated patients with schizophrenia and healthy controls, dorsolateral frontal flow was not specifically evaluated.

The NIMH rCBF laboratory has reported data linking dorsolateral prefrontal CBF reduction (and by inference neuronal hypometabolism) with cognitive deficts referrable to the same cortical region (Weinberger, Berman, & Zec, in press). Like Mathews *et al.* and Gur *et al.*, Weinberger *et al.* found no resting state differences in prefrontal flow. However, patients were also tested while performing in counterbalanced sequence a number-matching task and an automated version of the Wisconsin Card Sorting (WCS) test. Although the former test is very simple and involves minimal problem solving and abstraction, the latter has been shown to depend on normal dorsolateral prefrontal cortical processing (Milner, 1963). In this paradigm, the numbers task controls for activation of the nondorsolateral prefrontal areas coincidentally activated by the WCS procedure (e.g., visual cortex). rCBF topography did not differ significantly on the numbers tests between patients and controls. On the WCS, however, although controls increased dorsolateral frontal flow as predicted, the patients failed to do so and, in fact, showed a reduction in flow to that region. The group differences were qualitatively apparent in addition to being statistically significant. As a further indication of the physiological–cognitive relationship, these investigators found a significant correlation between the degree of impairment of WCS performance and the magnitude of reduced prefrontal flow.

These data appear to localize a dysfunctional area of cortex in schizophrenia and to link the physiological aberration with cognitive impairment. Of course, nonspecific factors have yet to be conclusively excluded, such as attention deficits, ongoing symptoms, and other state variables. Nevertheless, the results do not appear to be primarily related to such nonspecific factors (Berman, Zec, & Weinberger, in press). Rather, it appears that patients with schizophrenia have a disorder of dorsolateral frontal activation which manifests itself in clinical deficits reminiscent of patients with lesions of this cortical region. The deficit is particularly apparent in the presence of dorsolateral frontal cortical cognitive demand (i.e., the WCS).

Returning to the earlier question of structural CNS pathology, we might wonder how these cortical changes relate to findings in the limbic system. Are the blood flow observations indicative of structural degeneration in the frontal cortex in schizophrenia, as suggested by neuropathologists at the turn of the century (Dastur, 1959) and by some CT studies (Weinberger *et al.*, 1983)? Although the answer is unknown, the CBF pattern is not typical of patients with intrinsic cortical disease. Such patients tend to be "hypofrontal" at rest (Ingvar & Gustafson, 1970). The patients with schizophrenia seem to have physiological difficulty with a "switch" mechanism necessary to bring dorsolateral cortex "on line" at relevant times. This hypothesis brings the discussion back to the question of limbic pathology. It is interesting to note that the regions mentioned as being sites of possible quantitative pathology in schizophrenia—temporal cortex, amygdala, substantia innominata, septal region, hypothalamus, reticular formation, thalamus, and hipocampus are intimately linked to prefrontal cortex (Fuster, 1980). Pathology in these regions may critically deafferent prefrontal cortex.

Though highly speculative, the data summarized here suggest that schizophrenia is a disorder of this circuitry, of the regulation of dorsolateral frontal cortex involved in cognitive behavior by certain connected limbic sites involved in the regulation of affective and emotional behavior. If this is the underlying pathophysiology, then the multiplicity of potential etiologies that could disrupt the system, plus variations in the degree of pathology and the time of insult, may help explain clinical heterogeneity.

REFERENCES

Ariel, R. N., Golden, C. J., Berg, R. A., Quaife, M. A., Dirksen, J. W., Forsell, T., Wilson, J., & Graber, B. (1983). Regional cerebral blood flow in schizophrenia with the Xenon ^{133}Xe inhalation method. *Archives of General Psychiatry, 40*, 258–263.

Berman, K. F., Zec, R. F., & Weinberger, D. R. (in press). Dysfunction of dorsolateral prefrontal cortex in schizophrenia. II. Implications of neuroleptic medication and of attention. *Archives of General Psychiatry.*

Blumer, D. (1975). Temporal lobe epilepsy and its psychiatric significance. In D. F. Benson & D. Blumer (Eds.), *Psychiatric aspects of neurological disease* (pp. 171–198). New York: Grune & Stratton.

Bogerts, B., Hantsch, J., & Herzer, M. (1983) A morphometric study of the dopamine containing cell groups in the mesencephalon of normals, Parkinson patients, and schizophrenics. *Biological psychiatry,18*, 951-969.

Bogerts, B., Mertz, E., & Schonfeldt-Bausch, R. (in press). Basal ganglia and limbic system pathology in schizophrenia: A morphometric study. *Archives of General Psychiatry.*

Buchsbaum, M. S., Ingvar, D. H., Kessler, R., Waters, R. N., Cappelletti, J., van Kammen, D. P., King, A. C., Johnson, J. L., Manning, R. G., Flynn, R. N., Mann, L. S.,

Bunney, W. E., & Sokoloff, L. (1982) Cerebral glucography with positron tomography. *Archives of General Psychiatry*, *39*, 251-259.

Carlen, P. L., Wortzman, G., Holgate, R. C., Wilkinson, D. A., & Rankin, J. G. (1978). Reversible cerebral atrophy in recently abstinent chronic alchololics measured by computed tomography scans. *Science*, *200*, 1076–1078.

Chapman, J. (1966). The early symptoms of schizophrenia. *British Journal of Psychiatry*, *112*, 225–251.

Dastur, D. K. (1959). The pathology of schizophrenia. *Archives of Neurology and Psychiatry*, *81*, 601-614.

Davison, K., & Bagley, C. R. (1969). Schizophrenic-like psychoses associated with organic disorders of the central nervous system. *British Journal of Psychiatry, Supplement, 4*, 113–184.

Franzen, G., & Ingvar, D. H. (1975). Absence of activation in frontal structures during psychological testing of chronic schizophrenics. *Journal of Neurology, Neurosurgery and Psychiatry*, *38*, 1027–1032.

Fuster, J. (1980). *The prefrontal cortex*. New York: Raven Press.

Gloor, P., Olivier, A., Quesney, L. F., Anderman, F., & Horowitz. S. (1982). The role of the limbic system in experiental phenomena of temporal lobe epilepsy. *Annals of Neurology*, *12*, 129–144.

Gur, R. E., Shalnick, R. E., Gur, R. C., Caroff, S., Rieger, W., Obrist, W. D., Younkin, D., & Reivich, M. (1983). Brain function in psychiatric disorders. I. Regional cerebral blood flow in medicated schizophrenics. *Archives of General Psychiatry*, *40*, 1250–1254.

Halgren, E., Walter, R. D., Cherlow, D. G., & Crandall, P. H. (1978). Mental phenomena evoked by electrical stimulation of the human hippocampal formation and amygdala. *Brain*, *101*, 83–117.

Heinz, R., Martinez, J., & Haenggeli, A. (1977). Reversibility of cerebral atrophy in anorexia nervosa and Cushing's syndrome. *Journal of Computer Assisted Tomography*, *1*, 415–418.

Ingvar, D. H., & Franzen, G. (1974). Distribution of cerebral activity in chronic schizophrenia. *Lancet*, *2*, 1484–1486.

Ingvar, D. H., & Gustafson, L. (1970). Regional cerebral blood flow in organic dementia with early onset. *Acta Neurologica Scandinavica, Supplementum*, *43*, 42–73.

Isaacson, R. L. (1982). *The limbic system* (2nd ed.). New York: Plenum Press.

Johnstone, E. C., Crow, T. J., Frith, C. D., Stevens, M., Kreel, L., & Husband, J. (1978). The dementia of dementia praecox. *Acta Psychiatrica Scandinavica*, *57*, 305–324.

Kling, A. S., Kuhl, D. E., Metter, E. J., Kurtz, N., Phelps, M. E., Reiger, W., & Hullet, J. (1984). *Positron computed tomography and CT scans in schizophrenia and depression* (NR Abstract No. 102). American Psychiatric Association annual meeting, Los Angeles.

Luchins, D. J., Jackman, H., & Meltzer, H. Y. (1983). Lateral ventricular size and drug-induced Parkinsonism. *Psychiatry Research*, *9*, 9–16.

Mathew, R. J., Duncan, G. C., Weinman, M. L., & Barr, D. L. (1982). Regional cerebral blood flow in schizophrenia. *Archives of General Psychiatry*, *39*, 1121–1124.

Meltzer, H. Y., & Stahl, S. E. (1976). The dopamine hypothesis of schizophrenia: A review. *Schizophrenia Bulletin*, *2*, 19–76.

Mialet, J. P., & Pichot, P. (1981). Eye tracking patterns in schizophrenia. *Archives of General Psychiatry*, *38*, 183–186.

Milner, B. (1963). Effects of different brain lesions on card sorting. *Archives of Neurology*, *9*, 90–100.

Morihisa, J. M., Duffy, F. H., & Wyatt, R. J. (1983). Brain electrical activity mapping (BEAM) in schizophrenic patients. *Archives of General Psychiatry*, *40*, 719–728.

Nauta, W. J. H., & Domesick, V. B. (1982). Neural associations of the limbic system. In *The neural basis of behavior* (pp. 175–206). New York: Spectrum.

Nieto, D., & Escobar, A. (1972). Major psychoses. In J. Minkler (Ed.), *Pathology of the nervous system* (pp. 2654-2665). New York: McGraw-Hill.

Nyback, H., Wiesel, F. A., Berggren, B.-M., & Hindmarsh, T. (1982). Computed tomography of the brain in patients with acute psychosis and in healthy volunteers. *Acta Psychiatrica Scandinavica*, *65*, 403–414.

Rodeck, C. H., & Campbell, S. (1979). Reversible cerebral atrophy caused by corticotrophin. *Lancet*, *1*, 1246–1247.

Rosenblum, W. I. (1965). Cerebral microcirculation: A review emphasizing the interrelationship of local blood flow and neuronal function. *Angiology*, *16*, 485–507.

Schultz, S. C., Koller, M. M., Kishore, P. R., Hamer, R. M., Gehl, J. J., & Friedel, R. O. (1983). Ventricular enlargement in teenage patients with schizophrenia spectrum disorder. *American Journal of Psychiatry*, *140*, 1592–1595.

Sheppard, G., Gruzelier, J., Manchanda, R., Hirsch, J. R., Wise, R., Frackowiak, R., & Jones, T. (1983). 150 positron emission tomography scanning in predominantly never treated acute schizophrenic patients. *Lancet*, *2*, 1448–1452.

Stevens, J. R. (1982). Neuropathology of schizophrenia. *Archives of General Psychiatry*, *39*, 1131–1139.

Stuss, D. T., & Benson, D. F. (1984). Neuropsychological studies of the frontal lobes. *Psychological Bulletin*, *95*, 3–28.

Weinberger, D. R. (1984). CAT scan finds in schizophrenia: Speculation on the meaning of it all. *Journal of Psychiatric Research*.

Weinberger, D. R., Berman, K. F., & Zec, R. F. (in press). Dysfunction of dorsolateral prefrontal cortex in schizophrenia. I. Regional cerebral blood flow evidence. *Archives of General Psychiatry*.

Weinberger, D. R., Bigelow, L. B., Kleinman, J. E., Klein, S. T., Rosenblatt, J. E., & Wyatt, R. J. (1980). Cerebral ventricular enlargement in chronic schizophrenia: Association with poor response to treatment. *Archives of General Psychiatry*, *37*, 11–14.

Weinberger, D. R., Cannon-Spoor, H. E., Potkin, S. G., & Wyatt, R. J. (1980). Poor premorbid adjustment and CT scan abnormalities in chronic schizophrenia. *American Journal of Psychiatry*, *137*, 1410–1413.

Weinberger, D. R., DeLisi, L. E., Perman, G., Targum, S., & Wyatt, R. J. (1982). CT scans in schizophreniform disorder and other acute psychiatric patients. *Archives of General Psychiatry*, *39*, 778–783.

Weinberger, D. R., Kleinman, J. E., Luchins, D. J., Bigelow, L. B., & Wyatt, R. J. (1980). Cerebellar pathology in schizophrenia: A controlled post-mortem study. *American Jornal of Psychiatry*, *137*, 359–361.

Weinberger, D. R., Wagner, R. L., & Wyatt, R. J. (1983). Neuropathological studies of schizophrenia: A selective review. *Schizophrenia Bulletin*, *9*, 193–212.

Weinberger, D. R., & Wyatt, R. J. (1982). Cerebral ventricular size: A biological marker for subtyping chronic schizophrenia. In E. Usdin & I. Hanin (Eds.), *Biological markers in psychiatry and neurology* (pp. 505–512). Oxford: Pergamon Press.

COMMENTARY

Dr. Malcolm Bowers:* Any questions for Dr. Weinberger?

Dr. Nina R. Schooler†: I just wanted to comment that I think your statement that the enlarged ventricles can't possibly be progressive and

* New Haven, Connecticut.

† Bethesda, Maryland.

clearly predate the diagnostic symptomatology is probably a little overstated. It would seem to me that the data you presented may be suggestive, but that without progressive studies where the same individuals are followed over time, that we would not really, some of us at any rate, be comfortable with that statement.

Dr. Weinberger: I'm glad you asked that question, and I want to address another issue that I think the blood flow studies speak to, some studies of yours. If I said whatever the words you used, if those were my words, they are certainly overstated. I don't remember using exactly those words, but maybe I did.

Let me say first that I don't think you have to follow the same individual over time. I think the data is so overwhelmingly consistent in terms of there not being a relationship between length of illness and size of ventricles. In normals, age correlates with size of ventricles. Why wouldn't length of illness, if it were a factor? You don't need to do single individuals agewise to show that age correlates significantly. Every study that has ever looked at age in the same way across decades, not in the same individual, has shown that age correlates with ventricular size. In addition, if the change were more than age, these patients would have a degenerative brain disease. They would end up with paraplegia in flexion in front of our eyes in 20 years. They don't have a progressive degenerative brain disease. We know that from having spent time with them. They don't continually deteriorate neurologically in front of our eyes. I think that, if you can show the correlation for age, you should be able to show it with length of illness.

The other point was related to the blood-flow data. It speaks to a study of yours. One of your follow-up studies pointed to the impact of various kinds of treatment on relapse rates in schizophrenia, and one of the interesting observations you made was that the more structured the environment, and the more occupational therapy someone had and the less insight-oriented psychotherapy and perhaps dorsolateral cortical functional demand placed on them, the better they did.

One of the things that appealed to us about this finding was that it seemed to speak to something that is clinically familiar in schizophrenia, which is that schizophrenic patients don't only do badly when you put them in situations that demand stressful problem solving and high-level cognitive function, they do worse than they did before you put them in that situation. This may be a sort of mini-metabolic correlate of that observation.

Dr. Robert Rose:* I would like to offer initially my compliments to Dr. Weinberger for a clear, engrossing, exciting review of this topic, and if a little bit of exaggeration or overstatement was necessary in order to achieve clarity, that's okay. I thought it was very good.

* Galveston, Texas.

I have a question for you to comment on. Could you relate some of your findings to the observations from PET studies on hypofrontality in schizophrenia. You mentioned that at rest there is evidence for hyperfrontality using xenon-133 techniques, whereas the PET findings show a hypofrontality. Would you try to comment?

Dr. Weinberger: First, Dr. Buchsbaum's PET study, which was a small sample of eight patients, found hypofrontality with 2-deoxyglucose. The best way I can understand that is that 2-deoxyglucose has a time resolution of about 40 minutes, approximately, so that what you are doing is compressing 40 minutes of mental activity into a cross-sectional metabolic landscape. So what went on in the first 10 minutes is averaged with what went on in the next 30-minutes.

The study from England by Sheppard *et al.* using oxygen-15, which has a much shorter half-life, although the scanning time was still 40 minutes. They did not find hypofrontality. The time resolution in terms of the mathematics of the inhalation xenon-133 blood-flow technique is in order of a couple of minutes. The whole study takes 12 minutes, but the actual mathematics, derived gray-matter flow, occurs in the first few minutes. So it may be that we are viewing more transient mental phenomenon and that if you compress the whole thing into a longer time frame, you may miss something that occurs from moment to moment.

Dr. Eugene Lebensohn:* In your work at St. Elizabeths, did you find any fingerprints on the pineal?

Dr. Weinberger: We have not. Frankly, I don't know how much that has been looked at recently. There are some old studies that have raised questions about the pineal, but I don't know of any data implicating that recently.

Dr. Elaine Walker†: At the expense of sounding perseverative, I want to make one other comment about the issue of age at onset and degeneration. The problem is that age is so much more reliably measured than age at onset, that it is much easier to get a significant correlation between age and degeneration. It has been my experience that it is difficult to reliably estimate age at onset of symptoms, and the potential for error variance there is great.

Dr. Weinberger: But it would seem to me that the error variance on age of onset is going to be a couple of years. When you are looking at a spectrum of people across three decades of length of illness, that would seem to me to be a much more powerful determinant of the variance than just the two or three years that may be the difference between actual age of onset versus nonactual age of onset, and I don't see any systematic reason

* Washington, D.C.

† Ithaca, New York.

why people with large ventricles should be more likely to misreport their age of onset than the other patients.

Dr. Walker: I think all tend to misreport, and perhaps patients with more degeneration are more subject to cognitive impairment. Again, I'm not arguing that the data are not compelling. I think they are, but I would just hope that a relationship between age at onset and degeneration is not discounted altogether as a possibility, because it has etiological implications.

Dr. Weinberger: I think the last point about that is critical. Even if you didn't find it on CAT scans, I would be very suspicious of it being progressive, because clinically, the patients don't have a progressive neurological disorder. So what would we make of it if we found it? I would be very leery that it had any meaning. If we found that it was progressive, I would be more concerned that it was an artifact of the experience either of being schizophrenic or of the treatment, because the patients do not have a progressive neurological condition that is slowly but inexorably destroying their brain at a greater rate than is aging.

Dr. Walker: I'm not sure I agree.

7

Dopamine and Negative Symptoms in Schizophrenia: Critique of the Type I–II Hypothesis

HERBERT Y. MELTZER
*University of Chicago Pritzker School of Medicine
and Illinois State Psychiatric Institute*

INTRODUCTION

During the last two decades, there has been considerable interest in the role of dopamine (DA) in the etiology of schizophrenia. Briefly, pharmacologic evidence concerning the mechanisms of action of antipsychotic drugs and psychotomimetic drugs, such as phencyclidine and *d*-amphetamine, led to the hypothesis that increased dopaminergic activity may be involved in the etiology of schizophrenia. However, very little direct biochemical, neuroendocrine or electrophysiologic evidence to support this hypothesis has been published, except for a few reports of increased numbers of DA receptors in the basal ganglia and nucleus accumbens of deceased schizophrenics (Lee *et al.*, 1978; Owen *et al.*, 1978). Even these findings are controversial because such increases could be the result of previous treatment with neuroleptic drugs or secondary to decreased dopaminergic activity (Mackay *et al.*, 1982). In addition, the specificity of an abnormality of dopaminergic transmission for schizophrenia has been challenged because of psychopharmacologic and neurochemical evidence that suggests abnormalities in dopaminergic activity may be etiologically important for some aspects, or types, of depression and mania (Randrup *et al.*, 1975). Like the evidence for the role of DA in schizophrenia, such evidence is mainly inferential, that is, it is largely based on the presumptive mechanism of action of antidepressant or anti-manic drugs. These and other considerations have led to a widespread consensus that increased dopaminergic activity in an absolute sense, or relative to other neurotransmitters that can influence dopaminergic neurons (e.g., acetylcholine or GABA), may be involved in the "acute psychosis" syndrome that is common to schizophrenia, the affective psychoses, and some drug-induced psychoses (Meltzer & Stahl, 1976).

Because of the inability to establish direct evidence for increased dopaminergic activity in schizophrenia and the apparent lack of specificity of an abnormality in dopaminergic activity for schizophrenia, Meltzer and colleagues proposed that the DA hypothesis of schizophrenia be revised in three ways:

1. Some patients with the schizophrenic phenotype may have an entirely non-DA-dependent disorder.
2. Dopaminergic activity may be involved only in the early (acute) stages of the disorder.
3. Some aspects of schizophrenia, particularly negative symptoms (e.g., flat affect, poverty of thought content, and social withdrawal) could be due to decreased dopaminergic activity (Meltzer, 1979a, 1979b; Meltzer & Stahl, 1976).

It was proposed that viral infections, autoimmune mechanisms, cell-mediated toxicity, plastic changes in monoamine neurons such as branching or sprouting, or dysregulation of normally integrated neuronal systems should be considered as the primary etiologic factors. Increased or decreased dopaminergic activity was suggested to be secondary to one or more of these factors (Meltzer, 1979a, 1979b; Meltzer & Stahl, 1976).

A particularly useful variation of these concepts was offered by Crow (1980a, 1980b), who delineated a DA-related syndrome within schizophrenia (Type I) and a non-DA-related syndrome (Type II). Crow considers positive symptoms, such as hallucinations and delusions, during both the acute and the chronic phases of schizophrenia, good response to neuroleptics, and no intellectual impairment to be characteristic of the Type I syndrome. The etiology of the Type I syndrome was postulated to be increased dopaminergic activity, due to increased numbers of D_2-type DA receptors (Crow, 1980a, 1980b; Owen, Cross, Crow, Lofthouse, & Poulter, 1981). According to Crow, the Type II syndrome is characterized by negative symptoms (e.g., flat affect, poverty of thought and speech content, and loss of volition, as well as poor response to neuroleptics, irreversibility, and intellectual impairment). The etiology was postulated to be micro- and macroscopic morphological brain abnormalities. Crow proposed that the Type II syndrome was associated with ventricular enlargement and brain atrophy as seen by pneumoencephalography (PEG) or computed tomography (CT) in some chronic schizophrenics (Johnstone, Frith, Crow, Husband, & Kreel, 1976). He subsequently attributed these abnormalities to viral infections and suggested that the phenomenology of the Type II syndrome might be due to the loss from the brain of cholecystokinin (CCK), a neuropeptide (Ferrier *et al.*, 1983). This suggestion was based on a study that demonstrated a negative correlation between levels of CCK in the brain and the presence of negative symptoms in evaluations carried out some time prior the death (Ferrier *et al.*, 1983).

The concepts of Type I and Type II syndromes can be seen to be a reformulation of the major dimensions of schizophrenic subtyping. It clusters together acuteness, functional DA-related etiology, remission, positive symptoms, and good outcome, and contrasts these with chronicity, negative symptoms, a structural etiology unrelated to DA, neuroleptic resistance, and poor outcome. The major conceptual feature of this theory can be seen to be a sharp delimitation of the role of DA in schizophrenia and the specific linkage between CT scan abnormalities and a specific subtype of schizophrenia that was associated with a CCK deficiency. This theory, more so than any previous version of the DA hypothesis, emphasized that the phenomenology represented by the Type I and Type II syndromes, were "independent dimensions reflecting different underlying pathological processes" (Crow, 1980a). The diminished significance of DA in schizophrenia, the importance attached to the CT scan abnormalities (Johnstone *et al.*, 1976, Maser & Keith, 1983; Weinberger, Torrey, Neophytides, & Wyatt, 1979a, 1979b), and the increased emphasis on negative symptoms in this model has aroused considerable interest in the research community (Ashcroft, Blackwood, Besson, Palomo, & Waring, 1981; Freeman, 1981; Marsden, 1984).

A critical evaluation of some of the important concepts of the Type I and II syndromes will be the subject of the rest of this review. Specifically, we will examine (1) the responsiveness of negative symptoms to neuroleptic or L-Dopa treatment and hence their irreversibility; (2) the association between CT scan abnormalities and negative symptoms; (3) the relationship between CT scan abnormalities and catecholamines; and (4) the relationship between CCK, as well as other neuropeptides, and DA.

PSYCHOPHARMACOLOGIC STUDIES AND NEGATIVE SYMPTOMS

The evidence cited by Crow (1980a) for the unresponsiveness of negative symptoms to neuroleptics was (*a*) the ineffectiveness of *cis*-flupenthixol, a potent neuroleptic, for the treatment of negative symptoms compared to its effect on positive symptoms (Johnstone, Frith, Crow, Carney, & Price, 1978); and (*b*) the study of Angrist, Rotrosen, and Gershon (1980) in which negative symptoms defined as emotional withdrawal, motor retardation, and blunted affect subscales of the Brief Psychiatric Rating Scale (BPRS; Overall & Gorham, 1962), were less affected by neuroleptic treatment for 1–6 weeks, or by the administration of 0.5 mg/kg *d*-amphetamine in a drug-free state, than were the following positive symptoms: (1) thought disturbance, (2) activation, and (3) hostile–suspiciousness. On close examination, this evidence does not appear persuasive (see also Ashcroft *et al.*, 1981; Mackay, 1981). In the study from Crow's group (Johnstone *et al.*, 1978), 45 patients were randomly assigned to one of three treatments: *cis*-flupenthixol, *trans*-flupenthixol (which lacks significant DA receptor blocking properties at the dose used), and placebo. Thus, there were only 15 patients in each group. First, this is, as evidence to be presented suggests, probably an insufficient number of subjects to detect a drug effect if there is heterogeneity within the group with regard to responsiveness to neuroleptic treatment. Second, virtually no information was given as to the subjects' age, duration of illness, or number of previous episodes. These factors can strongly influence the response of negative symptoms to neuroleptic treatment (H. Y. Meltzer, unpublished data). Third, the dose of *cis*-flupenthixol, 6–9 mg/day, is relatively low, comparable to approximately 5–15 mg haloperidol/day if one uses the ability of both drugs to displace [^{3}H]-haloperidol from bovine or rat striatal membranes (Seeman, 1981) as a reference. Fourth, patients were evaluated after only 28 days. Although positive symptoms responded during the 4-week trial, negative symptoms may require longer periods of treatment. A fifth, and perhaps the most important critique of this study, is that the mean initial ratings of negative symptoms in the three groups of subjects was approximately 1, out of a maximum of 4. No indication of how many subjects had any negative symptoms was provided. In addition, only two negative symptoms were examined and these were examined separately rather than as part of a subscale. By contrast, positive symptoms were near maximal for the scale used, suggesting that the sample included a number of patients experiencing severe acute exacerbations, with few negative symptoms. In all, this study cannot be taken as significant evidence to support the *generalization* that negative symptoms do not respond to neuroleptic treatment and therefore have a different etiology.

The other study cited by Crow (1980b), that of Angrist *et al.* (1980), utilized the withdrawal–retardation factor of the BPRS to assess change in negative symptoms. Neither neuroleptic treatment or *d*-amphetamine had any effect on its components, motor retardation and blunted affect; however, the emotional withdrawal item did improve with neuroleptic treatment, whereas it worsened with *d*-amphetamine, suggesting it might be affected by changes in dopaminergic activity. Angrist *et al.* (1980; B. Angrist, personal communication, 1984) believe that ratings of the emotional withdrawal item of the BPRS do not assess inadequate capacity for emotional response but, rather, any incongruity between emotional and cognitive states, that is, inappropriate affect. Even if this is true in this study, some authors do accept inappropriate affect as a negative symptom (Andreasen, 1982; Lewine, Fogg, & Meltzer, 1983). Thus, this study as well as that of Johnstone *et al.* (1978) do not appear to provide strong support for the lack of responsiveness of negative symptoms to neuroleptics.

Neuroleptic Treatment and Negative Symptoms

Review of the literature on negative symptoms and neuroleptic treatment in schizophrenia reveals considerable evidence that indicates that such clinical symptoms as flat affect; poverty of thought and speech content; indifference to environment; impaired social participation; and slowed speech and movements, do respond to neuroleptic treatment in a significant proportion of schizophrenic patients at various phases of their illness (Meltzer, in preparation). It is beyond the scope of this article to review this literature in detail here. However, it will be of value to mention four types of evidence to support the above conclusions: (1) the NIMH Collaborative Study of the effect of phenothiazines (Goldberg, Klerman, & Cole, 1965); (2) the effect of pimozide and other diphenylbutylpiperidine (DPBP) neuroleptics on negative symptoms; (3) the effect of clozapine on negative symptoms; and (4) the effect of sulpiride on negative symptoms.

THE NIMH COLLABORATIVE STUDY

Goldberg *et al.* (1965) randomly assigned 340 acute schizophrenic patients to placebo, chlorpromazine (CPZ), thioridazine, or fluphenazine. The duration of treatment was 6 weeks and the dose was equivalent to 650 mg/day CPZ. The major rating instrument was the Ward Behavior Rating Scale (WBRS; Burdock, Hakerem, Hardesty, & Zubin, 1959) and the Inpatient Multidimensional Psychiatric Rating Scale (IMPS; Lorr, Klett, McNair, & Laskey, 1962). Ratings were done blindly. Drug-treated patients showed significantly more improvement than placebo-treated patients in such apparent negative symptoms as hebephrenic symptoms, social participation, indifference to environment, and slowed speech and movement. It must be noted that 50% of the patients in the NIMH Collaborative Study were experiencing their first psychotic episode, 60% were experiencing their first hospitalization, and a high proportion had an acute onset following a precipitating event. Thus, this study does not specifically bear upon the issue of the responsiveness of negative symptoms to neuroleptic treatment in the most chronic patients.

DIPHENYLBUTYLPIPERIDINE NEUROLEPTIC DRUGS

There have been a variety of controlled and uncontrolled comparisons, involving in the aggregate large numbers of schizophrenic patients, in which pimozide, clopimozide, fluspiriline, and penfluridol, all of which are DPBP-type drugs, have been compared to phenothiazines or butyrophenones with regard to their overall efficacy as antipsychotic drugs and their ability to diminish negative and positive symptoms (Frangos *et al.*, 1978; Gallant, Mielke, Spirtes, Swanson, & Bost, 1974; Haas & Beckmann, 1982; Kudo, 1972; Lapierre, 1978; Lapierre & Lavalle, 1975; Shopsin, Klein, Gerbino, & Selzer, 1977; Singh,. 1973). A large proportion of these studies report significant advantages, or trends, in the direction of the DPBP drugs producing greater improvement than other types of neuroleptics in emotional withdrawal, anergia, blunted affect, and social interaction, while having equivalent efficacy in treating positive symptoms. For example, Haas and Beckmann (1982) treated 15 schizophrenics with haloperidol (40–60 mg/day) or pimozide (40–60 mg/day) for 30 days. Two-thirds of the patients in both groups had a good or very good response but only the pimozide-treated patients had a significant decrease in emotional withdrawal and blunted affect on the BPRS. Further controlled study of pimozide versus non-DPBP neuroleptics with more sophisticated means of assessing negative symptoms would be of interest. Gould, Murphy, Reynolds, and Snyder (1983) recently proposed that the greater ability of DPBP drugs to diminish negative symptoms might be related to their greater potency in blocking calcium channels. This is an intriguing suggestion but there is no direct evidence to support this as yet.

EFFECT OF CLOZAPINE ON NEGATIVE SYMPTOMS

Clozapine, a dibenzodiazepine, is another antipsychotic drug for which there is some evidence that it is superior to standard neuroleptics in treating negative symptoms. In a multicenter, double blind, collaborative study, 150 schizophrenic patients were randomly assigned to clozapine or CPZ at median doses of clozapine (300–450 mg/day) or CPZ (450–900 mg/day) for an 8-week period. Clozapine was superior to CPZ in nearly all categories of symptoms, but particularly in diminishing emotional withdrawal and blunted affect, as rated with the BPRS at the end of both 2 and 8 weeks of treatment (Honigfeld, Patin, Belendiuk, & Singer, 1983). Clozapine was also superior to CPZ in decreasing anergia in a European collaborative study (Honigfeld *et al.*, 1983). Similar results were reported by Gelenberg and Doller (1979). In the study of I. Gerlach, Koppelhus, Helweg, and Monrad (1974), there was a trend for clozapine to be superior to CPZ in the reduction of BPRS withdrawal. However, both Nisikanen *et al.* (1974) and Guirguis, Voinesko, Gray, and Schlieman (1977) reported that clozapine and chlorpromazine had comparable effects on negative symptoms. Further investigation of the effect of clozapine versus standard neuroleptics on negative symptoms is clearly necessary.

EFFECT OF SULPIRIDE ON NEGATIVE SYMPTOMS

Sulpiride is a substituted benzamide which, like clozapine, has a profile of low extrapyramidal side effects and has been claimed to be especially effective in defect-stage schizophrenics (Elizur, Davidson, & Psych, 1975; Haase, Floru, & Ulrich, 1974; Harnryd *et al.*, 1984; Nishiura, 1976). For example, Harnryd *et al.* (1984) compared the effect of chlorpromazine versus sulpiride on 50 schizophrenics on an "autism" scale that consisted of (1) inability to feel; (2) lassitude; (3) withdrawal; (4) reduced speech; and (5) slowness of movement. Sulpiride produced significantly greater improvement than chlorpromazine at 1–8 weeks in this subscale despite no overall difference in the change in positive symptoms or global ratings.

Preliminary Report of Neuroleptic Treatment of Schizophrenia: Effect on Negative Symptoms

We have carried out a retrospective analysis of the effects of neuroleptic treatment, mainly with CPZ or trifluroperazine, on negative and positive symptoms in schizophrenics. The method of the study and its results will be briefly reported here because of its relevance to the issue at hand. Patients admitted to the Mental Health Clinical Research Center of the University of Chicago–Illinois State Psychiatric Institute were diagnosed according to Research Diagnosis Criteria (RDC, Spitzer, Endicott, & Robins, 1978) based on the Present State Examination (Wing, Cooper, & Sartorius, 1974) and additional data (Meltzer, Perline, & Lewine, 1982). Patients were rated weekly with the Schedule for Affective Disorder–Change (SADS–C; Endicott & Spitzer, 1978). Patients were also rated with the (NOSIE, Honigfeld, Gillis, & Klett, 1966) by nursing staff at admission and discharge. There were 169 patients admitted between September 1977 and June 1983 who met the RDC for schizophrenia. The mean age was 27.0 ± 7.6 years; 60% were male, 40% were female. The number of previous admissions was 3.6 ± 2.9 and the duration of illness was 6.1 ± 4.5 years. The duration of treatment was 10.0 ± 5.1 weeks (range 2–44 weeks). The mean peak dose of neuroleptic in chlorpromazine equivalents was 727 ± 432 mg/day.

Negative and positive symptoms were assessed by means of scales derived by our laboratory from the SADS–C (Lewine *et al.*, 1983). The Negative Symptom Scale (NSS) consists of 11 items. Eight of the 11 items are also included in the Scale for the Assessment of Negative Symptoms (SANS, Andreasen, 1982). These are blunted affect, inappropriate affect, poverty of content, loss of interest, loss of sexual interest, slowed speech, slowed body movements, and fatigue. The other three items are incoherence, loose associations, and depressed appearance. The first two items were included in the NSS based on Bleuler's inclusion of them in the core characteristics of schizophrenia; depressed appearance was included after empirical testing indicated it belonged within the group (Lewine *et al.*, 1983). The Positive Symptom Scale (PSS) consists of 23 SADS–C items concerning delusions and hallucinations only. The total NSS and Positive Symptom Scale (PSS) scores were tallied by summing up the items present, regardless of severity. Median PSS and NSS scale scores were 5 and 4, respectively.

Only the issue of the response of positive and negative symptoms to treatment will be discussed here. Significant decreases in both PSS and

Table 1. ANCOVA of Positive and Negative Symptoms in Male and Female Schizophrenics

	Adjusted means							
	Positive				Negative			
Sex	*N*	Adm.	Disch.	Δ	*N*	Adm.	Disch.	Δ
Male	103	4.71	2.44	2.27	103	3.62	2.86	0.78
Female	68	4.74	2.34	2.40	68	4.00	2.41	1.59

ANCOVA table	*F*	*p*	ANCOVA table	*F*	*p*
Sex	0.00	0.95	Sex	0.020	0.875
Time	52.76	0.000	Time	3.83	0.05
Time × Sex	0.11	0.75	Time × Sex	2.78	0.007

Hebephrenic and Nonhebephrenic Negative Symptoms in Male and Female Schizophrenics

	Hebephrenic				Nonhebephrenic			
Sex	*N*	Adm.	Disch.	Δ	*N*	Adm.	Disch.	Δ
Male	103	1.26	0.66	0.60	105	2.51	1.74	0.77
Female	66	1.29	0.52	0.77	68	2.66	1.92	0.74

ANOVA table	*F*	*p*	ANOVA table	*F*	*p*
Sex	.19	.66	Sex	.016	.90
Time	42.85	0	Time	22.34	0
Time × Sex	.66	.42	Time × Sex	3.97	.048

NSS symptom scores between admission and discharge were observed (Table 1). An analysis of covariance demonstrated that the decrease in PSS and NSS was significant even after covarying out the influence of the change in one on the change in the other. The improvement in PSS was the same in both sexes but improvement in NSS was significantly greater in females than males. Thus, there was a 22% decrease in NSS in male schizophrenics compared to a 40% decrease in female schizophrenics. The latter figure compares closely to the 48% and 51% decreases in PSS scores observed in male and female schizophrenics. Positive symptoms, while treatment responsive, did not clear completely by any means. At discharge, 60/169 (35.5%) patients had 0 or 1 NSS ratings, compared to 100/169 (59.2%) with 0 or 1 PSS ratings. Of the patients with NSS or PSS ratings of at least 5 at admission, we identified those who had an improvement in PSS or NSS scores of at least 5. There were 21/55 (38.2%) such patients with improvement in NSS of at least 5 as well as 44/78 (56.4%) with improvement in PSS of at least 5 ($\chi^2 = 4.32, p < .05$). Thus, marked improvement in NSS as well as PSS was possible but such change was more common in PSS. These results indicate that significant improvement in negative as well as positive symptoms is possible in schizophrenic patients, at least in the milieu of our unit, with our patients, and with the duration of treatment and dosage of drugs we utilized. However, negative symptoms were less treatment-responsive than positive symptoms, especially in 5 male schizophrenics.

The patients in this study usually had admixtures of positive and negative symptoms at admission, and lesser amounts of both at discharge. Only 21/165 (12.7%) of the patients had zero PSS ratings at admission; another 13 (7.9%) had only one positive symptom. This may have contributed to the significant effect of neuroleptic treatment on negative symptoms in this study. It could be that a study that includes only in-patients with residual schizophrenia, who could approximate the clinical profile of the Type II syndrome, will not show a neuroleptic effect. Overall and Rhodes (1982) found no evidence for neuroleptic effect in a reanalysis of data from 473 patients, most of whom can be assumed to be schizophrenic, who had the withdrawn–disorganized profile on the BPRS (high on emotional withdrawal, motor retardation, blunted affect, and disorganization; low on hallucinations, unusual thought content, hostility, suspiciousness, anxiety, and excitement). However, neuroleptic effects were apparent in 965 probable schizophrenic patients with three other syndromes: florid thinking disorder, agitation–excitement, and hostility–suspiciousness. These syndromes included high ratings on one or more of the following symptoms but not all of them: emotional withdrawal, motor retardation, blunted affect, or disorganization. There was no way to determine specifically from the published data if neuroleptics affected these symptoms in a significant proportion of these patients, but given the 25%–39% incidence of at least 50% reduction in BPRS total score between admission and 6 weeks of neuroleptic treatment in these patients, compared to 6%–29% improvement in placebo-treated patients, it is likely that some, if not all, of these symptoms also improved in these patients.

The data from the NIMH Collaborative Study, DPBP drug studies, and clozapine versus standard neuroleptics, as well as our data, strongly indicate that negative symptoms are not irreversible and may respond during neuroleptic treatment. It will require more controlled studies to determine if this improvement is due to the DA receptor blocking action of neuroleptics and whatever adaptive changes in the dopaminergic system that are the consequence of DA receptor blockade.

EFFECT OF L-DOPA ON NEGATIVE SYMPTOMS

The ability of neuroleptic treatment to diminish negative symptoms would appear to indicate a role of DA in the genesis of negative symptoms. However, it would be premature to conclude from these studies that the improvement in negative symptoms is related to the ability of the neuroleptics to block postsynaptic DA receptors. Effects of these drugs on DA neurons may be relevant (e.g., blockade of DA autoreceptors). It has already been suggested that the ability of DPBP drugs to diminish negative symptoms is due to calcium channel blockade. It is also possible that effects on other neurotransmitters or neuromodulators, including peptidergic neurons, might mediate neuroleptic effects on negative symptoms. We and others have suggested decreased dopaminergic activity may be relevant to the treatment of negative symptoms (Chouinard & Jones, 1978; Mackay, 1981; Meltzer, 1979a, 1979b; Meltzer & Stahl, 1976). This issue may be, in part, addressed pharmacologically. L-Dopa, the precursor of DA, in doses of .5–6.0 g/day, produced little or no improvement in negative symptoms in a small number of schizophrenic patients in most open studies (Angrist, Sathananthan, & Gershon, 1973; Calil, Yesavage, & Hollister, 1977; Yayura-Tobias, Diamond, & Merlis, 1970). However, other studies, both uncontrolled (Inanaga *et al.*, 1975; Ogura, Kishimato, & Nakao, 1976) and controlled (Alpert, Friedhoff, Marcos, & Diamond, 1978; Buchanan, Parton, & Warren, 1975; J. Gerlach & Luhdorf, 1975; Inanaga *et al.*, 1975) have provided evidence that L-dopa, in doses of 0.5–5.0 gm/day, when given to patients who have also usually been receiving neuroleptics, may improve negative symptoms without exacerbation of positive symptoms. In these studies, L-dopa was particularly effective in schizophrenics who were ill for no more than 10 years.

We have administered L-dopa or L-dopa and carbidopa to 6 schizophrenic patients receiving neuroleptics who had received a course of neuroleptic drug treatment alone following admission to the hospital (H. Meltzer, unpublished data). Five of the six patients still had marked negative symptoms at the end of treatment with neuroleptic alone. Of the six patients, two had a slight or moderate decrease in NSS scores during the neuroleptic alone phase. L-Dopa was added to the neuroleptic treatment without changing the dose of neuroleptic. The mean dose of neuroleptic alone was 733 ± *SD* 50 mg/day CPZ equivalent. The mean duration of neuroleptic alone treatment was 31.8 ± 12.4 days (range 15–47 days). The mean dose of L-dopa or L-dopa and carbidopa expressed as L-dopa equivalents was 1400 ± 692 mg/day (range 400–2000 mg/day). The mean duration of neuroleptic plus L-dopa was 31.3 ± 18.4 days (range 18–65 days).

Five of the six patients had a slight reduction in NSS scores following the addition of L-dopa. One of the six L-dopa-treated patients had none of the symptoms included in the NSS score at the end of the L-dopa trial. The four others who improved still had considerable symptoms as indicated by a mean NSS scores of 4.0 ± *SD* 0.8, compared to 6.0 ± 1.4 prior to the addition of L-dopa/carbidopa. Clinically meaningful improvement in social functioning, interest and participation in ward activities, social interaction, self-grooming, and spontaneous activity occurred following L-dopa administration in three of the five patients who improved after L-dopa. One of the five responders, a female, had no positive symptoms at any time during this study but the other four had hallucinations, delusions, and thought disorder. L-dopa did not induce or exacerbate positive symptoms in five of the six subjects. As mentioned above, one of the subjects had an increase in auditory hallucinations and delusions while receiving L-dopa.

The improvement in NSS scores in five of six patients following the addition of L-dopa could have been a placebo effect or the result of the additional weeks of treatment with neuroleptics. Further placebo-controlled studies appear to be indicated.

Space considerations permit only a brief discussion of the biological basis for the improvement in negative symptoms due to L-dopa, and to reconcile the apparent paradox of two classes of drugs with opposite modes of action, DA antagonists and DA agonists, producing improvement, in this set of symptoms. An indirect DA agonist, *d*-amphetamine, can also produce improvement in positive symptoms in some schizophrenics (van Kammen, 1981; van Kammen *et al.*, 1982). Direct-acting DA agonists, such as bromocriptine, at low doses can also produce improvement in schizophrenia, possibly by autoreceptor stimulation (Meltzer, 1982); we have also observed improvement with high doses of bromocriptine in some patients, in uncontrolled trials (H. Meltzer, unpublished data). The possible biological basis for the therapeutic benefit of both DA agonists and antagonists on positive and negative symptoms could be the existence of two DA pathways (e.g., prefrontal cortex and mesolimbic) that have an inhibitory effect on the other. Diminished activity of one of the pathways (e.g., the prefrontal cortex) could be involved in the etiology of negative symptoms, whereas increased activity of the other pathway could be involved in the pathophysiology of the positive symptoms. The therapeutic benefits of DA agonists would be due to stimulation of the dopamine receptors in the prefrontal cortex, which would then lead to inhibition of the subcortical DA pathways. Neuroleptics would act by blocking postsynaptic receptors of the subcortical pathway (Bannon & Roth, 1983). Differences in DA receptor affinity for agonists and antagonists in the two areas could provide the biological basis for the selective action of the agonists or antagonists. Regional differences in DA agonist and antagonist binding-site density and affinity on a genetic basis have been described (Boehme & Ciaranello, 1981). Other mechanisms are certainly possible to explain the DA agonist and antagonist efficacy and will be discussed elsewhere (Meltzer, in preparation).

If, indeed, negative symptoms are responsive to neuroleptics and DA agonists, regardless of mechanism and regardless of whether the improvement is a direct effect or secondary to the improvement in positive symptoms, then two basic concepts of Crow's model, which argued against a role of

DA in the etiology of negative symptoms, will clearly have been invalidated. However, even if the irreversibility and failure to respond to neuroleptics (or L-dopa) of negative symptoms were established facts, would they provide valid reasons for drawing the conclusion that DA is not involved in the etiology of the Type II syndrome? It is generally accepted that treatment response is rarely a valid reason for either assuming or rejecting basic etiology. The classic example in neuropsychiatry of where clinical response is not a valid indication of etiology is Parkinson's disease, in which the responsiveness of early Parkinson's disease to anticholinergic drugs would lead to the erroneous conclusion that increased cholinergic activity was the cause of Parkinson's disease. Similarly, if one examined only severe endstage Parkinson's disease in which L-dopa responsiveness disappears altogether, one would draw the erroneous conclusion that DA was irrevelant to the pathophysiology of that disorder. The same error might occur with severe tardive dyskinesia when it becomes irreversible and totally unresponsive to suppression by neuroleptic drugs, obscuring the high probability that DA is involved in its pathophysiology. Thus, reasoning from lack of treatment response can lead to erroneous conclusions concerning pathogenesis. Negative symptoms in some patients may be unresponsive to increases or decreases in dopaminergic activity at the time of study for reasons such as structural changes in dopaminergic neurons or because other neurotransmitters or neuromodulators exert a more powerful influence on symptom expression (Meltzer, 1979a).

BIOLOGICAL MEASURES AND NEGATIVE SYMPTOMS

Negative Symptoms and Platelet MAO Activity

We examined the relationship between platelet MAO activity and NSS in schizophrenia because of the possibility that both negative symptoms and platelet MAO activity could be related to decreased dopaminergic activity and that platelet MAO might be a marker for brain dopaminergic activity.

Platelet MAO activity was determined in 42 male and 17 female schizophrenic patients of whom all but two had ratings of at least 1 on the NSS. A significant positive Spearman correlation ($\rho = 0.53, N = 42, p = .0003$) was found in the male schizophrenics; split half correlations were .49 ($p = .023$) and .61 ($p = .003$). The correlation between platelet MAO and NSS scores was not significant in female schizophrenics ($\rho = -.30, N = 17, p =$ NS). Platelet MAO activity did not significantly correlate with PSS scores for either men or women ($\rho = -0.21$ and 0.27, respectively). Contributing to the correlation between NSS scores and platelet MAO activity in the male schizophrenics were significant correlations between platelet MAO and fatigue, slowed speech, loosening of associations.

The biological basis and significance of the correlation between platelet MAO activity and NSS scores in male schizophrenics has been discussed in detail elsewhere (Lewine & Meltzer, 1984). The relationship we have observed between platelet MAO activity and negative symptoms will have to be replicated in an independent sample and with more detailed ratings of negative symptoms than was possible in our retrospective study. Nevertheless, it is of interest that the symptoms associated with the Type II syndrome were related to an enzyme that is intimately involved in the metabolism of DA. There is evidence that brain DA is metabolized by both MAO A and B (Glover, Elsworth, & Sandler, 1980; Glover, Sandler, Owen, & Riley, 1977; O'Carroll, Fowler, Phillips, Tobbia, & Tipton, 1983). Platelet MAO is the type B form. It is possible that high MAO B activity in some areas of the brain might lead to a DA deficiency. It is of interest that platelet MAO activity is significantly correlated with CSF HVA concentrations in patients with Parkinson's disease (Mann, Stanley, Kaplan, Sweeney, & Neophytides, 1983). Thus, increased brain MAO activity may be a factor through which a decrease in dopaminergic activity leads to negative symptoms.

Ventricular Brain Ratio, Negative Symptoms, and Dopamine

An integral part of Crow's argument for the differentiation of Type I and Type II schizophrenia is that the Type II syndrome was associated with structural changes in the brain on both the microscopic (cell loss) and gross levels (enlarged ventricles as demonstrable in CT scans) and that this was associated with negative symptoms (Johnstone *et al.*, 1976, 1978). A number of pneumoencephalographic studies had previously reported ventricular enlargement in patients with marked deficit state symptoms (Asano, 1967; Haug, 1962; Huber, 1957; Huber, Gross, & Schutter, 1975; Nagy, 1963). Numerous research groups have sought to validate the CT findings reported by Johnstone *et al.* (1976). Most investigators have found increased ventricle-to-brain ratios (VBR) in some chronic schizophrenics (Andreasan, Olsen, Dennent, & Smith, 1982; Golden *et al.*, 1980; Luchins, Lewine, & Meltzer, 1984; Nasrallah, Jacoby, McCalley-Whitters, & Kuperman, 1982; Nasrallah, McCalley-Whitters, & Jacoby, 1982; Okasha & Madkour, 1982; Weinberger, Torrey, Neophytides, & Wyatt, 1979), but the percentage of abnormal scans observed in most of these studies was far less than that reported by Crow's group (Johnstone *et al.*, 1976). Several investigators have found no such increase (Benes *et al.*, 1982; Jernigan, Zatz, Moses, & Berger, 1982) but there are legitimate concerns over the nature of the patient populations in both studies. Furthermore, some groups found the incidence of enlarged ventricles in schizophrenics and affective disorders to be not significantly different (Luchins *et al.*, 1984; Nasrallah, McCalley-Whitters & Jacoby, 1982; Pearlson & Veroff, 1981; Rieder, Mann, Weinberger, van Kammen, & Post, 1983). Kling, Kurtz, Tachiki, and Orzeck (1982–1983) found that alcoholics and patients with migraine or seizure disorders, as well as schizophrenics, had significantly larger VBRs than normal controls. This indicates that increased VBR is not specific to patients with the Type II syndrome and may be present in psychotic patients with largely a Type I clinical picture plus affective symptoms.

Studies of the relationship between increased VBR (or other morphological abnormalities such as sulcal widening and cerebral asymmetry), and negative symptoms or cognitive impairment in patients who meet criteria for schizophrenia, have produced mixed results. Takahashi *et al.* (1981) found a relationship between CT abnormalities (including enlarged ventricles) and blunted affect and conceptual disorganization in 280 schizophrenics. Andreasen *et al.* (1982) found a slight, nonsignificant tendency toward increased negative symptoms (especially alogia, anhedonia, and attention deficit, but not flat affect or decreased volition) in 16 patients with ventricles 1 *SD* above the control mean, compared to 16 patients with the smallest ventricles. Patients with large ventricles had significantly fewer positive symptoms than patients with small ventricles. Patients with large ventricles also had significantly lower mean scores on the Mini-Mental Status Exam than did patients with small ventricles. Kling *et al.* (1982–1983) recently reported that, in a group of 26 chronic schizophrenic patients who were nonresponsive to neuroleptic treatment, those who met DSM-III criteria for residual schizophrenia had large VBRs compared to the paranoid schizophrenics and normal controls. They noted that the patients with larger VBRs were characterized by blunted affect but that Type I and II symptoms were common to both groups of patients. However, Bishop *et al.* (1983) found a *negative* correlation between VBR and discharge BPRS ratings of emotional withdrawal, depression, and blunted affect in 46 schizophrenic patients, whereas Nasrallah, Jacoby *et al.* (1982) found no relationship between negative symptoms and VBR or sulcal widening but the negative symptoms were assessed from a chart review and may not have been reliable. Golden *et al.* (1980) also found more neuropsychological impairment using the Luria–Nebraska Neuropsychological Battery in schizophrenics with large ventricles.

Weinberger *et al.* (1980) found no significant clinical response to neuroleptics in patients with large ventricles, whereas those with normal ventricles had a good response. However, several other studies have been unable to replicate the relationship between poor clinical response to neuroleptic drugs and increased VBR in schizophrenia (Boronow, Pickar, & Ninan, 1985; Luchins *et al.*, 1984; van Kammen *et al.*, 1983). Thus, the conclusion that Type II schizophrenics specifically have large ventricles or that large ventricles are associated with poor response to neuroleptics must be considered as in doubt. The specific clinical profile, if any, of the schizophrenics with large ventricles has yet to be identified.

There is, however, some evidence that relates VBR to the dopaminergic system and other biogenic amines. Nyback, Berggren, and Hindmarsh (1983) found a significant negative correlation between the size of the lateral ventricles and the levels of the DA metabolite homovanillac acid (HVA) and the serotonin metabolite, 5-hydroxyindoleacetic acid (5-HIAA), in the CSF. This was not so for normal controls. These results were interpreted to indicate decreased dopaminergic and serotonergic activity, or a decreased number of brain 5-HT or DA neurons, in the brains of patients with large ventricles. Second, van Kammen *et al.* (1983) found lower CSF HVA levels and dopamine-β-hydroxylase (DBH) activity in schizophrenic patients with CT evidence of brain atrophy compared to patients with normal CT scans. Finally, we have reported (Luchins, Jackman, & Meltzer, in press) that during a 5-week period of treatment with CPZ, the VBR of 8 schizophrenic patients who required antiparkinsonian medication for treatment of rigidity was greater than that of 12 such patients who did not require antiparkinsonian medication, or a control group. This is further evidence that increased VBR may be associated with decreased dopaminergic activity, since the tendency to develop parkinsonian side effects with neuroleptic treatment is known to be associated with decreased dopaminergic activity assessed by measurement of CSF (van Praag, 1977) or urinary HVA (Crowley *et al.*, 1978). Kleinman *et al.* (1982) found no relationship between VBR and serum prolactin levels in 17 drug-free schizophrenic patients, but found a significant negative correlation between serum prolactin and total BPRS or thought disturbance in normal ventricle, but not large ventricle patients, perhaps suggesting that enlarged ventricles interfere with dopaminergic activity. We were unable to confirm this (Luchins, Robertson, & Meltzer, in press).

Thus, CT studies provide some evidence that schizophrenic patients with a Type II characteristic (i.e., large ventricles) may have decreased rather than normal dopaminergic activity.

Cholecystokinin, Negative Symptoms, and Dopamine

As part of the argument that DA is not involved in the defect state, Crow presented evidence that the peptide CCK is deficient in schizophrenic brains and that a significant negative correlation between defect-state ratings prior to death and postmortem CCK levels was present in schizophrenia (Crow, 1981). On this basis, Crow proposed that loss of CCK containing neurons, possibly through viral infections, might be the basis of the defect state.

In order to evaluate the hypothesis that CCK is involved in a nondopaminergic etiology of the defect state, it is necessary to consider whether there is any evidence for an abnormality of CCK in schizophrenia and whether CCK and DA are independent of each other. Perry *et al.* (1981) measured CCK concentrations by radioimmunoassay in the entorhinal cortex of 5 schizophrenic patients, 12 normal controls, 9 patients with depression, and 10 with Alzheimer's disease. Although no significant differences were noted between any of the 4 groups, there was a trend for higher levels in the schizophrenics versus the other three groups (e.g., 271 ± *SE* 99 pmol/g CCK equivalents vs. 18.2 ± *SE* 25 pmol/g for the controls). The two highest levels in the 36 subjects studied, 400 and 600 pmol/g, were found in schizophrenics. Crow's group (Ferrier *et al.*, 1983) subsequently studied CCK levels in four cortical regions, the amygdala, hippocampus, thalamus, globus pallidus and putamen of 14 schizophrenics and 12 control subjects. The schizophrenics were evaluated for negative and positive symptoms sometime prior to death. Seven had only positive symptoms (Type I group), 7 had both positive and negative symptoms (Type II group). A multivariate analysis of variance revealed a significant decrease in CCK levels in the temporal cortex of all schizophrenics with no difference between Type I and Type II schizophrenics. Type II schizophrenics had significantly lower CCK levels in the hippocampus and amygdala than Type I schizophrenics or normal controls. No correlations between CCK and negative symptoms were significant in any brain area.

The reasons for the discrepancy between the studies of Perry *et al.* (1981) and Ferrier *et al.* (1983) are unclear at the present time. Post mortem studies of CCK levels are difficult to interpret because of the absence of information about CCK turnover, receptor sensitivity, influence of cotransmitters, drug effects, and agonal changes. Determination of CCK is dependent upon radioimmunoassay methods, which can differ markedly in sensitivity and specificity between laboratories. The approach taken by Crow to rate positive and negative symptoms prior to death is noteworthy. However, the significance of such cross-sectional ratings is questionable. It is also surprising that half of Crow's sample had less than two negative symptoms. The Type I patients in Crow's sample were significantly younger than the controls and the difference in ages between Type I and Type II patients also approached significance. No information about the duration of illness of the Type I patients was given. It is unusual that a group of schizophrenics who were 48 ± 7 years old would have so few negative symptoms, given that they were selected from a group of 14 chronically hospitalized schizophrenic patients.

Verbanck *et al.* (1984) reported decreased CSF CCK levels in 9 untreated schizophrenics (2.6 ± *SE* .8 pmol/liter) compared to 51 normal controls (5.4 ± .8 pmol/liter, $p < .05$). Bipolar depressed patients also had decreased CSF CCK levels. Gerner and Yamada (1982) reported no significant difference in CSF CCK levels between untreated schizophrenics and normal controls. The study by Verbanck *et al.* (1984) does indicate a possible deficiency in

CCK in schizophrenia but it appears to be shared by bipolar patients. If both findings are verified, it might indicate that any CCK deficiency in schizophrenia is unrelated to negative symptoms.

Caerulein, a decapeptide chemically related to CCK-8, was administered intramuscularly to 20 chronic schizophrenic patients on stable doses of neuroleptics. Improvement in BPRS ratings were noted, including emotional withdrawal, blunted affect, uncooperativeness, and mannerisms and posturing; the effect lasted for at least several weeks (Moroji, Watanabe, Auki, & Itoh, 1982). Nair, Bloom, and Nestoros (1982) reported that CCK produced a marked improvement in positive and negative symptoms in chronic schizophrenic patients receiving neuroleptic treatment. However, C. Tamminga (personal communication, 1984) and Hommer *et al.* (in press) have not been able to replicate the caerulein results. Hommer *et al.* (in press) also found no effect of an intravenous infusion of CCK itself in 4 schizophrenic patients. The reasons for these discrepancies are unknown. It could reflect genuine differences in patient populations, based, in part, on ethnic differences. The lack of clinical efficacy of CCK would not rule out a deficiency of CCK in schizophrenia. It could be that little of the CCK injected actually reaches the brain. Further clinical study is indicated.

However, even if the relationship between a deficiency of CCK and the defect state were to be established, this would not rule out an important role for DA in the defect state because of the extensive evidence that DA and CCK have critically important interactions. Hokfelt, Rehfeld *et al.* (1980) were the first to provide histochemical evidence that CCK and DA coexist in mesolimbic neurons. The presence of CCK in the cell bodies and terminal areas of the mesolimbic and striatal DA system has been strongly supported by subsequent histochemical and lesion studies (Beinfeld, Meyer, Eskay, Jensen, & Brownstein, 1981; Fallon *et al.*, 1983; Studler *et al.*, 1981; Vanderhaegen, Lotstra, DeMey, & Gillis, 1980; Williams, Gayton, Zhu, & Dockray, 1981).

There is extensive behavioral evidence that CCK-8 has neuroleptic-like properties. CCK induces catalepsy in mice (Zetler, 1981). In rats, CCK reduces conditioned avoidance (CA), potentiates the haloperidol-induced blockade of CA, facilitates avoidance extinction, and diminishes apomorphine-induced stereotypy, but failed to produce catalepsy (Cohen, Knight, Tamminga, & Chase, 1982). The intracerebral injection of CCK-8 or ceruletide, or both, was found to have neuroleptic-like effects in some but not all paradigms, including blockade of the decrease in locomotor activity due to low dose apomorphine and the increase in locomotor activity due to high dose apomorphine (Van Ree, Gaffori, & DeWied, 1983). The nucleus accumbens, which is rich in DA terminals, appeared in these studies to be much more sensitive to CCK than was the caudate nucleus. However, Widerlov, Kalivas, Lewis, Prange, and Breese (1983) found no specific effect of an injection of CCK into the ventral tegmental area or of intracerebral CCK on apomorphine- or amphetamine-induced stereotypy.

CCK was reported to produce DA autoreceptor supersensitivity (Hommer & Skirboll, 1983). CCK has also been shown to increase the firing rate of the mesencephalic neurons, which contain both CCK and DA (Skirboll *et al.*, 1981). Zetler (1983) suggested that presynaptic DA autoreceptors are involved in the interaction of CCK-like peptides and apomorphine with respect to ptosis.

Agnati *et al.* (1983) reported that CCK-8 *in vitro* can modulate the kinetic characteristics of [^{3}H]–DA antagonist binding sites; the B_{max} and K_D of [^{3}H]spiperone binding sites in striatal membranes were both decreased by 10%. Murphy and Schuster (1982) reported that CCK-8 had complicated *in vitro* and *in vivo* effects on the binding of [^{3}H]–DA to striatal and olfactory tubercle (OT) homogenates. Specifically, systemic administration of 20 μg/kg CCK for 4 days decreased [^{3}H]–DA binding sites in the striatum and enhanced them in the OT. Chang, Lotti, Martin, and Chen (1983) found that three different procedures that reduce dopaminergic function of the brain (chronic haloperidol, intracisternal 6-hydroxydopamine, and unilateral radiofrequency lesions of the ventral tegmentum) enhanced CCK binding to limbic and frontal cortical regions but not to striatum, hippocampus, or posterior. Frey (1983) reported that CCK-8-sulfate concentrations were increased in the striatum and mesolimbic system after 2 and 4 weeks of treatment with haloperidol, chlorpromazine, or clozapine.

The data on the effect of CCK on DA turnover is mixed. One group has reported CCK-8 increases DA turnover in several regions of rat brain (Fekete, Kadar, Penke, Kovacs, & Telegdy, 1981). Widerlov *et al.* (1983) found no effect of intracerebroventricular CCK-8 on DA turnover in the limbic areas or the striatum. They did note a significant decrease in CSF 5-HIAA, which is consistent with other evidence that CCK may decrease 5-HT turnover (see Widerlov *et al.*, 1983, for references). Meyer and Krauss (1983) have obtained evidence that suggests that the release of endogenous DA enhances the secretion of CCK. The reason for these discrepancies is not clear and will require further study. Nevertheless, behavioral, biochemical, electrophysiological, and neuroendocrine data suggest that CCK-8 has neuroleptic-like properties in rodent brain, acting at both autoreceptors and postsynaptic DA receptors.

This selected review of the literature strongly suggests that CCK may have important effects on DA neurons and vice versa, and further, that both substances may coexist in the same neurons. The investigation of the interaction between CCK and DA is certainly in its infancy. Nevertheless, it would appear to be premature to rule out a role for DA in the etiology of negative symptoms just because CCK also may be involved. The same reasoning would apply for other peptides that may have behavioral effects such as TRH, substance P, endogenous opiate peptides, ACTH, and neurotensin, all of which have been shown to have important effects on DA or vice versa (Cools, Wiegant, & Gispen, 1978; Haubrich, Martin, Pflueger, & Williams, 1982; Heal & Green, 1979; Hokfelt, Johansson, Ljungdahl, Lundberg, & Schultzberg, 1980a; Hong, Yang, Fratta, & Costa, 1978; Nemeroff *et al.*, 1983; Waldmeier, Karn, & Stocklin, 1978).

It is beyond the scope of this review to consider the argument of Crow (1983) and colleagues (Baker *et al.*, 1983) that schizophrenia may be an infectious disease, in particular a viral infection. Murray and Reveley (1983) have argued against Crow's interpretation of the evidence he has marshalled and we have reviewed some of the early evidence elsewhere (Meltzer, 1979b). It appears doubtful that viral infections, of either the slow virus or short latency type, play a significant etiologic role in more than a very small proportion of patients who meet modern diagnostic criteria for schizophrenia.

CONCLUSIONS

We have reviewed some of the evidence for and against the Type I–II hypothesis of schizophrenia (Crow, 1980b). The evidence for increased numbers of D_2 DA receptors as the basis for delusions and hallucinations was not considered here because it has been thoroughly reviewed by us and others elsewhere (Mackay *et al.*, 1982; Meltzer, 1980). It is possible that positron emission tomography will enable quantitative studies of brain DA receptors in never-medicated schizophrenic patients (Wagner *et al.*, 1983). At this juncture, the evidence for a non-drug-induced increase in DA receptors in schizophrenics is not compelling nor has it been related to positive symptoms satisfactorily. Indeed, Mackay (1980) has argued that because mainly chronic, older schizophrenics have been found to have increased numbers of DA receptors, if this increase is not due to drugs, it is more likely to be related to Type II schizophrenia. It is also possible that it is related to decreased dopaminergic activity, as would occur following lesions of the substantia nigra or ventral tegemental area. Increased dopaminergic activity in schizophrenia has recently been attributed to greater coupling of D_1 DA receptors to adenylate cyclase (Memo, Kleinman, & Haubauer, 1983). There is little question that delusions and hallucinations do respond well to neuroleptic treatment, but this model fails to account for the large proportion of schizophrenics in whom such treatment fails to diminish positive symptoms completely. In the 169 patients we reported on previously, only 73 (43.2%) were entirely free of delusions or hallucinations at discharge from hospital, despite intensive state-of-the-art application of neuroleptic treatment plus psychosocial rehabilitation over a 3–5 month period.

The evidence for a lack of involvement of DA in the etiology of the Type II syndrome must be regarded as much less secure than the evidence for the role of DA in the Type I syndrome. Although the main clinical features of the Type II syndrome (flat affect, loss of volition, and poverty of speech and thought content) are well-recognized aspects of schizophrenia, it appears unlikely that they are *qualitatively* different from positive symptoms with regard to irreversibility, response to neuroleptic treatment, or relation to enlarged ventricles and other PEG- or CT-detectable structural abnormalities, and that they therefore are not related to DA.

The issue of how negative symptoms are related to DA will not be discussed in detail here because of limitations of space. Newer evidence to support the view that negative symptoms are related to decreased dopaminergic activity (Mackay, 1980; Meltzer, 1979b; Meltzer & Stahl, 1976) will be presented elsewhere. This argument suggests that increased dopaminergic activity in some pathways contributes to positive symptoms, whereas decreased dopaminergic activity in others leads to negative symptoms.

The emphasis on the importance of DA in the etiology of positive and negative symptoms is not meant to exclude the possible importance of other neurotransmitters or neuromodulators in producing various aspects of the psychopathology of schizophrenia. Given the heterogeneity of schizophrenia, it is possible that abnormalities in other neurotransmitters can produce similar psychopathology as abnormalities in DA, or that dopaminergic pathways may be a final common pathway for the disturbances in some of the other neurotransmitters or neuromodulators.

ACKNOWLEDGMENT

Supported, in part, by the USPHS MH 30059, MH 25116 and by the Department of Mental Health, State of Illinois. HYM is recipient of USPHS Research Career Scientist Award MH 47808.

REFERENCES

Agnati, L. F., Fuxe, K., Benfenati, F., Celani, M. F., Battistini, N., Mutt, V., Cauicchioli, L., Galli, G., & Hokfelt, T. (1983). Differential modulation by CCK-8 and CCK-4 of ^{3}H-spiperone binding sites linked to dopamine and 5-hydroxytryptamine receptors in the brain of the rat. *Neuroscience Letters*, *35*, 179–183.

Alpert, M., Friedhoff, A. J., Marcos, L. R., & Diamond, F. (1978). Paradoxical reaction to L-DOPA in schizophrenic patients. *American Journal of Psychiatry*, *135*, 1329–1332.

Andreasen, N. C. (1982). Negative symptoms in schizophrenia: Definition and reliability. *Archives of General Psychiatry*, *39*, 784–788.

Andreasen, N. C., Olsen, S. A., Dennert, J. W., & Smith, M. R. (1982). Ventricular enlargement in schizophrenia: Relationship to positive and negative symptoms. *American Journal of Psychiatry*, *139*, 297–302.

Angrist, B., Rotrosen, H., & Gershon, S. (1980). Differential effects of amphetamine and neuroleptics on negative vs positive symptoms in schizophrenia. *Psychopharmacology*, *72*, 12–19.

Angrist, B., Sathananthan, G., & Gershon, S. (1973). Behavioral effects of L-DOPA in schizophrenic patients. *Psychopharmacologia, 31*, 1–12.

Asano, N. (1967). Pneumoencephalographic study of schizophrenia. In H. Mitsuda (Ed.), *Clinical genetics in psychiatry. Problems in nosological classification*. Tokyo: Igaku Shoin.

Ashcroft, G. W., Blackwood, G. W., Besson, J. A. O., Palomo, T., & Waring, H. L. (1981). Positive and negative symptoms and the role of dopamine. *British Journal of Psychiatry, 138*, 268–269.

Baker, H. F., Ridley, R. M., Crow, T. J., Bloxham, R. A., Parry, R. P., & Tyrell, D. A. (1983). An investigation of the effects of intracerebral injection in the marmoset of cytopathic cerebrospinal fluid from patients with schizophrenia or neurological disease. *Psychological Medicine, 13*, 499–511.

Bannon, M. J., & Roth, R. H. (1983). Pharmacology of mesocortical dopamine neurons. *Pharmacological Reviews, 35*, 53–68.

Beinfeld, M. C., Meyer, D. K., Eskay, R. L., Jensen, R. I., & Brownstein, M. J. (1981). The distribution of cholecystokinin immunoreactivity in the central nervous system of the rat as determined by radioimmunoassay. *Brain Research, 212*, 51–57.

Benes, F., Sunderland, P., Jones, B., Lemay, M., Cohen, B. M., & Lipinski, J. (1982). Normal ventricles in young schizophrenics. *British Journal of Psychiatry, 141*, 90–93.

Bishop, R. J., Golden, C. J., Macinnes, W. D., Chu, C.-C., Ruedrich, S. L., & Wilson, J. (1983). The BPRS assessing symptom correlates of cerebral ventricular enlargement in acute and chronic schizophrenia. *Psychiatry Research, 9*, 225–231.

Boehme, R. E., & Ciaranello, R. D. (1981). Dopamine receptor binding in inbred mice. Strain differences in mesolimbic and nigrostriatal dopamine binding sites. *Proceedings of the National Academy of Sciences of the U.S.A., 78*, 3255–3259.

Boronow, J., Pickar, D., & Ninan, P. T. (1985). Atrophy limited to IIIrd ventricle only in chronic schizophrenic patients: Report of a controlled series. *Archives of General Psychiaty 42*, 266–271.

Buchanan, F. H., Parton, R. V., & Warren, J. W. (1975). Double-blind trial of L-DOPA in chronic schizophrenia. *Australian and New Zealand Journal of Psychiatry, 9*, 269–271.

Burdock, E. I., Hakerem, G., Hardesty, A. S., & Zubin, J. (1959). *Ward Behavior Rating Scale*.

Calil, H. M., Yesavage, J. A., & Hollister, L. F. (1977). Low dose levodopa in schizophrenia. *Communications in Psychopharmacology, 1*, 593–596.

Chang, R. S. L., Lotti, J., Martin, G. E., & Chen, T. B. (1983). Increase in brain ^{125}I-cholecystokinin (CCK) receptor binding following chronic haloperidol treatment, intracisternal 6-hydroxydopamine or ventral tegmental lesions. *Life Sciences, 32*, 871–878.

Chouinard, G., & Jones, B. D. (1978). Schizophrenia as a dopamine deficiency disease. *Lancet, 2*, 99–100.

Cohen, S. L., Knight, M., Tamminga, C. A., & Chase, T. N. (1982). Cholecystokinin-octapeptide effects on conditioned avoidance behavior, stereotypy and catalepsy. *European Journal of Pharmacology, 83*, 213–222.

Cools, A. R., Wiegant, V. M., & Gispen, W. H. (1978). Distinct dopaminergic systems in ACTH-induced grooming. *European Journal of Pharmacology, 50*, 265–268.

Crow, T. J. (1980a). Molecular pathology of schizophrenia: More than one disease process. *British Medical Journal, 280*, 66–68.

Crow, T. J. (1980b). Positive and negative schizophrenic symptoms and the role of dopamine. *British Journal of Psychiatry, 139*, 379–386.

Crow, T. J. (1981). Positive and negative symptoms and the role of dopamine. *British Journal of Psychiatry*, *139*, 251–254.

Crow, T. J. (1983). Is Schizophrenia an infectious disease? *Lancet*, *1*, 173–175.

Crowley, T. J., Hoehn, M. M., Rutledge, C. O., Stahling, M. A., Heaton, R. H., Sundell, S., & Stilson, D. (1978). Dopamine excretion and vulnerability to drug-induced parkinsonism. *Archives of General Psychiatry*, *35*, 97–104.

Elizur, A., Davidson, S., & Psych, F. R. C. (1975). The evaluation of the antibiotic activity of sulpiride. *Current Therapeutic Research*, *18*, 578–584.

Endicott, J., & Spitzer, R. (1978). A diagnostic interview. A schedule for affective disorders and schizophrenia. *Archives of General Psychiatry*, *35*, 837–844.

Fallon, J. H., Wang, C., Kim, Y., Canepa, N., Loughlin, S., & Seroogy, K. (1983). Dopamine- and cholecystokinin-containing neurons of the crossed mesostriatal projection. *Neuroscience Letters*, *40*, 233–238.

Fekete, M. T., Kadar, B., Penke, K., Kovacs, K., & Telegdy, G. (1981). Influence of cholecystokinin octapeptide sulfate ester on brain monoamine metabolism in rats. *Journal of Neural Transmission*, *50*, 81–88.

Ferrier, I. N., Roberts, G. W., Crow, T. J., Johnstone, E., Owens, D. G. C., Lee, Y. C., O'Shaughnessy, D., Adrian, T. E., Polak, J. M., & Bloom, S. R. (1983). Reduced cholecystokinin-like and somatostatin-like immunoreactivity in limbic lobe is associated with negative symptoms in schizophrenia. *Life Sciences*, *33*, 475–482.

Frangos, H., Zissis, N. P., Leontopoulos, I., Diamantas, N., Tsitouridis, S., Gavriel, I., & Tsolis, K. (1978). Double-blind therapeutic evaluation of fluspirilene compared with fluphenazine decanoate in chronic schizophrenics. *Acta Psychiatrica Scandinavica*, *57*, 436–446.

Freeman, T. (1981). Positive and negative symptoms in schizophrenia. *British Journal of Psychiatry*, *13*, 210–211.

Frey, P. (1983). Cholecystkinin octapeptide levels in rat brain are changed after subchronic neuroleptic treatment. *European Journal of Pharmacology*, *95*, 87–92.

Gallant, D. M., Mielke, D. H., Spirtes, M. A., Swanson, W. C., & Bost, R. (1974). Penfluridol: An efficacious long-acting oral antipsychotic compound. *American Journal of Psychiatry*, *131*, 699–702.

Gelenberg, A. J., & Doller, J. C. (1979). Clozapine versus chlorpromazine for the treatment of schizophrenia: Preliminary results from a double-blind study. *Journal of Clinical Psychiatry*, *40*, 238–240.

Gerlach, J., Koppelhus, P., Helweg, E., & Monrad, A. (1974). Clozapine and haloperidol in a single-blind cross-over trial: Therapeutic and biochemical aspects in the treatment of schizophrenia. *Acta Psychiatrica Scandinavica*, *50*, 410–424.

Gerlach, J., & Luhdorf, K. (1975). The effect of L DOPA on young patients with simple schizophrenic treated with neuroleptic drugs. *Psychopharmacologia*, *44*, 105–110.

Gerner, R. H., & Yamada, K. (1982). Altered neuropeptide concentrations in cerebrospinal fluid of psychiatric patients. *Brain Research*, *238*, 298–302.

Glover, V., Elsworth, J. D., & Sandler, M. (1980). Dopamine oxidation and its inhibition by (−) deprenyl in man. *Journal of Neural Transmission*, *16*, 163–172.

Glover, V., Sandler, M., Owen, F., & Riley, G. J. (1977). Dopamine is a monoamine oxidase B substrate in man. *Nature (London)*, *265*, 80–81.

Goldberg, S. C., Klerman, G. L., & Cole, J. O. (1965). Changes in schizophrenic psychopathology and ward behavior as a function of phenothiazine treatment. *British Journal of Psychiatry*, *111*, 120–135.

Golden, C. J., Moses, J. A., Zelanzowski, R., Graber, B., Zatz, L. M., Horvath, T. B., & Berger, P. A. (1980). Cerebral ventricular size and neuropsychological impairment in young schizophrenics. *Archives of General Psychiatry*, *37*, 619–623.

Gould, R. J., Murphy, K. M. M., Reynolds, I. J., & Snyder, S. H. (1983). Antischizophrenic drugs of the diphenylbutylpiperidine type act as calcium channel antagonists. *Proceedings of the National Academy of Sciences of the U.S.A.*, *80*, 5122–5125.

Guirguis, E., Voinesko, G., Gray, J., & Schlieman, E. (1977). Clozapine (Leponex) vs chlorpromazine (Largactil) in acute schizophrenia. (A double-blind controlled study). *Current Therapeutic Research*, *21*, 707–719.

Haas, S., & Beckmann, H. (1982). Pimozide versus haloperidol in acute schizophrenia. A double-blind controlled study. *Pharmacopsychiatry*, *15*, 70–74.

Haase, H. J., Floru, L., & Ulrich, F. (1974). Klinisch neuroteptische untersuchung des n- (1-athyl-pyrrolidin-2-YL)-methyl-2 methoxy-5-sulfamoyl-benzamide-neurolepticums sulprid (Dogmatil) an akut erkrankten schizofren. *International Pharmacopsychiatry*, *9*, 77–94.

Harnryd, C., Bjerkenstedt, L., Bjork, K., Gullberg, B., Oxenstierna, G., Sedvall, G., Wiesel, F.-A., Wik, G., & Asberg-Wistedt, A. (1984). Clinical evaluation of sulpiride in schizophrenic patients—A double-blind comparison with chlorpromazine. *Acta Psychiatrica Scandinavica*, *69*, 7–30.

Haubrich, D. R., Martin, G. E., Pflueger, A. B., & Williams, M. (1982). Neurotensin effects on brain dopaminergic systems. *Brain Research*, *231*, 216–221.

Haug, J. O. (1962). Pneumoencephalographic studies in mental disease. *Acta Psychiatrica Scandinavica*, *38*, 1–114.

Heal, D. J., & Green, A. R. (1979). Administration of thyrotropin releasing hormone (TRH) to rats releases dopamine in N accumbens but not N caudateus. *Neuropharmacology*, *18*, 23–31.

Hokfelt, T., Johansson, O., Ljungdahl, A., Lundberg, M., & Schultzberg, M. (1980). Peptidergic neurones. *Nature (London)*, *284*, 515–521.

Hokfelt, T., Rehfeld, J. F., Skirboll, L., Ivermark, B., Goldstein, M., & Markey, K. (1980). Evidence for coexistence of dopamine and CCK in mesolimbic neurones. *Nature (London)*, *285*, 476–478.

Hommer, D. W., Pickar, D., Roy, A. Ninan, P., Boronow, J., & Paul, S. M. (in press). The effects of ceruletide in schizophrenia. *Archives of General Psychiatry*.

Hommer, D. W., & Skirboll, L. R. (1983). Cholecystokinin-like peptides potentiate apomorphine-Induced inhibition of dopamine neurons. *European Journal of Pharmacology*, *91*, 151–152.

Hong, J. S., Yang, H. Y. T., Fratta, W., & Costa, E. (1978). Rat striatal methionineenkephalin content after chronic treatment with cataleptogenic and noncataleptogenic antischizophrenic drugs. *Journal of Pharmacology and Experimental Therapeutics*, *205*, 141–147.

Honigfeld, G., Gillis, R., & Klett, J. (1966). A treatment-sensitive ward behavior scale. *Psychological Reports*, *19*, 180–182.

Honigfeld, G., Patin, J., Belendiuk, G., & Singer, J. (1983). Efficacy. In G. Honigfeld & J. Singer (Eds.), *The clozapine monograph: A summary of safety and antipsychotic efficacy findings*. East Hanover, NJ: Sandoz Pharmaceuticals.

Huber, G. (1957). *Pneumoencephalographische und psychopathologische: Bilder bei Eendogen psychosen*. Berlin: Springer-Verlag.

Huber, G., Gross, G., & Schutter, R. (1975). A long-term follow-up study of schizophrenia: Psychiatric course of illness and prognosis. *Acta Psychiatrica Scandinavica*, *52*, 49–57.

Inanaga, K., Nakazawa, Y., Inoue, K., Tachibana, H., Oshima, M., Lotoril, J., Tanaka, M., & Ogawa, N. (1975). Double-blind controlled study of L-DOPA therapy in schizophrenia. *Folia Psychiatrica et Neurologica Japonica*, *29*, 123–143.

Jernigan, T. L., Zatz, L. M., Moses, J. A., & Berger, P. A. (1982). Computed tomography in schizophrenics and normal volunteers. I. Fluid volume. *Archives of General Psychiatry*, *39*, 765–770.

Johnstone, E. C., Frith, C. D., Crow, T. J., Husband, J., & Kreel, L. (1976). Cerebral ventricular size and cognitive impairment in chronic schizophrenia. *Lancet*, *2*, 824–826.

Johnstone, E. C., Frith, C. D., Crow, T. J., Carney, M. W. P., & Price, J. S. (1978). Mechanism of the antipsychotic effect in the treatment of acute schizophrenia. *Lancet*, *1*, 848–851.

Kleinman, J. E., Weinberger, D. R., Rogol, A. D., Bigelow, L. B., Klein, S. T., Gillin, J. C., & Wyatt, R. J. (1982). Plasma prolactin concentration and psychopathology in chronic schizophrenia. *Archives of General Psychiatry*, *39*, 655–657.

Kling, A. S., Kurtz, N., Tachiki, K., & Orzeck, A. (1982–1983). CT scans in subgroups of chronic schizophrenics. *Journal of Psychiatric Research*, *17*, 375–384.

Kudo, Y. (1972). A double-blind comparison of pimozide with carpipramine in schizophrenic patients. *Acta Psychiatrica Belgica*, *72*, 685–697.

Lapierre, Y. D. (1978). A controlled study of penfluridol in the treatment of chronic schizophrenia. *American Journal of Psychiatry*, *135*, 956–959.

Lapierre, Y. D., & Lavalle, J. (1975). Pimozide and the social behaviors of schizophrenics. *Current Therapeutic Research*, *18*, 181–188.

Lewine, R. J., Fogg, L., & Meltzer, H. Y. (1983). Assessment of negative and positive symptoms in schizophrenia. *Schizophrenia Bulletin*, *9*, 368–376.

Lewine, R. J., & Meltzer, H. Y. (1984). Negative symptoms and platelet monoamine oxidase activity in male schizophrenic patients. *Psychiatry Research*, *12*, 99–111.

Lorr, M., Klett, C. J., McNair, D. M., & Laskey, J. J. (1962). *Inpatient multidimensional psychiatric scale (IMPS) manual*. Copyright: Maurice Lorr.

Luchins, D. J., Jackman, H., & Meltzer, H. Y. (1984). Lateral ventricular size and drug-induced parkinsonism. *Psychiatry Research*, *9*, 9–16.

Luchins, D. J., Lewine, R. R. J., & Meltzer, H. Y. (1984). Lateral ventricular size, psychopathology and medication response in the psychoses. *Biological Psychiatry*, *19*, 29–44.

Luchins, D. J., Robertson, A. G., & Meltzer, H. Y. (1984). Serum prolactin, psychopathology and ventricular size in chronic schizophrenics. *Psychiatry Research*, *12*, 149–153.

Mackay, A. V. P. (1981). Positive and negative schizophrenic symptoms and the role of dopamine. *British Journal of Psychiatry*, *137*, 379–383.

Mackay, A. V. P., Iversen, L. L., Lassor, M., Spokes, E., Bird, E., Arrequi, A., Cruse, I., & Snyder, S. H. (1982). Increased brain dopamine and dopamine receptors in schizophrenia. *Archives of General Psychiatry*, *39*, 991–997.

Mann, J. J., Stanley, M., Kaplan, R. D., Sweeney, J., & Neophytides, A. (1983). Central catecholamine metabolism *in vivo* and the cognitive and motor deficits in parkinson's disease. *Journal of Neurology, Neurosurgery and Psychiatry*, *46*, 905–910.

Marsden, C. M. (1984). Dopamine hypothesis in acute psychosis. *British Journal of Psychiatry*, *138*, 268–272.

Maser, J. D., & Keith, S. J. (1983). CT scans and schizophrenia—Report on a workshop. *Schizophrenia Bulletin*, *9*, 265–283.

Meltzer, H. Y. (1979a). Biochemical studies in schizophrenia. In L. Bellak (Ed.), *Disorders of the schizophrenic syndrome*. New York: Basic Books.

Meltzer, H. Y. (1979b). Biology of schizophrenic subtypes. A review and proposal for method of study. *Schizophrenia Bulletin*, *5*, 460–479.

Meltzer, H. Y. (1982). Dopamine autoreceptor stimulation: Clinical significance. *Pharmacology, Biochemistry, and Behavior*, *17*, 1–10.

Meltzer, H. Y., Perline, R., & Lewine, R. (1982). Biological studies of DSM-III psychotic disorders. 1. Platelet measures of apomorphine-induced growth hormone response. *Journal of Nervous and Mental Disease*, *170*, 758–765.

Meltzer, H. Y., Stahl, S. (1976). The dopamine hypothesis: A review. *Schizophrenia Bulletin*, *2*, 19–76.

Memo, M., Kleinman, J. E., & Haubauer, I. (1983). Coupling of dopamine D_1 recognition sites with adenylate cyclase in nuclei accumbens and caudatus of schizophrenics. *Science*, *221*, 1304–1307.

Meyer, D. K., & Krauss, J. (1983). Dopamine modulates cholecystokinin release in neostriatum. *Nature (London)*, *301*, 338–340.

Moroji, T., Watanabe, N., Aoki, N., & Itoh, S. (1982). Antipsychotic effects of caerulein, a decapeptide chemically related to cholecystokinin octapeptide, on schizophrenia. *International Pharmacopsychiatry*, *17*, 255–273.

Murphy, R. B. & Schusker, D. I. (1982). Modulation of [^{3}H]-dopamine binding by cholecystokinin octapeptide (CCK-8). *Peptides*, *3*, 539–543.

Murray, R. M., & Reveley, A. M. (1983). Schizophrenia as an infection. *Lancet*, *1*, 583.

Nagy, K. (1963). Pneumoencephalographische befunde ber endogen psychosen. *Nervenarzt*, *34*, 543–548.

Nair, N. P., Bloom, D. M., & Nestoros, J. M. (1982). Cholecystokinin appears to have antipsychotic properties. *Progress in Neuropsychopharmacology and Biological Psychiatry*, *6*, 509–512.

Nasrallah, H. A., Jacoby, C. G., McCalley-Whitters, M., & Kuperman, S. (1982). Cerebral ventricular enlargement in subtypes of chronic schizophrenia. *Archives of General Psychiatry*, *39*, 774–777.

Nasrallah, H. A., McCalley-Whitters, M., & Jacoby, C. G. (1982). Cerebral ventricular enlargement in young manic males. A controlled CT study. *Journal of Affective Disorders*, *4*, 15–19.

Nemeroff, C. B., Luttinger, D., Hernandez, D. E., Mailman, R. B., Mason, G. A., Davis, S. D., Widerlov, E., Frye, D., Kilts, A., Beaumont, K., Breese, G. R., & Prange, A. J., Jr. (1983). Interactions of neurotensin with brain dopamine systems: Biochemical and behavioral studies. *Journal of Pharmacology and Experimental Therapeutics*, *225*, 337–345.

Nishiura, M. (1976). Clinico-pharmacological studies of sulpiride. *Current Therapeutic Research*, *20*, 164–172.

Nisikanen, P., Achte, K., Jaskari, M., Karesoja, M., Meisted, B., Nilsson, L. B., Routavaara, M., Tamminen, T., Tienari, P., & Vogel, G. (1974). Results of a comparative double-blind study with clozapine and chlorpromazine in the treatment of schizophrenic patients. *Psychiatria Fennica*, pp. 307–313.

Nyback, H., Berggren, B.-M., & Hindmarsh, T. (1983). Cerebroventricular size and cerebrospinal fluid monoamine metabolites in schizophrenic patients and healthy volunteers. *Psychiatry Research*, *9*, 301–308.

O'Carroll, A. M., Fowler, C. J., Phillips, J. P., Tobbia, I., & Tipton, K. F. (1983). The deamination of dopamine by human brain monoamine oxidase: Specificity for the two enzyme forms in seven brain regions. *Naunyn-Schmiedeberg's Archives of Pharmacology*, *322*, 198–202.

Ogura, C., Kishimato, H., & Nakao, T. (1976). Clinical effects of L-DOPA on schizophrenia. *Current Therapeutic Research*, *20*, 308–318.

Okasha, A., & Madkour, O. (1982). Cortical and central atrophy in chronic schizophrenia. *Acta Psychiatrica Scandinavica*, *65*, 29–34.

Overall, J. E., & Gorham, D. R. (1962). Brief psychiatric rating scale (BPRS). *Psychological Reports*, *10*, 799–812.

Overall, J. E., & Rhoades, J. V. (1982). Refinement of phenomenological classification in clinical psychopharmacology research. *Psychopharmacology*, *77*, 24–30.

Owen, F., Cross, A. J., Crow, T. J., Lofthouse, R. & Poulter, M. (1981). Neurotransmitter receptors in brain in schizophrenia. *Acta Psychiatrica Scandinavica*, *63 Suppl. 291*, 20–26.

Owen, F., Cross, A. J., Crow, T. J., Longden, A., Poulter, M., & Riley, G. J. (1978). Increased dopamine receptor sensitivity in schizophrenia. *Lancet*, *2*, 223–225.

Pearlson, G. H., & Veroff, A. E. (1981). Computerized tomographic scan changes in manic-depressive illness. *Lancet, 2*, 470.

Perry, R. H., Dockray, G. J., Dimaline, R., Perry, E. K., Blessed, G., & Tomlinson, B. E. (1981). Neuropetides in Alzheimer's disease, depression and schizophrenia. *Journal of Neurological Sciences, 51*, 465–472.

Randrup, A., Munkvad, I., Fog, R., Gerlach, J., Molander, L., Kjellberg, B., & Scheel-Kruger, J. (1975). Mania, depression and brain dopamine. In W. B. Essman & L. Valzelli (Eds.), *Current developments in psychopharmacology* (pp. 206–248). New York: Halstead Press.

Rieder, R. O., Mann, L. S., Weinberger, D. R., van Kammen, D. P., & Post, R. M. (1983). Computed tomographic scans in patients with schizophrenia, schizoaffective and bipolar affective disorder. *Archives of General Psychiatry, 40*, 735–739.

Seeman, P. (1981). Brain dopamine receptors. *Pharmacological Reviews, 32*, 229–313.

Shopsin, B., Klein, H., Gerbino, L., & Selzer, G. (1977). Penfluridol: An open phase III study in acute newly admitted hospitalized schizophrenic patients. *Psychopharmacology, 55*, 157–164.

Singh, A. N. (1973). Clinical evaluation of fluspirilene as a maintenance therapy in chronic schizophrenic patients. *Canadian Psychiatric Association Journal, 18*, 415–419.

Skirboll, L. R., Grace, A. A., Hammer, D. W., Rehfeld, J., Goldstein, M., Hokfelt, T., & Bunney, B. S. (1981). Peptide-monoamine coexistence: Studies of actions of cholecystokinin-like peptides on the electrical activity of midbrain dopamine neurons. *Neuroscience, 6*, 2111–2124.

Spitzer, R. L., Endicott, J., & Robins, E. (1978). Research diagnostic criteria: Rationality and reliability. *Archives of General Psychiatry, 35*, 773–782.

Studler, J. M., Simon, H., Cesselin, F., Legrand, J. C., Glowinski, J., & Tassin, J. P. (1981). Biochemical investigation on the localization of the cholecystokinin octapeptide in dopaminergic neurons originating from the ventral tegmental area of the rat. *Neuropeptides (Edinburgh), 2*, 131–139.

Takahashi, R., Inaba, Y., Inanaga, K., Kato, N., Kumashiro, H., Nishimura, T., Okuma, T., Otsuki, S., Sakai, T., Sato, T., & Shimazono, Y. (1981). CT scanning and the investigation of schizophrenia. In C. Perris, G. Struwe, & B. Jansson (Eds.), *Biological psychiatry* (pp. 259–268). Amsterdam: Elsevier/North-Holland Biomedical Press.

Vanderhaeghen, J. J., Lotstra, F., DeMey, J., & Gilllis, C. (1980). Immunohistochemical localization of cholecystokinin and gastrin-like peptides in the brain and hypophysis of the rat. *Proceedings of the National Academy of Sciences of the U.S.A., 77*, 1190–1194.

van Kammen, D. P. (1981). *d*-Amphetamine and schizophrenia: Behavioral, pharmacological and physiological evaluations. *Advances in the Biosciences, 31*, 43–47.

van Kammen, D. P., Docherty, J. P., Marder, S. R., Schulz, S. C., Dalton, L. A., & Bunney, W. E., Jr. (1982). Antipsychotic effects of pimozide in schizophrenia treatment response prediction with acute dextroamphetamine response. *Archives of General Psychiatry, 39*, 261–266.

van Kammen, D. P., Mann, L. S., Sternberg, D. E., Scheinen, M., Ninan, P. T., Marder, S. R., van Kammen, W. B., Rieder, R. O., & Linnoila, M. (1983). Dopamine-β-hydroxylase activity and homovanillac acid in spinal fluid of patients with brain atrophy. *Science, 220*, 974–977.

van Praag, H. M. (1977). The significance of dopamine for the mode of action of neuroleptics and the pathogenes is of schizophrenia. *British Journal of Psychiatry, 130*, 463–474.

Van Ree, J. M., Gaffori, O., & DeWied, D. (1983). In rats, the behavioral profile of CCK-8 related peptides resembles that of antipsychotic agents. *European Journal of Pharmacology, 93*, 63–78.

Verbanck, P. M. P., Lotstra, F., Gillis, C., Linkowski, P., Mendlewicz, J., & Vanderhaeghen, J. J. (1984). Reduced cholecystokinin immunoreactivity in the cerebrospinal fluid of patients with psychiatric disorders. *Life Sciences*, *34*, 67–72.

Wagner, H. N., Jr., Burns, H. D., Dannals, R. F., Wong, D. F., Langstrom, B., Duelfer, T., Frost, J. J., Ravert, H. T., Links, J. M., Rosenbloom, S. B., Lukas, S. E., Kramer, A. V., & Kuhar, M. J. (1983). Imaging dopamine receptors in the human brain by positron tomography. *Science*, *221*, 1264–1266.

Waldmeier, P. C., Kam, R., & Stocklin, K. (1978). Increased dopamine metabolism in rat striatum after infusions of substance P into the substantia nigra. *Brain Research*, *159*, 223–227.

Weinberger, D. R., Bigelow, L. B., Kleinman, J. E., Klein, S. T., Rosenblatt, J. E., & Wyatt, R. J. (1980). Cerebral ventricular enlargement in chronic schizophrenia: Its association with poor response to treatment. *Archives of General Psychiatry*, *37*, 11–13.

Weinberger, D. R., Torrey, F., Neophytides, A. N., & Wyatt, R. J. (1979a). Lateral cerebral ventricular enlargement in chronic schizophrenia. *Archives of General Psychiatry*, *36*, 735–739.

Weinberger, D. R., Torrey, E. F., Neophytides, A. N., & Wyatt, R. J. (1979b). Structural abnormalities in the cerebral cortex of chronic schizophrenic patients. *Archives of General Psychiatry*, *36*, 935–939.

Widerlov, E., Kalivas, P. W., Lewis, M. H., Prange, A. J., Jr., & Breese, G. R. (1983). Influence of cholecystokinin on central monoaminergic pathways. *Regulatory Peptides*, *6*, 99–109.

Williams, R. G., Gayton, R. J., Zhu, W., & Dockray, G. J. (1981). Changes in brain cholecystokinin octapeptide following lesions of the medial fore brain bundle. *Brain Research*, *213*, 227–230.

Wing, J. K., Cooper, J. E., & Sartorius, N. (1974). *The measurement and classification of psychiatric symptoms*. London & New York: Cambridge University Press.

Yayhura-Tobias, J. E., Diamond, B., & Merlis, S. (1970). The action of L-DOPA on schizophrenic patients. *Current Therapeutic Research*, *12*, 528–533.

Zetler, G. (1981). Central depressant effects of caerulein and cholecystokinin octapeptide (CCK-8) differ from those of diazepam and haloperidol. *Neuropharmacology*, *26*, 277–283.

Zetler, G. (1983). Neuroleptic-like effects of ceruletide and cholecystokinin and cholecystokinin octapeptide: Interactions with apomorphine, methylphenidate and picrotoin. *European Journal of Pharmacology*, *94*, 261–270.

8

Restitutive Processes in the Regulation of Behavior

ARNOLD J. FRIEDHOFF
New York University School of Medicine

Little attention has been paid to the integration of new discoveries in neurobiology, molecular genetics, and neuropharmacology into a modern concept of mental illness. This lack of advance in the theoretical sphere probably derives from the failure to discover the primary etiological factor in any of the major mental illnesses. Despite the lack of specific knowledge of genetic or biological lesions in schizophrenia or the major affective disorders, sufficient new information has been discovered to make new insights possible. The correct formulation of a concept of psychiatric disorder is of more than philosophical interest. As will be shown later, the concept of the nature of mental disease, whether implicit or explicit, shapes the kinds of pharmacological agents we develop, and undoubtedly also influences the nature of psychological approaches to treatment.

The common wisdom has it that psychiatric disease is a distrubance in adaptation; someone with a mental disorder is often referred to as being "maladjusted." By this it is meant that, put into a situation that requires accommodation or adaptation, the disturbed person cannot cope in a normal fashion. Is this layman's view, reflected in lay terminology, supported by any body of evidence? Curiously, as is now well known, both the antidepressant drugs and the antipsychotic drugs exercise their primary therapeutic effect only after a rather long lag period, often of several weeks. One would surmise that during that time adaptive changes were occurring and that it was these adaptive processes that were responsible for the therapeutic effect. We now know that in the case of the tricyclic antidepressants an adaptive change occurs in the beta-noradrenergic and serotonergic systems that are believed to mediate the therapeutic action of these drugs. In the case of neuroleptic antipsychotic drugs, compensatory adaptations occur in the dopaminergic system, believed to be more related to side effects of these agents, so that the mechanisms for delayed therapeutic effect is not known.

The fact that drugs useful in treatment produce therapeutic effects by inducing adaptive changes does not, of course, provide definitive evidence that the disorders being treated are the result of disturbances in adaptation; however it will be shown later that there is evidence to support this view. What is particularly anachronistic is that, until recently, little attention has been paid to the nature of the adaptive changes produced by psychotropic drugs. Investigations of pharmacological effects at the synapse have been directed toward on-line functions and moment-to-moment operational aspects. As has been pointed out, both neuroleptic and antidepressant drugs almost certainly exert their therapeutic action through some kind of compensatory mechanism, although we do not know all the details of compensatory changes produced. In this report, I would like to propose a new concept of the therapeutic action of neuroleptics, and demonstrate that the action of both neuroletptics and antidepressants point toward the presence of important stabilizing or restitutive systems in the brain.

Many of the known functional units of the biogenic amine synapse have an adaptive aspect, and are in some kind of dynamic equilibrium with each other. For instance, if the postsynaptic dopamine receptor is blocked, one of the first adaptive responses is an outpouring of dopamine from the presynaptic terminal (Seeman, 1977, 1980), a response geared toward overcoming the blockade. There are also adaptive aspects of the mechanism that couples the postsynaptic recognition site to the enzyme adenylate cyclase (Memo, Kleinman, & Hanbauer, 1983). The postsynaptic dopaminergic neuron has other elements known to be capable of adaptive responses. Most of these changes are homeostatic in character; that is, they are designed to produce changes that maintain the status quo of the synapse. Thus, if dopamine receptors are blocked by neuroleptics, new sites emerge in an attempt to overcome the blockade. In the brain of the postnatal animal the homeostatic principle appears to dominate. As will be shown later, this is not the case during gestation, when a principle of accommodation prevails. Both of these adaptive modes appear to have survival value to the animal, as will be discussed later.

At least two kinds of dopamine receptor sites have been established, called D_1 and D_2 receptors. The D_2 sites probably regulate ion channels, whereas the D_1 sites are coupled to the enzyme adenylate cyclase via regulatory proteins (Clement-Cormier, Parrish, Petzold, Kebabian, & Greengard, 1975; Costa, Gnegy, & Uzunov, 1977; Creese, Usdin, & Snyder, 1979). When dopamine impinges on the D_1 recognition sites, more cyclic AMP is made. When D_1 receptors are blocked, the formation of cyclic AMP by adenylate cyclase is inhibited. When D_2 sites are blocked for a time, the number of D_2 sites is increased, as a compensatory response (Friedhoff, Bonnet, & Rosengarten, 1977). D_1 receptors do not as readily upregulate in response to blockade as do D_2 sites (H. Rosengarten & A. J. Friedhoff, unpublished observation).

In an experiment carried out a number ot years ago, we gave haloperidol to rats for three weeks and then measured the change in various aspects of dopaminergic function. We found that chronic haloperidol, which blocked access of dopamine to dopamine receptors, produced an increase in the number of dopaminergic binding sites and in the activity of the enzyme adenylate cyclase. There was also an increase in a dopamine-dependent behavior, apomorphine-induced stereotypy. When the haloperidol treatment was followed by administration of L-dopa as sinemet, all three measures rapidly returned to normal, presumably because L-dopa was converted to dopamine in the brain so that an over supply of dopamine was produced. This served to reverse the effects of the dopamine blocker, haloperidol, and downregulated the dopaminergic system to its normal set point (Friedhoff *et al.*, 1977). Thus, we have found that the dopaminergic system is an example of a neuronal system that has the capacity to adapt in a biphasic manner.

Let us consider for a moment the role of the dopaminergic system in mediating the therapeutic effects of antipsychotic drugs. When dopaminergic activity is reduced by the blocking action of neuroleptics, psychotic symptoms often disappear; that is, downregulation of the system increases resistance to the etiological factors producing the psychosis, resulting in improved mental state. Is it likely that this wonderfully adaptive system evolved only in anticipation of the discovery of antipsychotic drugs? Put another way, it seems likely that this regulatable aspect of the dopaminergic system has a physiological role in mediating some normal aspect of mental function. What is the probable role of a system that produces increased resistance to psychotic destabilization of mental function? It seems more than reasonable that this system functions in everyday life to protect us from the variety of psychological or biological insults that would otherwise puch us over the edge. Psychosis may occur only when both the requisite etiological factors are present and this restitutive dopaminergic down regulating system is not functioning properly.

As mentioned earlier, the dopaminergic–synaptic complex has many components that are capable of making compensatory responses and that may be involved in a restitutive system. One well-studied relationship, the balance between the dopaminergic and cholinergic systems in the caudate nucleus, was earlier discussed by Friedhoff and Alpert (1973), who pointed out that Parkinsonism responds either to dopaminergic stimulation or cholinergic inhibition, and that, similarly, psychosis can be relieved by dopaminergic inhibition or, temporarily at least, by cholinergic stimulation. We now know that this balance occurs by means of inhibitory dopamine receptors located on cholinergic cells in the candate. In studies carried out by Miller and Friedhoff (1979), it was found that this balance between the dopaminergic and cholinergic systems is also subject to adaptive change. We found that when rats were given neuroleptics for 3 weeks, and the drug was then allowed to wash out, the release of acetylcholine from striatal brain slices was inhibited by significantly lower concentrations of dopamine.

Another interactional aspect of the dopaminergic system subject to compensatory change is the relationship between the D_1 and D_2 systems. The D_2 system has been found to inhibit the D_1 system (Stoof & Kebabian, 1981); that is, stimulation of the D_2 system inhibits the formation of cAMP initiated by dopamine impinging on the D_1 receptors. Thus a balance exists between the D_1 and D_2 systems, not unlike the balance between the D_2 and cholinergic systems.

Although a number of D_2-dependent behaviors have been described, prior to some recent studies we have carried out, no one was able to demonstrate a D_1-mediated behavior. After the seminal publication of Stoof and Kebabian (1981) showing D_2 inhibition of the D_1 system, we thought that we might be able to elicit a D_1 behavior if we could disinhibit the D_1 system. First, we gave very low doses of spiroperidol, which blocks only D_2 and serotonin receptors and not D_1 receptors. We also gave spiroperidol with apomorphine, a dopaminergic agonist. Apomorphine stimulates both the D_1 and the D_2 system, but with low-dose spiroperidol blockade of D_2, only D_1 receptors were stimulated. This selective D_1 stimulation produced a very peculiar behavior. The rats opened and closed their jaws at a very fast rate, producing the "pac man" syndrome (Rosengarten & Friedhoff, 1983). When apomorphine was given with sulpiride, another selective D_2 blocker, the jaw activity could also be produced. Finally the activity could be produced by a specific D_1 agonist, and inhibited by a specific D_2 agonist.

We also have found that the adaptive capacity of the dopaminergic system can be fine-tuned during gestation. In some studies that Rosengarten and I carried out, we found that the number of D_2 receptors, and thus the inhibitory tone of the dopaminergic system, is determined by the extent of exposure of developing D_2 receptors to dopamine during a critical period of prenatal life (Rosengarten & Friedhoff, 1979). In the mature animal, reduction of the dopamine impinging on postnatal receptors results in a compensatory increase in the number of these receptors. As mentioned earlier, in mature animals the response is of a homeostatic nature. In the prenatal animal, however, a different principle operates. Reducing access of dopamine to postnatal receptors results in an enduring decrease in the number of D_2 receptors. In the prenatal animal, instead of homeostasis, accommodation occurs.

Miller and I have also shown that the ratio of dopaminergic to cholingergic receptors can be fine-tuned during prenatal life; curiously, the fewer dopamine receptors that are produced during gestation the more cholinergic receptors (Friedhoff & Miller, 1983). Thus, by administering neuroleptics during gestation, the number of D_2 receptors is decreased, the number of cholinergic receptors increased, and a dominantly high-cholinergic rat results.

Another interesting phenomenon results from exposure to neuroleptics in utero; the dopaminergic system loses its capacity to adapt. It no longer responds to neuroleptic intervention by producing more receptors. Thus, if a rat is exposed to neuroleptics in utero, it tends to be more cholinergic by having a greater ratio of cholinergic to dopaminergic receptors and by losing its ability to increase D_2 inhibition of the cholinergic system as an adaptive response. The behavioral implications of this loss of adaptive capacity and cholinergic dominance are as yet unknown, but should be of great interest.

We see, through several examples, that in the prenatal animal accommodations to the cellular environment occur in systems that respond with typical homeostatic adaptations postnatally. It is my view that these two kinds of responses are of great importance to the survival of the organism and for optimal function in interactions with environmental forces.

We have shown, in the prenatal animal, that reduction of the dopamine impinging on the developing brain produces a decrease in the number of dopamine receptors. We have shown that dopamine has a limited ability to cross the placenta (A. J. Friedhoff & J. C. Miller, unpublished data). In the fetus no blood–brain barrier exists. Both of these circumstances facilitate the transfer of information from the environment to the fetus via the mother. The principle in the prenatal animal is to be as much like the mother as possible, inasmuch as the mother has survived in the environment into which the fetus will be born. Thus the fetus accommodates to the environment. Once having survived birth, however, nature attempts to sustain this success, by involving homeostatic mechanisms in response to environmental pressures.

Having been personally concerned in the early 1960s with the formulation of the so-called dopamine hypothesis of schizophrenia (Friedhoff & Van Winkle, 1964), I have continued my interest in the possible relationship between dopamine and schizophrenia. Originally, we proposed that dopamine had an etiological role in schizophrenia, because reduction of dopaminergic activity by neuroleptic blockade improved the symptoms of this illness. Later it became clear that an etiological role was not possible, because dopamine-blocking agents have therapeutic effects in many types of psychosis, and dopamine cannot be an etiological factor in all of them. There is no question, however, that dopamine is somehow involved in the mediation of a neuroleptic drug.

I have proposed a new concept of the role of dopamine in psychosis that appears to reconcile many of the known facts. The concept is that the dopaminergic system serves as a restitutive system whose purpose is to maintain mental normalcy in the face of biological or psychological insult. This model implies that there is a dynamic equilibrium between predisposing, precipitating, and restitutive factors. It also proposes that the reduction in dopaminergic activity produced by the receptor-blocking action of neuroleptics, which produce remission in psychiatric symptoms, is a drug model of a normal physiological function.

It seems logical that the dopaminergic system did not evolve in anticipation of neuroleptics. Thus, what would be the expected effect of a physiologically produced reduction in dopaminergic activity? I have previously proposed that the dopaminergic system spontaneously regulates its output when events occur that tend to destabilize mental function in the direction of psychosis (Friedhoff, 1983). Clinical psychosis occurs only when the downregulating system is not efficient enough to produce an adequate compensatory or restitutive response. Schizophrenia in a patient with low dopaminergic activity would signify that the dopaminergic restitutive system had been maximally involved, but that the etiological forces were so great that this was not sufficient to stave off psychosis. One would predict that such patients would be poor neuroleptic responders, inasmuch as they had already maximally reduced dopaminergic activity so that neuroleptics could not produce a further reduction. In contrast, schizophrenic patients with evidence of high dopaminergic activity should be good responders to neuroleptic treatment.

Both Alpert and Bowers, in separate experiments, have found evidence for this premise. Alpert found that the sensitivity to extrapyramidal (EPS)-producing effects of neuroleptics is negatively correlated with the therapeutic efforts of these drugs (Alpert, Diamond, & Kesselman, 1977). If a subject already has low dopaminergic activity or a poorly responsive dopaminergic system and is given a neuroleptic, he is more likely to get EPS, because the dopaminergic system cannot compensate. Thus, in Alpert's studies, patients with evidence of hypodopaminergia had a poor therapeutic response.

Bowers, studying plasma HVA, the principal brain metabolite of dopamine, also found that patients with high baseline HVA and a vigorous increase after treatment was initiated, were the ones that responded well (Bowers, Swigar, Jatlow, & Goicoechea, 1984). Thus the dopaminergic system appears to mediate a restitutive system, whose downregulation prevents the expression of psychotic symptoms. In most cases this probably occurs successfully before an individual comes to psychiatric notice. In other cases the adaptation is not successful, either because the system did not get tuned down efficiently, in which case neuroleptics will help, or because maximal spontaneous downregulation was not enough to offset the etiological forces, in which case neuroleptics will not help. These latter patients may be the so-called deficit-symptom schizophrenics who are nonresponders to neuroleptics. It is of great interest that a primary deficit symptom is flat affect, which is also found in Parkinson patients, known to be suffering from low central dopaminergic activity.

This model has more than theoretical interest. From the standpoint of this conceptualization it is clear that we ought to be studying the regulatory aspects of the dopaminergic system, and how it gets tuned up and down. It may be possible to develop drugs that can up- or downregulate the system, perhaps even beyond the capacity of the system to regulate itself. Understanding the regulation should provide the basis for developing new kinds of pharmacological agents, not only for the treatment of psychosis but for enhancement of the restitutive capacity of unstable nonpsychotics.

REFERENCES

Alpert, M., Diamond, F., & Kesselman, M. (1977). Correlation between extrapyramidal and therapeutic effects of neuroleptics. *Comprehensive Psychiatry, 18,* 333–336.

Bowers, M. B., Jr., Swigar, M. E., Jatlow, P. I., & Goicoechea, N. (1984). Plasma catecholamine metabolites and early response to haloperiodol. *Journal of Clinical Psychiatry, 45,* 248–251.

Clement-Cormier, Y. C., Parrish, R. G., Petzold, G. L., Kebabian, J. W., & Greengard, P. (1975). Characterization of a dopamine sensitive adenylate cyclase in the rat caudate nucleus. *Journal of Neurochemistry, 25,* 143–149.

Costa, E., Gnegy, M. E., & Uzunov, P. (1977). Regulation of dopamine receptor sensitivity by an endogenous protein activator or adenylate cyclase. *Naunyn-Schmiedeberg's Archives of Pharmacology, 297,* 547–548.

Creese, I., Usdin, T., & Snyder S. H. (1979). Guanine nuclotides distinguish between two dopamine receptors. *Nature (London), 278,* 577–578.

Friedhoff, A. J. (1983). A strategy for developing novel drugs for the treatment of schizophrenia. *Schizophrenic Bulletin, 9,* 656–662.

Friedhoff, A. J., & Alpert, M. (1973). A dopaminergic-cholinergic mechanism in production of psychotic symptoms. *Biological Psychiatry, 6,* 165–169.

Friedhoff, A. J., Bonnet, K. A., & Rosengarten, H. (1977). Reversal of two manifestations of dopamine receptor sensitivity by administration of L-dopa. *Research Communications in Chemical Pathology and Pharmacology, 16,* 411–423.

Friedhoff, A. J., & Miller, J. C. (1983). Prenatal psychotropic drug exposure and the development of central dopaminergic and cholinergic neurotransmitter systems. *Monographs in Neural Sciences, 9,* 91–98.

Friedhoff, A. J., & Van Winkle, E. (1964). Biological o-methylation and schizophrenia. *Psychiatric Research Reports, 19,* 149–153.

Memo, M., Kleinman, J. E., & Hanbauer, I. (1983). Coupling of dopamine D_1 recognition sites with adenylate cyclase in nuclei accumbens and caudatus of schizophrenics. *Science, 221,* 1304–1307.

Miller, J. C., & Friedhoff, A. J. (1979). Dopamine receptor-coupled modulation of the K^+-depolarized overflow of ^{3}H-acetylcholine from rat striatal slices. Alteration after chronic haloperidol and alpha-methyl-p-tyropine pretreatment. *Life Sciences, 25,* 1249–1256.

Rosengarten, H., & Friedhoff, A. J. (1979). Enduring changes in dopamine receptor cells of pups from drug administration to pregnant and nursing rats. *Science, 203,* 1133–1135.

Rosengarten, H., & Friedhoff, A. J. (1983). Induction of oral dyskinesias in naive rats by D_1 stimulation. *Life Sciences, 33,* 2479–2482.

Seeman, P. (1977). Anti-schizophrenic drugs: Membrane receptor sites of action. *Biochemical Pharmacology, 26,* 1741–1748.

Seeman, P. (1980). Brain dopamine receptors. *Pharmacological Reviews, 32,* 229–313.

Stoof, J. C., & Kebabian, J. W. (1981). Opposing roles for D_1 and D_2 dopamine receptors in effux of cyclic AMP from rat neostriatum. *Nature (London), 294,* 366–368.

General Discussion

Dr. Malcolm Bowers:* What is exciting to me is that increasingly it seems that individuals with different expertise in nosology, chemistry, and pathology are somehow trying to pull things together. I think that some of the ideas we have heard this afternoon suggest that it is going to occur and that we have better ideas now than we used to have.

I just want to make a couple of points. I think one of the by-products of this kind of activity where we increasingly try to relate the behavior to the pathology, whether it's neuropathology or chemical pathology, has to do with an increased focus on the clinical processes. It seems to me that the clinical concept that has been highlighted is the deficit state or the defect symptoms, and I think that is going to be in our focus for a long time, so I'd like to say something briefly about this idea.

First, I think that is a very complicated concept, from the point of view of a clinician, at least. Will Carpenter alluded to that this morning, suggesting already that he's made a division between negative symptoms and deficit state. From the point of view of a clinician, people who become psychotic often have, as many of you know, problems in their lives, defects if you will, before they are ill, and once they are ill, it doesn't get better. That is, new deficits accrue. Someone said this is not a true dementia. It may not be a dementia, but when you become ill at a time when psychosocially your peers are on a kind of log scale of development, what you have is a kind of relative deficit in what you've been able to do. They're marrying, they're having children, and you are still trying to get a job at age 30. That may not be dementia, but it nevertheless represents over time an accrued deficit, a psychosocial deficit state.

I think negative symptoms also help us focus upon the existential plight of the patient. I don't want to sentimentalize this, but the facts are, if you are psychotic at a young age, if you must take neuroleptic drugs, if you have any sense at all of the future, it doesn't take a lot of insight to get

* New Haven, Connecticut.

discouraged from time to time and to have little hope. Will Carpenter has stressed that.

In other words, in my opinion the concept of negative symptoms and deficit state is much more complicated than we have yet realized and is going to challenge us from here on, making it even more important for us to characterize clinically what we are comparing neuroantomically and psychopathologically.

Dr. Burt Angrist:* Dr. Meltzer cited the amphetamine–neuroleptic data of mine to indicate some improvement of negative symptoms with neuroleptic treatment, but particularly I would like to underline one problem. Item 3 on the BPRS is a difficult one for the rater, at least for me. The specific instructions are to "rate the degree to which the patient is out of emotional contact during the interview." I think any psychiatrist is impressed by grossly *incongruent* behavior. For example, "Good morning, Mr. Jones," and he punches you. That is extreme lack of emotional contact during the interview, and I would score it accordingly, but that is not deficit, nor is it deficient emotionality. It's strong but incongruent emotionality. I don't have a solution. Personally, what I am doing is I am writing "deficit and incongruence" under that item and scoring them separately.

Incongruence, I suspect, is a positive symptom. That's why it behaves as a positive symptom pharmacologically.

If I can add just one more comment here, you made some sanguine comments about CCK, and I know our own preliminary data are dismal, and I think I know three or four other people with ongoing studies who would concur.

Dr. Meltzer: The only comment I'd make about the ratings is, as we've heard all today, that we are still in the process of developing better means to assess them. I think that the issue should best be addressed by a wide range of techniques to assess them. It clearly can be defined; the negative symptom or deficit state could be defined to exclude only those that never change, and then we will prove the consequences of that. But I think if we take a broader view at this point, an open-ended point of view and most importantly, assess in different kinds of ways, we may find some associations that we hadn't expected, like the ones I found. I have some of the same problems in using the BPRS that you do, and I think that does make a number of the pharmacological studies in the past less easy to interpret, but I think that Dr. Goldberg might comment more. When you read the kind of assessment that went into the NIMH Collaborative Study, where you didn't use the BPRS and did use the broad behavior-rating scale and the IMPS, one gets the sense that you were describing changes in what I

* New York, New York.

think most people in this group would consider the deficit state or defect state. Would you comment on that?

Dr. Solomon C. Goldberg:* I have nothing much further to say except yes. In a symptom we called "indifference to environment," which is pretty close to blunted affect, there was a very large drug effect of 1 standard deviation between drug and placebo, but there are others as well, such as lack of social participation.

Dr. Meltzer: It's hard to imagine that that study will ever be replicated as well because of the need for placebo controls, and so it would be critically important to even go back to that data and to try to tease this out.

Dr. Goldberg: With my apologies to Dr. van Kammen whose place in line I have just taken, I would like to say that associated with enlarged ventricles, there are certain symptoms that do not respond to neuroleptic treatment in comparison to placebo, but they are not what everybody is calling negative symptoms. I would point to a number of symptoms that sound more like organicity, such as disorientation for time, place, and person; memory deficit; and visual and olfactory hallucinations. In the sense that these fail to respond to neuroleptics, they are part of the deficit state.

Dr. Daniel R. Weinberger†: I'd like to make a brief comment on that. This may have been discussed this morning, and I missed this morning's session, so I apologize if this is redundant, but I can't help making the observation in listening to this discussion that there are really two issues that seem to crop up about defect symptoms. The first is, how do you define them, and that I see as a real conundrum. There's a million ways to approach defining. The second question is, is there any validity to them in terms of the neurobiology of the illness, and I think the irony of the second point is that it is intuitively obvious to most people that there is some inherent validity to them. It's not that surprising to me that we have trouble defining them because, for example, inattentiveness to one's environment can be the result of a number of psychic states of the patient. Some patients, for example, don't attend to their environment because they are convinced if they open their mouth, they are going to be struck dead in an instant. Now, that might be a positive symptom, as opposed to somebody who is inattentive to their environment for reasons of being mildly demented.

I think we all are familiar with the fact that in patients treated with drugs, there are certain symptoms that seem to hang on, and they tend not to be the auditory hallucinations. They tend not to be the florid preoccupied delusions. They tend to be what Kraepelin called the "mental enfeeblement."

So I guess my concern is that we could get very bogged down, and we obviously have to find ways to quantify these things, but I think it is a

* Richmond, Virginia.
† Washington, D.C.

mistake to take findings in the literature as necessarily facts. They are observations based on the limitations of the instruments that are used to observe them. We can't forget our clinical experience, which I think speaks to some neurobiological validity to this concept.

Dr. Eugene Lebensohn:* My question is addressed to Dr. Meltzer. In your series of negative symptoms schizophrenics who have failed to respond to neuroleptics, have you had any experience with them responding to ECT, and would you comment, please?

Dr. Meltzer: I don't have any experience with their responding to ECT. The people in the L-dopa trial who had not responded to neuroleptics alone and had high negative symptoms were people who had predominantly failed to respond to neuroleptics. So it, I think, would go along with Arnie [Friedhoff's] notions about exhaustion or inability to adapt and that those particularly would be people in whom one would want to enhance dopaminergic activity.

There is some evidence in the literature that ECT will enhance dopamine receptor supersensitivity, for example. So I think it is possible that a course of ECT would be useful. In our state system, it is frowned upon, unfortunately. So it is not something that we readily try.

Dr. Daniel P. van Kammen†: This was for me a very exciting afternoon because it seems that, in both Dr. Meltzer's and Dr. Friedhoff's presentations, we are getting away from the concept of too much dopamine causing schizophrenia. Now we are getting into more dynamic phenomena of a dysregulation. I agree with Dan Weinberger that if there is a lesion, we probably are much more dealing with lesions in a regulatory system, such as the limbic system, than a clearly identifiable and localized deficit. In other words, schizophrenia is a disorder of regulation of the DA system, which is out of phase with environmental demands. In terms of CSF HVA, we have now data from 56 patients where we find an extremely significant difference between the patients with brain atrophy who have low CSF HVA and DOPAC. We also find in the group with brain atrophy *increased* CSF dopamine sulfate. When we make a total dopamine metabolites over dopamine sulfate ratio, as a measure of total DA utilization, we get highly significant decreased dopamine turnover in the group with brain atrophy (D. P. van Kammen, M. Linnoila, L. Mann, M. Scheinin, P. T. Ninan, W. B. van Kammen, in preparation).

We also find a stronger correlation between DA metabolites and cortical atrophy than with the ventricular enlargement. I think that relates very much to the cortical DA problems in schizophrenia that Dr. Weinberger was pointing to.

Second, what I also find very exciting are your MAO data. I think we are dusting off the MAO findings that we have been struggling with for

* Washington, D.C.

† Pittsburgh, Pennsylvania.

years. We found the same correlation that you found, Dr. Meltzer, but people seem to be somewhat tired of low-platelet MAO activity in schizophrenia because neuroleptics decrease MAO activity in some schizophrenic patients. However, both your and our patient groups were off drugs for a long time. I do believe that we need to look again at state-dependent factors interacting with MAO activity.

Third, with the negative symptoms we have a similar perceptual problem. People either say it has already been shown for years that neuroleptics do affect negative symptoms or you get comments stating that everyone knows neuroleptics do not change negative symptoms. So, it is being said again, loud and clear, that neuroleptics decrease negative symptoms, which makes me feel very good. With Dr. Hommer we analyzed our pimozide data and found negative symptoms to decrease with the positive symptoms.

A final comment about your talk saying that maybe the subcortical dopamine system gets turned up by neuroleptics; that may help to interpret our findings that those patients who improved with IV amphetamine were also the ones who responded the most to pimozide, and I think that is something that really leads to a rethinking of our concept of too much dopamine. Dopamine blockage may be relevant mostly in acute studies. Chronic treatment response relates to an adaptational process that takes place over time. Not all patients improve after the first dose of neuroleptics, obviously, and it takes weeks before we get an optimal effect and even longer sometimes to get an effect with the negative symptoms. Improvement with neuroleptics occurs mostly after adaptational processes and biochemical stabilization.

Finally, there is a report by van Praag and Korf (1973), who showed that decreased CSF HVA accumulation after probenecid was associated with extrapyamidal side effects and also that people with higher HVA tended to respond more to meuroleptics. Interestingly, low CSF HVA is also associated with brain atrophy, so maybe we are putting it all together in a clinically meaningful way. It seems that we are getting a lot of findings from the past, which did not fit easily in a linear dopamine model, finally back into focus again with a concept of stabilization of regulatory mechanisms.

*Dr. William T. Carpenter, Jr.**: We should avoid tautologic resolution of questions requiring empiric study. I suggest distinguishing negative from deficit symptoms, and testing pharmacologic responsivity of each. Using the differentiation between negative and deficit symptoms, I believe both Herb Meltzer and Sol Goldberg have demonstrated that negative symptoms improve during neuroleptic treatment in cases where there is also improvement in positive symptoms. The literature is rather consistent on this point, but it cannot be discerned whether improvement is primary or secondary. Similar

* Baltimore, Maryland.

observations led Sol Snyder to hypothesize that antipsychotics which block calcium flow channels are efficacious for negative symptoms. All of this is quite different from demonstrating efficacy of drugs in treating the deficit syndrome. Here the task is to demonstrate specific drug effect independent of general improvement in psychosis.

Dr. Donald F. Klein:* I think that I may be beating a dead horse here, but there is a real confusion of terminology between negative, positive, and deficit, and this is doubly confounded by the distinction necessary between the symptomatology that occurs in the acute state and the symptomatology that occurs at the chronic state.

In the acute schizophrenia, it has been known for a long time that there are patients who approximate but do not have full-blown catatonia. These people are withdrawn. They don't speak very much. They speak very low if at all. If you want to say that is a negative state, well, it sure is, but it also has the best prognosis of any of the acute schizophrenic psychoses. So the mere fact these people are in a "negative state" doesn't mean they can't get better.

That's in the context of acute illness. In my own studies with schizophrenia placebo-controlled studies, we have the same thing as Sol Goldberg. The patients who present with massive perplexity, withdrawal, referential states, and marked thought disorder did extremely well on the phenothiazines in a normalizing way as compared to placebo, and as well as those who have positive symptomatology, which I think simply means loud, fast, and threatening.

Now, Merv Clark did a very nice study in chronic schizophrenics that is not often referred to and related the degree of agitation of the patient to the degree of phenothiazine effect. He found that the more positive view, if you will, the more agitated these chronic schizophrenic patients were, the worse they did on antipsychotics, not the better.

But I would submit that the agitation that occurs in the chronic, demented schizophrenic is a lot different than the agitation that occurs in the acutely disorganized schizophrenic.

There ought to be some biological or pharmacological intervention to help dissect out what is the negative state that is probably due to a chronic dementing process and the negative state due to the actual, apparently inhibitory, processes that go on during states that approximate catatonia or retarded schizo-affected disease. It has been known for a long time that intravenous sodium amytal is extremely effective in waking up catatonics and bring retarded schizo-affected people back into contact. I don't know of any real data indicating that intravenous sodium amytol has much to do with any of the catecholaminergic systems. That plus the other reports of

* New York, New York.

5% carbon dioxide waking up retarded and catatonic schizophrenics indicates there is a lot more to be understood that is not catecholaminergic.

Dr. Weinberger: I just want to underscore Dr. Klein's comments. I think those are very important points. It brings to mind again, I think that this notion of negative is really sort of misbegotten from—it's attributed to Hughlings Jackson and it is really not the way Hughlings Jackson meant the word at all. In fact, Hughlings Jackson would have considered a massive absence in a petit mal seizure to be positive symptoms; he was talking about neurophysiological mechanisms and not the behavior or the most distant manifestations of the behavior itself. I think that there is a real problem here in defining these terms, and maybe, as Herb [Meltzer] said, it is best to define them operationally in terms of what responds to something like medicine and what doesn't. But that, of course, creates a major bias in what the criteria are for definition. I think the point is very well made that aimless agitation in somebody who is a very poor prognosis, chronically institutionalized patient would not be a positive symptom in the sense of this person's having or not having a defect state. It becomes sort of redundant.

Dr. George Winokur:* I have two points to make, one for Dr. Weinberger, a question, and the other for Dr. Meltzer. First, Dr. Weinberger makes a very good point with the idea that the ventricle changes are in Nolan Lewis's concept probably aplastic rather than atrophic. They remain much the same over the course of time. But the fact happens to be that although there is no increasing neurological deficit, there is a marked change in psychiatric deficit over time, so that a psychiatric patient with hebephrenic catatonic schizophrenia will have an equal amount of negative and positive symptoms at the beginning of the illness, but after about 6 years have passed, the positive symptoms will have left, and the negative symptoms will continue on and on for another 12 to 30 years. Why do not the ventricles reflect the active psychiatric process?

As regards Dr. Meltzer's paper I'd like to report data from a study of chronic hebephrenic catatonic schizophrenics who had been ill for 12 to 30 years. They became ill long before the time of neuroleptics, but somewhere along the line they were put on neuroleptics, and after having been put on neuroleptics, they didn't improve at all with their negative symptoms, which was mostly what remained of their illness. Also, there's another very, very good study by Lettemendia and Harris in England, where about 28 chronic schizophrenic patients living on a back ward were put on chlorpromazine. The doses were relatively low, and that may be a problem. These were about 300 milligrams a day, but the time that the patients were kept on the medication was very long for one or two years. At the end of that study, I

* Iowa City, Iowa.

can tell you what happened to the schizophrenic patients as regard their negative and positive symptoms: nothing happened.

Dr. Meltzer: What I had to rush at the end of my talk was the concept of the importance of the temporal dimension, which none of the speakers really had a chance to address adequately. I don't think that the dopaminergic system nor any other, really, in the brains of schizophrenics, is that constant over time. Dan [Weinberger] made the point that we don't have a progressive neurological disease here. I'm not so sure I would make that case. I mean, I know the way you mean it in the sense of MS or motorneuron disease growing and changing, but I don't feel that the final word is in terms of the concepts that I'm talking about, which is the fine structure of innovation, and I hope I was careful enough to make the point that I was dealing with a group of 18- to 35-year-old patients, basically. The modal age was 27 with an illness of 5 or 6 years, and in that group of patients in that period of time—and by the way, like many other people, I don't see catatonia anymore—if there are two catatonics in that sample of 175 patients, there are a lot, and I don't think there were two. So let's leave that out.

But people who had been ill for 30 years and then got minimal treatment with neuroleptics, as in the Lettemendia study, and did not respond, doesn't speak to my point. I think not only are we going to have to get sharper in terms of our assessment of symptoms; we really are going to have to look at the phase of the illness we are talking about, and age, or age at onset, may not be the only, the best way to get at that handle. The processes that we are talking about—I am sure in the childhood schizophrenic, they begin at birth, and then in some others, that might not begin until age 29. So I don't think we can necessarily rule out these concepts that I think perhaps Arnie [Friedhoff] and I most identified with today simply on the basis of a single population that may not have acted in accord with some of the predictions of those.

Dr. Weinberger: Let me just briefly respond. I think that there are two issues in the model that I proposed that really challenge the model. One is how do we understand a static deficit that exists perhaps early in development, only manifesting itself, at least dramatically, in late adolescence. Although it may actually manifest itself all of the life of the individual, it may only be in late adolescence that the demands of the system are such that the deficit becomes much more dramatic. But how do we explain the fact that it has an age of onset in late adolescence, which is certainly one of the striking aspects about schizophrenia. I think that is a problem we have to ask about every model that we propose to explain this illness. Let me suggest a way to view that we can recall analogies from what we do know about how certain diseases affect the brain. For example, there are many people who are born with static lesions that don't do anything for the first 15 years of life and all of a sudden they develop seizures in adolescence from a lesion that existed at birth. There are obviously maturation of certain inhibitory systems, changes in receptors, regression of other inhibitory systems, and so forth, that result in an expression of a lesion that existed for a long time.

On the other hand, it is also very common for people with static brain lesions to have decompensations in a lesion, and once they decompensate, the striking thing is, it takes a very long time for them to recompensate. This is very typically seen in dementia. So I don't think that those observations in themselves invalidate the model—because I think even in your studies, most of the patients seem to stabilize after a while. The slope is not the same. There are periods of stabilization, and I think that that is not inconsistent with what is seen in a host of static brain conditions.

Dr. John Nurnberger:* I think part of the confusion in the definition of negative symptoms and the defect state may result from the inclusion of patients with affective-type symdromes in the group of schizophrenic patients. I am referring to the talk by Dr. Meltzer, and if I understood your slide correctly, there was an inclusion of RDC schizoaffective patients, affective type, along with the schizophrenic?

Dr. Meltzer: No, absolutely not.

Dr. Nurnberger: Those patients were excluded?

Dr. Meltzer: Yes.

Dr. Nurnberger: So the people you were describing had chronic schizophrenic-like illnesses?

Dr. Meltzer: Right.

Dr. Nurnberger: I see. I am mistaken. In any case, the symptom complex that you described as consisting of negative symptoms looked a lot like depression in a lot of its symptoms, and I think it is probably quite different from what Crow would describe as the defect state.

Dr. Meltzer: Let me just refer you to the paper in the *Schizophrenic Bulletin* where we described the development of that scale and discussed the issues of those items that looked like depression. It is not a depression scale. It doesn't relate at all to Hamilton items, and in fact, in terms of the frequency of the items that most people have, they are predominantly items such as flat affect and emotional withdrawal and the like rather than some of the more depressive-like items.

Dr. Smadar Levin†: I want to point out that we haven't heard very much today about attention. Perhaps we will tomorrow, but it is interesting to note that the markers for vulnerability that Dr. Zubin mentioned, such as the crossover effect, the cross-modal effect, and the eye movement findings, can all be interpreted as related to a dysregulation of an attentional system

* Bethesda, Maryland.

† Boston, Massachusetts.

that modulates ongoing behavior in terms of changes in the external environment and in internal conditions. In reviewing the literature on frontal lobe dysfunctions in humans and animals, it is interesting to find that they have dysfunctions that are very similar to the reaction time, the eye movement, and the autonomic nervous system abnormalities described in schizophrenics. So the neuroanatomy suggests a tie-up in schizophrenia between the clinical disruptions of affect and attention, and the behavioral measures that we've all talked about for so many years; but had earlier felt were neither specific nor very informative. In the context of a frontal lobe dysfunction about which we've heard so much today, a lot of these old findings become much more understandable.

Dr. Nina Schooler:* I just wanted to natter on a bit more about the negative symptoms. One of the things that Sol Goldberg didn't mention in his comment was that in a study following the one from which the data that Herb [Meltzer] cited were drawn, when patients were followed for a longer period of time, same rater same hospitals, what appeared was that symptoms of withdrawal stopped improving. I think it was after 13 weeks—5 weeks, where paranoid symptoms continued to improve for the entire 26 weeks of the study.

Last year, I had the opportunity to review a whole series of old studies of neuroleptic versus placebo in a range of patient populations—inpatient, outpatient, acute, and chronic—and what seemed to me to be the integrating feature in terms of whether negative or withdrawal symptoms seemed to show improvement was the degree of chronicity of the patient population that was being looked at, and I think this is the thing that Herb was referring to earlier, and that in the acute context, those symptoms do improve and show fairly dramatic improvements. As the patient population becomes more chronic, the ability to detect a difference between drug and placebo in those symptoms seems to fade, and I think that the analysis that Sol Goldberg did that simply looked at symptoms over time in that context is very cogent in pointing to that.

Comment from audience: I think we shouldn't forget that some of the so-called deficit or negative symptoms are manifestations of the treatment of neuroleptics themselves and that they may in fact result from a decrement in dopaminergic activity, either produced by neuroleptics or spontaneously produced in an attempt to compensate. They may be the price you pay for downregulating your dopaminergic system: flat affect, loss of motivation, blunting of affect, and so on. They are all manifestations of neuroleptic treatment.

* Bethesda, Maryland.

SECTION THREE

COGNITIVE ASPECTS

9

Psychosis Proneness

LOREN J. CHAPMAN AND JEAN P. CHAPMAN
University of Wisconsin–Madison

Knowledge of psychosis would accrue more rapidly if researchers could identify persons who are at high risk for the disorder. Identification of such psychosis-prone persons would make it possible to study the development of psychosis, and to study the environmental events that either increase or decrease the probability of a psychotic break. Investigators would also be able to search more effectively for genetic markers of psychosis and for subgroups of psychotics who differ on these markers.

In collaboration with several of our students, we have been using specially designed psychological tests to screen large groups of young adults in order to identify and to study those persons who appear to be at high risk for psychosis. This method of mass screening young adults for signs of high risk has an advantage over the method of studying persons with a family history of psychosis because it should yield a more representative sample of future psychotics. After all, only about 5% to 10% of schizophrenics have a schizophrenic parent. The major disadvantage of the method of screening for signs of high risk is that there is available only tentative evidence concerning what measures should be useful in that screening.

We started by developing true–false scales for several traits of schizotypy as described by Meehl (1962, 1964) and of pseudoneurotic schizophrenia as described by P. Hoch and Cattell (1959). Both Meehl's schizotypy and Hoch and Cattell's pseudoneurotic schizophrenia resemble DSM-III schizotypal personality disorder. The traits that we have studied include physical and social anhedonia (L. J. Chapman, Chapman, & Raulin, 1976; Eckblad, Chapman, Chapman, & Mishlove, 1982); perceptual aberration (L. J. Chapman, Chapman, & Raulin, 1978); magical ideation (Eckblad & Chapman, 1983); and impulsive nonconformity (Chapman *et al.*, in press).

This research started as an attempt to measure proneness toward schizophrenia rather than psychosis, and to distinguish proneness toward different varieties of disorder within schizophrenia. Initially, this project used a broad definition of schizophrenia in keeping with the then-current

DSM-II system. Because DSM-III narrows the definition of schizophrenia and places many patients formerly called schizophrenic into other categories of psychosis, we have restated the goal of our project as measuring proneness toward psychosis, rather than schizophrenia only, and differentiating among psychotic disorders. We would like to differentiate proneness toward DSM-III schizophrenia from proneness to other psychoses.

Our initial studies were on perceptual aberration and on physical anhedonia. In developing scales for these traits, we followed the method of rational scale development as described by Jackson (1970). We started out by writing a trait specification that spelled out the nature of the trait we wished to measure. A number of item writers composed items consistent with the trait specification. Items were worded to refer to stable characteristics of the individual rather than current state. For example, the Perceptual Aberration Scale contains the following item: "Parts of my body have felt dead and unreal," rather than a wording that refers more to the present, such as "Parts of my body seem dead or unreal." The instructions ask the subject to indicate having had only those experiences they have had when not on drugs. Items were administered to subjects together with independent measures of acquiescence and social desirability in order to screen items, minimizing variance from those sources. Items were also selected for high item–scale correlation.

SCALES FOR PERCEPTUAL ABERRATION AND PHYSICAL ANHEDONIA

The 35-item Perceptual Aberration Scale includes items such as "Sometimes I've had the feeling that I am united with an object near me" (keyed true), "I have sometimes felt that some part of my body no longer belongs to me" (keyed true), and "My hands or feet have never seemed far away" (keyed false). Twenty-eight of our 35 perceptual aberration items, like these, refer to distortions in the perception of one's own body, and 7 refer to other perceptual changes, such as insensitivity to sights and sounds. The 61-item version of the Physical Anhedonia Scale contains such items as "The beauty of sunsets is greatly overrated" (keyed true), "I have seldom cared to sing in the shower" (keyed true), and "I have always loved having my back massaged" (keyed false).

The coefficient-alpha reliabilities of the scales are about 80 for the Physical Anhedonia Scale and about .90 for the Perceptual Aberration Scale. The test–retest reliabilities with 6 weeks intervening is about .79 for the Physical Anhedonia Scale and .75 for the Perceptual Aberration Scale. Mean scores on both scales are elevated in schizophrenia, but only a minority of patients have elevated scores. High scores on the Physical Anhedonia

Scale are found more often in patients labeled poor premorbid schizophrenia using the Phillips (1953) Scale of Premorbid Adjustment. Surprisingly, high scores on the two scales do not tend to occur in the same individuals. Rather, the two scales have a slightly negative correlation (L. J. Chapman, Chapman, & Miller, 1982). Thus, if both scales measure psychosis proneness they may measure proneness to different psychoses.

We use these and other scales for mass screening of approximately 3000 college students each year from introductory psychology classes. Subjects who score deviantly high on the scales are selected for further studies. A deviant score is defined here as one that is at least two standard deviations above the mean. Because the distributions are skewed toward high scores, this criterion labels about 4% or 5% of the subjects as deviant on each scale. We choose control subjects who are no more than half a standard deviation above the mean on all scales.

We have limited our systematic work to white subjects because we have too few subjects of other races to gather normative data. It is clear, however, that East Asian students at the University of Wisconsin score, as a group, substantially higher on the Physical Anhedonia Scale than white students, and that black students score higher on the Magical Ideation Scale (described subsequently) than white students. Because scores on these scales vary with the subculture, investigators in other locales should gather their own norms for the definition of deviant performance.

Validation of these scales as indicators of psychosis proneness will require a long-term follow-up study spanning many years. In the interim, we use several tentative criteria of psychosis proneness to guide us in evaluating predictive measures. The hypothesis that these subjects are truly psychosis prone is strengthened if they show other characteristics expected in the psychosis prone. Our tentative criteria are social isolation, psychotic-like symptoms, mild thought disorder, and incidence of psychosis at short-term follow-up.

We have interviewed our subjects for both current and past social adjustment and for history of various symptoms that are consistent with psychosis proneness. We assess social adjustment using the Weissman and Paykel (1974) Social Adjustment Scale interview, modified for use with college students. Published clinical reports (A. Hoch, 1910; Kretschmer, 1925; Millon, 1981) indicate that an extreme lack of interest in social interaction is consistent with psychosis proneness. For assessing symptoms, we use a modification of the Schedule for Affective Disorders and Schizophrenia—Lifetime Version (SADS–L) (Spitzer & Endicott, 1977). We have expanded the questions about psychotic experiences to ask also about psychotic-like experiences, which are attenuated versions of full-fledged psychotic experiences. The logic is that persons who have had psychotic-like experiences are likely to be at higher-than-normal risk for clinical psychosis in the future. This principle is based on clinical reports that psychotic patients often are found to have had less-deviant forms of their psychotic symptoms before their full-fledged psychotic illness (Bleuler, 1911/1950; J. Chapman, 1966; Gillies, 1958; Strauss, 1969). We test our groups for evidence of mild thought disorder—*cognitive slippage* to use Meehl's term—again because of reports that many schizophrenics have a history of such symptoms before they develop overt psychosis (P. Hoch & Cattell, 1959; Meehl, 1962, 1964).

Psychotic-like experiences can be ordered on degree of deviancy. For example, one DSM-III symptom of psychosis is transmission of thoughts in the Schneiderian sense of experiencing thoughts leaving one's head so that anyone in the area can hear them. A slightly less deviant experience of the same type is that strangers sometimes intrusively read one's mind and learn one's bad thoughts. Even less deviant is the experience that friends in distant places sometimes pick up one's thought waves, and less deviant yet is the experience that friends who are physically present sometimes read one's thoughts telepathically. These types of experiences fall on a continuum of deviancy between Schneiderian transmission of thoughts down to the suspicion that one or two people who know the person well receive his thoughts telepathically. Transmission of thoughts is one of six classes of experiences for each of which the experiences fall on a continuum of deviancy corresponding to a psychotic symptom. We rate each psychotic or psychotic-like experience on an 11-point scale of deviancy using a rating manual (L. J. Chapman & Chapman, 1980). Ratings of 6 to 11 are used for experiences that are judged to be of a psychotic degree of deviancy and ratings of 2 to 5 are used for experiences that are judged to be of a psychotic-like degree of deviancy. The other symptoms or continua are (1) passivity experiences, (2) voice experiences and other auditory hallucinations, (3) thought withdrawal, (4) personally relevant aberrant beliefs, and (5) visual experiences. Altogether, the manual provides rating values for 80 types of psychotic and psychotic-like experiences that fall into the six continua. The ratings provided by the manual for each type of experience are the median of the values suggested by six schizophrenia researchers. (The original judges who provided the ratings used in the manual were Will Carpenter, John Strauss, Nancy Andreasen, Martin Harrow, Lyman Wynne, and Loren Chapman.) The interviewer distinguishes whether the experiences occur only in a full waking state or in a sleepy state, and rules out drug experiences. Only experiences occurring after the 13th birthday are scored. For experiences that have religious content, the subject's religious background is taken into account. Full details of the scoring system are reported elsewhere (L. J. Chapman & Chapman, 1980).

Rating an experience as psychotic or psychotic-like in this system does not mean that the individual is clinically psychotic. Instead, the person is judged to have had an experience of the kind that characterizes clinical psychotics. A person may function fairly adequately in most aspects of living despite occasional or isolated psychotic or psychotic-like symptoms.

We will now present the findings in detail for one series of subjects and then summarize results for some other series. In the first series (L. J. Chapman, Edell, & Chapman, 1980), 50 physical anhedonics, 65 perceptual aberration subjects, and 66 control subjects were interviewed. All were college students. Each group was composed of roughly half males and half females, and the findings were much the same for the two sexes. The groups were matched on academic year and the subjects were mostly 18 or 19 years of age.

Both perceptual-aberration and anhedonic subjects showed symptoms consistent with psychosis proneness although they showed somewhat different symptoms. The perceptual aberration group reported many psychotic-like experiences, whereas the physically anhedonic group reported little interest in other people or in the opposite sex.

Psychotic-like Experiences

Combining results for the six classes of symptoms, it was found that the perceptual aberration group exceeded the control group both on number of subjects who reported psychotic experiences, $\chi^2 = 7.58$, $p < .01$, and on number of subjects who reported either psychotic or psychotic-like experiences, $\chi^2 = 26.69$, $p < .001$. The anhedonic subjects did not differ significantly from control subjects on either measure.

Thought-transmission experiences were reported by 25% of the perceptual aberration group and 6% of the control group. The perceptual aberration group exceeded the control group on mean deviancy score, $t = 2.89$, $p < .01$. Four subjects reported having directly experienced, with varying degrees of conviction, that other people could either hear or receive or experience their thoughts. An example is the belief or suspicion that strangers on the street hear one's bad thoughts. Three more reported that close friends occasionally receive their thoughts telepathically.

On passivity experiences, 28% of the perceptual aberration and 3% of the control subjects reported a scoreable experience and the difference between groups on mean score was again significant, $t = 4.56$, $p < .001$. These experiences were usually the belief or suspicion that thoughts or feelings are frequently put into their heads in ways that would be viewed as magical by conventional standards.

Scoreable voice experiences and other auditory hallucinations were reported by slightly more than half of the perceptual-aberration subjects but only 15% of the control subjects, and most of the control group's experiences were marginally scoreable "voice of conscience" experiences.

The difference between these two groups on mean score was significant, $t = 5.32$, $p < .001$. Most of these voice experiences, but not all, involved inner voices. An inner-voice experience received a score only if the subject found it more like a voice than like thoughts, and could distinguish this kind of experience from his usual thoughts.

The subjects showed very little thought withdrawal. Only two perceptual aberration subjects and no control subjects reported this.

Aberrant beliefs were scored only when the belief was personally relevant. For example, no score was given for the abstract belief that a stranger can hypnotize one by a glance of his eyes. However, a score was given to subjects who believed that this happened to themselves or who believed that they did this to other people. (Also, a score was not given for an aberrant belief that received a higher score on another one of these categories, for example, passivity experiences.) Using these criteria, 32% of the perceptual aberration subjects but only 5% of the control subjects reported an aberrant belief. The difference between mean scores was significant, $t = 4.53$, $p < .001$.

Visual experiences were less common. These experiences were brief hallucinations, striking illusions, and hypnogogic hallucinations. Eleven percent of the perceptual aberration subjects and none of the control subjects reported scoreable visual experiences, and the difference between mean scores was significant, $t = 2.56$, $p < .02$.

Lack of Heterosexual and Social Interest

On heterosexual adjustment, only the anhedonics, not the perceptual aberration subjects, differed from the control subjects. Each subject was asked to estimate the number of dates that he or she had had in each year of high school, starting with the 9th grade. A date was defined as getting together by prearrangement with a member of the opposite sex. The median total number of reported dates for the 4 years of high school was 53 for the anhedonics, 128 for the perceptual aberration subjects, and 139 for the control subjects, but the distributions were extremely skewed. Only the anhedonic group differed significantly from the control group as shown by a Mann–Whitney *U*-test, $p < .01$. We also asked about current interest in the opposite sex, to avoid mistaking late development for lack of interest. Among the anhedonics, 22% declared that they had not gone steady with a member of the opposite sex and did not currently have more interest in dating than they had in high school. Only 3% of the control subjects fell in this category and the difference between groups was significant, $\chi^2 = 8.47$, $p < .01$. Because the Physical Anhedonia Scale did not include any items that asked about heterosexual interest, the findings indicate that the trait of anhedonia has sufficient generality to predict heterosexual interest. We did not inquire about homosexual interest. However, the deficiency in social interactions of all kinds probably indicates that homosexuality is not the whole explanation of the anhedonic subjects' low heterosexual interest.

Both anhedonic and perceptual aberration subjects reported social withdrawal. Subjects were scored as socially withdrawn if they stated that they usually prefer to be by themselves, or if they declared that they seldom enjoyed the company of other people or that they had little need for social life. Altogether, 32% of the anhedonic group, 31% of the perceptual aberration group and 11% of the control subjects were rated as socially withdrawn. Both the anhedonic and the perceptual aberration group differed significantly from the control subjects, $p < .01$.

Schizotypal Features

Groups also were compared on RDC schizotypal features as defined by the Research Diagnostic Criteria (RDC) of Spitzer, Endicott, and Robins (1977). Unlike the RDC procedure, we rated all subjects on schizotypal features, regardless of their other symptoms. The RDC contains six clusters of schizotypal features with two of the six required for definite schizotypal features. One category, inadequate rapport, was omitted because of problems of interjudge reliability. At least two of the remaining five schizotypal features were shown by 18% of the anhedonics, 49% of the perceptual-aberration subjects, but only 3% of the control subjects. The difference from control subjects was significant for both the anhedonic group, Fisher exact test, $p < .01$, and for the perceptual aberration group, $\chi^2 = 34.01$, $p < .001$.

Affective Symptoms

A history of a major depressive syndrome was reported by 17% of the perceptual aberration group, 8% of the anhedonic group, and 3% of the control group. The difference between the perceptual aberration and control group was significant, $\chi^2 = 5.60$, $p < .02$. Similarly, hypomanic episodes were reported by 22% of the perceptual aberration group, 8% of the anhedonic group, and 6% of the control group. Again, the difference between the perceptual-aberration group and control group was significant, $\chi^2 = 5.38$, $p < .02$. These findings are consistent with the possibility that some of the perceptual-aberration group may be prone to affective disorder with psychosis, rather than schizophrenia.

THE MAGICAL IDEATION SCALE

Eckblad and Chapman (1983) developed a 30-item scale for magical ideation, a trait that is strongly emphasized by Paul Meehl as a precursor of schizophrenia. The method of scale development was like that described previously for the Physical Anhedonia Scale and Perceptual Aberration Scale. Magical ideation is defined as a belief in forms of causation that, by conventional standards of our society, are not valid but are magical. Examples of items are "I think I could learn to read other people's minds if I wanted to" (keyed true), "The hand motions that strangers make seem to influence me at times" (keyed true), and "I have never doubted that my dreams are the products of my own mind" (keyed false).

Many of the items inquire about the subject's interpretation of his or her own personal experiences, whereas other items ask about the belief in the theoretical possibility of magical forms of causation. These experiences, many of which enjoy some subcultural support, include thought transmission, psychokinetic effects, precognition, astrology, spirit influences, reincarnation, good luck charms, and the transfer of energies between people.

Subjects who score high on this scale tend to show the same kinds of psychotic-like, schizotypal, and affective symptoms as subjects who are high on the Perceptual Aberration Scale. The Perceptual Aberration Scale and the Magical Ideation Scale have been found to correlate about .70. Nevertheless, a group of 28 magical ideation subjects (half male and half female) who were selected for nondeviant scores on perceptual aberration was found to exceed a group of 27 control subjects on the highest score for any psychotic or psychotic-like experience ($t = 4.18, p < .001$). Because of these findings, we currently combine the two scales into a single scale, which we call the Perceptual Aberration–Magical Ideation Scale (Per–Mag Scale). A subject is defined as deviant on this scale who scores 2.0 *SD* above the mean on either of its two constituent scales or 3.0 on the sum of the two *Z*-scores.

THE IMPULSIVE NONCONFORMITY SCALE

Our project has also developed a 51-item true–false Impulsive Nonconformity Scale (L. J. Chapman *et al.*, in press). One might reasonably be skeptical of this trait as an indicator of psychosis proneness when used alone, because most impulsive nonconforming persons appear instead to be at risk for antisocial personality. Nevertheless, many clinical writers have reported impulsive, nonconforming, and antisocial behavior in the prepsychotic adjustment of some schizophrenics. These writers include P. Hoch and Cattell (1959), Dunaif and Hoch (1955), Kraepelin (1913/1919), Federn (1952), Bychowski (1953), Fenichel (1945), and Zilboorg (1941). More recent research reports with similar findings include those of Ricks and Berry (1970), Watt (1972), Watt and Lubensky (1976), Heston (1970), and Roff, Knight, and Wertheim (1976). We believe that only a subset of impulsive nonconforming persons are at risk for psychosis, and these might be identifiable by scores on other scales, such as our Per–Mag Scale.

The trait specification used for the development of the Impulsive Nonconformity Scale emphasized a lack of concern for other people's rights or feelings, a lack of respect for prevailing social and ethical standards of society and for conventional mores, hostility, a lack of empathy for the pain of others, impulsivity, and an unrestrained pursuit of self-gratification. Illustrative items are "I usually laugh out loud at clumsy people" (keyed true), "Being in debt would worry me" (keyed false), and "When I start out in the evening I seldom know what I'll end up doing" (keyed true).

Groups of 120 college students (38 male and 82 female) who scored high on the scale and 176 control subjects (82 male and 94 female) were interviewed. As expected, the experimental subjects reported more antisocial behavior, more drug and alcohol use, and more angry, distant relations with friends and family than did control subjects, thus supporting the construct validity of the scale as a measure of impulsive nonconformity. More relevant to our interest here is psychosis proneness. The experimental subjects received a higher mean rating on psychotic or psychotic-like experiences, $t = 2.95$, $p < .01$ for males and $t = 3.88$, $p < .001$ for females. They also exceeded control subjects on mean number of schizotypal experiences, $t = 5.50$, $p < .001$ for male subjects and $t = 5.74$, $p < .001$ for female subjects. Nevertheless, the deviancy of impulsive nonconformity subjects on psychotic, psychotic-like, and schizotypal symptoms was not as large as found for either the perceptual aberration or the magical ideation subjects.

The Impulsive Nonconformity Scale correlates in the .40s with both the Perceptual Aberration Scale and the Magical Ideation Scale. As will be seen below, the Impulsive Nonconformity Scale seems especially useful in identifying a subset of per–mag subjects who show cognitive slippage or mild thought disorder.

A 25-MONTH FOLLOW-UP OF HYPOTHETICALLY PSYCHOSIS-PRONE SUBJECTS

We are engaged in a long-term follow-up of subjects who score high on the scales of psychosis proneness, in order to determine the incidence of various kinds of psychosis. While waiting for these data, we have meanwhile done a short-term follow-up of groups of subjects falling in the per–mag group, the physical anhedonia group, and the impulsive nonconformity group, as well as a group of control subjects. We did an initial interview, followed by a second interview 25 months on the average after the first interview. We would, of course, expect only a small percentage of future psychotics to have their first psychotic break during this 25-month period. Exactly how many is hard to say. Using Slater and Cowie's (1971) data on age of first hospitalization for schizophrenia in England and Wales, only about 11% of future schizophrenics would be expected to have their first psychotic break during this 25-month interval. Using Loranger's (1984) data for first episode of DSM-III schizophrenia, one would expect about 12% of future schizophrenics to have their first episode during this 25-month period. The percentage of the lifetime incidence of first episode of affective psychosis that would be expected during this period might be expected to be lower because the subjects were young.

We followed up 161 per–mag subjects, 67 physical anhedonic subjects, 60 impulsive nonconformity subjects, and 144 control subjects. The reports of symptoms in their initial interviews were like those reported by the comparable groups in the earlier studies summarized above. We were able to find and reinterview about 94% of the subjects. Some of the subjects had left school and others were still at the university.

The per–mag group reported having experienced many more emotional problems of various kinds and problems of adjustment than the control group during the follow-up period; 22% of the per–mag group had sought professional help for their problems during the follow-up period, as compared to only 7% of the control group. Most of the problems for which subjects reported seeking help were problems of mild psychopathology and of maladjustment. Ten percent of the per–mag group and none of the control subjects reported having had symptoms during the 25-month follow-up period that were severe enough to be rated as psychotic, using our rating scale (L. J. Chapman & Chapman, 1980).

We were especially interested, however, in subjects who received their first clinical attention for psychosis during the 25-month period. Three of our subjects did so, and all three were in the per–mag group. One of these developed a clear-cut bipolar disorder. She was hospitalized once for a manic episode with psychosis and once for a major depressive episode with psychosis. Another subject became a DSM-III schizophrenic and was hospitalized twice. During the follow-up interview, he expressed disbelief that the interviewer could not hear his voices. He had been hospitalized after manifesting a range of bizarre psychotic symptoms, including religious delusions, grandiosity, hallucinations, and passivity experiences. A third per–mag subject did not receive hospitalization, but went into therapy for a paranoid delusion. She had found herself believing from time to time that two scientists had placed her in her local community in order to test her reactions on a day-to-day basis. She recognized this belief as aberrant and sought therapy. We diagnose her by DSM-III criteria as having had paranoia. In addition, one other subject in the per–mag group was hospitalized for depression without psychotic features during the follow-up period, and five others in this group named depression as a reason for out-patient therapy. Thus, the data indicate that the per–mag scale identifies individuals who are prone toward a variety of psychopathology including both affective disorder and schizophrenia, but does not by itself separate out persons prone toward a particular psychosis. This finding is a major impetus to our search for other measures that may help resolve the heterogeneity of the per–mag group. We wish to find ways both to reduce false positives who are not psychosis prone and to separate those who are prone to schizophrenia from those who are prone to affective disorder.

The follow-up data thus far do not support the hypothesis that the anhedonic and nonconformity subjects are psychosis prone. Nevertheless, we will continue to follow these groups because of the other findings consistent with their psychosis proneness.

STRATEGIES FOR REDUCING THE HETEROGENEITY OF SUBJECTS IN THE PER–MAG GROUP

The subjects who score high on the Per–Mag Scale appear to be our most deviant group. Nevertheless, not all of them report having had psychotic-like symptoms or being socially withdrawn, and the groups surely include many false positives. Moreover, the total number of deviant subjects is too great for all to become psychotic. Also, the Per–Mag Scale appears to identify persons prone toward either schizophrenia or affective disorder. We are using additional measures of traits and symptoms in an attempt to reduce the number of false positives as well as to separate the two kinds of high-risk subjects. One strategy is the measurement of other traits of per–mag subjects, such as impulsive nonconforming behavior, that are believed to be associated with psychosis proneness. Several recent studies indicate that per–mag subjects who are also somewhat high on the Impulsive Nonconformity Scale have a higher-than-normal incidence of cognitive slippage, but that the per–mag subjects who are low on impulsive nonconformity do not. This finding is consistent with the possibility that the first group may include more schizophrenia-prone subjects.

In one such study (Miller & Chapman, 1983), a continued word-association task was used to compare male per–mag subjects with control subjects. The subjects were given a single stimulus word, such as *king*, printed once at the top of the page, and were asked to write for 60 seconds as many words as the stimulus word called to mind. The per–mag subjects ($N = 22$) produced more idiosyncratic responses than control subjects ($N = 21$), $t = 2.09$, $p < .05$, as well as fewer common responses, $t = 2.48$, $p < .05$, and fewer popular responses, $t = 2.57$, $p < .05$.

Table 1 lists scores separately for those per–mag subjects who scored above and below their own group median on the Impulsive Nonconformity Scale. (This median value was 1.0 *SD* above the mean for the entire group tested.) As seen in Table 1, the differences in deviant word association were due to those per–mag subjects who were also high on the Impulsive

Table 1. Word Association Scores for Two Subgroups of Perceptual Aberration–Magical Ideation Subjects

	N	Idiosyncratic responses	Common responses	Popular responses
Per–Mag[a]				
Lo Non Con[b]	12	66.5	175.4	59.5
Hi Non Con	10	100.8	148.9	48.9
Control	21	54.7	177.4	63.8

[a] Per–Mag is the Perceptual Aberration–Magical Ideation group.
[b] Non Con is the score on the Impulsive Nonconformity Scale.

Nonconformity Scale. The per–mag subgroup that was high on impulsive nonconformity differed from the control group at the 1% significance level on the measures of idiosyncratic responses, popular responses, and response commonality. The per–mag subgroup that was low on impulsive nonconformity did not differ significantly from the control group on any of these measures.

Martin and Chapman (1982) obtained similar findings using the Rosenberg–Cohen Word-Communication Test, which is a measure of communication deviancy. The task is designed to measure a speaker's ability to take into account a listener's problems of understanding messages. Schizophrenics do especially badly on this task (Cohen & Camhi, 1967). A subject, acting in the speaker role, is given two words, one of which is arbitrarily designated as the referent. The subject is instructed to provide a one-word cue that would enable a listener to determine which of the two words is the referent, that is, which of the two is the word the speaker has in mind. For example, one word-pair is *lady* and *woman*, with the referent being *lady*. A good cue might be *Lord* or *Chatterley* or *bug*, because each of these has a higher associative strength to *lady* than to *woman*. The cue *female* would be poor. We gave our subjects 36 such word-pairs. The dependent variable was adequacy of the cue word, which was evaluated using the associative strength of the cue word to each of the two members of the word-pair. A group of 26 perceptual aberration subjects (13 male and 13 female) gave less effective cue words than a group of 26 control subjects (14 male and 12 female). We examined the mean scores, dividing the perceptual aberration group into those who were above and below the median for that group on the Impulsive Nonconformity Scale. The subgroup above the median on impulsive nonconformity again contributed all of the difference between the perceptual aberration group and the control group.

Another study in our laboratory (Fisher-Beckfield, 1982) found that per–mag subjects high on impulsive nonconformity are also deviant on a role-playing measure of social skill. Iglarsh (1983) found that this same group is deviant on the Halstead–Reitan Category Test. All of these findings are consistent with the hypothesis that this group is especially psychosis prone.

THE REVISED SOCIAL ANHEDONIA SCALE

In still another approach to resolving the heterogeneity of the per–mag group, we have recently been using a revision of our earlier Social Anhedonia Scale. The original Social Anhedonia Scale (L. J. Chapman *et al.*, 1976) distinguished schizophrenic from control subjects but did not have, among nonpsychotic subjects, a strong relationship to other symptoms and traits expected in the psychosis prone. This scale, however, included items that measure social anxiety as well as items that measure schizoid lack of interest in social interaction. The latter trait should have the greater relevance to psychosis proneness (A. Hoch, 1910; Kretschmer, 1925; Millon, 1981). A recent 40-item revision of the Social Anhedonia Scale (Eckblad *et al.*, 1982) excludes the social-anxiety items and includes additional items that measure schizoid lack of interest in social relationships. Illustrative items are "People sometimes think I am shy when I really just want to be left alone" (keyed true) and "I sometimes become deeply attached to people I spend a lot of time with" (keyed false). Mishlove and Chapman (in press) have found that among male subjects, those per–mag subjects who also score at least 1.0 *SD* above the mean on the Revised Social Anhedonia Scale report more psychotic and psychotic-like symptoms, $t = 2.94$, $p < .01$, as well as more schizotypal symptoms, $t = 2.39$, $p < .05$, than those who do not. The corresponding differences were not significant for female subjects. Thus the scale may be useful in reducing the heterogeneity of the perceptual aberration–magical ideation group for male subjects. We are puzzled by the inconsistency of the findings for the two sexes, and we plan to explore the correlates of this scale in greater detail.

MEASURES OF LATERALIZED DYSFUNCTION

We are also exploring the resolution of the heterogeneity of the per–mag group through the use of measures of lateralized cerebral dysfunction. Considerable literature indicates the possibility that schizophrenics have defects of left-hemisphere functioning and that patients with major depression have defects of right-hemisphere functioning. The literature is difficult to interpret, however, because of psychometric problems concerning the measurement of the lateralization of defect. We believe we have made some progress in resolving these psychometric problems, but that is too long a tale to relate in the present context. Our research group is also in the process of developing psychometrically matched neuropsychological tests of left-hemisphere functioning and of right-hemisphere functioning and will use these tests to seek syndromes of disorder both in hypothetically psychosis-prone subjects and in psychotic patients. There is now sufficient evidence of the cognitive deviancy of the per–mag subjects who are also high on impulsive nonconformity that future studies of this group should use the matched-task design (L. J. Chapman & Chapman, 1973a, 1973b, 1978) to rule out the possibility that the findings are attributable to generalized deficit.

ACKNOWLEDGMENTS

This research was supported by a research grant (MH-31067) from the National Institute of Mental Health, United States Public Health Service.

The authors are indebted to Terry Fujioka, Michael Mishlove, Mark Eckblad, Eric Miller, Judith Iglarsh, and Laurie Frost for their critical comments on an earlier draft of the manuscript.

REFERENCES

Bleuler, E. (1950). *Dementia praecox, or the group of schizophrenias* (J. Zinkin, Trans.). New York: International Universities Press. (Original work published 1911)

Bychowski, G. (1953). The problem of latent psychosis. *Journal of the American Psychoanalytic Association, 1*, 484–503.

Chapman, J. (1966). The early symptoms of schizophrenia. *British Journal of Psychiatry, 112*, 225–251.

Chapman, L. J., & Chapman, J. P. (1973a). *Disordered thought in schizophrenia*. New York: Appleton-Century-Crofts.

Chapman, L. J., & Chapman, J. P. (1973b). Problems in the measurement of cognitive deficit. *Psychological Bulletin, 79*, 380–385.

Chapman, L. J., & Chapman, J. P. (1978). The measurement of differential deficit. *Journal of Psychiatric Research, 14*, 321–325.

Chapman, L. J., & Chapman, J. P. (1980). Scales for rating psychotic and psychoticlike experiences as continua. *Schizophrenia Bulletin, 6*, 476–489.

Chapman, L. J., Chapman, J. P., & Miller, E. G. (1982). Reliabilities and intercorrelations of eight measures of proneness to psychosis. *Journal of Consulting and Clinical Psychology, 50*, 187–195.

Chapman, L. J., Chapman, J. P., Numbers, J. S., Edell, W. S., Carpenter, B. N., & Beckfield, D. (in press). Impulsive nonconformity as an indicator of psychosis proneness. *Journal of Nervous and Mental Disease*.

Chapman, L. J., Chapman, J. P., & Raulin, M. L. (1976). Scales for physical and social anhedonia. *Journal of Abnormal Psychology, 85*, 374–382.

Chapman, L. J., Chapman, J. P., & Raulin, M. L. (1978). Body-image aberration in schizophrenia. *Journal of Abnormal Psychology, 87*, 399–407.

Chapman, L. J., Edell, W. S., & Chapman, J. P. (1980). Physical anhedonia, perceptual aberration, and psychosis proneness. *Schizophrenia Bulletin, 6*, 639–653.

Cohen, B. D., & Camhi, J. (1967). Schizophrenic performance in a word-communication task. *Journal of Abnormal Psychology, 72*, 240–246.

Dunaif, S. L., & Hoch, P. H. (1955). Pseudopsychopathic schizophrenia. In P. H. Hoch & J. Zubin (Eds.), *Psychiatry and the law* (pp. 169–175).New York: Grune & Stratton.

Eckblad, M. L., & Chapman, L. J. (1983). Magical ideation as an indicator of schizotypy. *Journal of Consulting and Clinical Psychology, 51*, 215–225.

Eckblad, M. L., Chapman, L. J., Chapman, J. P., & Mishlove, M. (1982). *The revised social anhedonia scale*. Unpublished test.

Federn, P. (1952). *Ego psychology and the psychoses*. New York: Basic Books.

Fenichel, O. (1945). *The psychoanalytic theory of neurosis*. New York: Norton.

Fisher-Beckfield, D. (1982). *Interpersonal and problem-solving competence among college males hypothesized to be at risk for schizophrenia*. Unpublished doctoral dissertation, University of Wisconsin, Madison.

Gillies, H. (1958). The clinical diagnosis of early schizophrenia. In T. F. Rodger, R. M. Mowbray, & J. R. Roy (Eds.), *Topics in psychiatry* (pp. 47–56). London: Cassell.

Heston, L. L. (1970). The genetics of schizophrenic and schizoid disease. *Science, 167*, 249–256.

Hoch, A. (1910). Constitutional factors in the Dementia Praecox group. *Review of Neurology and Psychiatry, 8*, 463–475.

Hoch, P., & Cattell, J. (1959). The diagnosis of pseudoneurotic schizophrenia. *Psychiatric Quarterly, 33*, 17–43.

Iglarsh, J. N. (1983). *Neurological impairment in hypothetically psychosis-prone college students*. Unpublished master's thesis, University of Wisconsin, Madison.

Jackson, D. N. (1970). A sequential system for personality scale development. In C. N. Speilberger (Ed.), *Current Topics in Clinical and Community Psychology* (Vol. 2, pp. 61–96).New York: Academic Press.

Kraepelin E. (1919). *Dementia praecox and paraphrenia*. Edinburgh: E. & S. Livingstone. (Original work published 1913)

Kretschmer, E. (1925). *Physique and character*. New York: Harcourt, Brace & World.

Loranger, A. W. (1984). Sex difference in age at onset of schizophrenia. *Archives of General Psychiatry, 41*, 157–161.

Martin, E. M., & Chapman, L. J. (1982). Communication effectiveness in hypothetically psychosis-prone college students. *Journal of Abnormal Psychology, 91*, 420–425.

Meehl, P. E. (1962). Schizotaxia, schizotypy, schizophrenia. *American Psychologist, 17*, 827–838.

Meehl, P. E. (1964). *Manual for use with checklist of schizotypic signs*. Unpublished manuscript, University of Minnesota, Minneapolis.

Miller, E. N., & Chapman, L. J. (1983). Continued word association in hypothetically psychosis-prone college students. *Journal of Abnormal Psychology, 92*, 468–478.

Millon, T. (1981). Schizoid personality: The asocial pattern. In T. Millon (Ed.), *Disorders of personality, DSM III: Axis II* (pp. 273–296). New York: Wiley.

Mishlove, M., & Chapman, L. J. (in press). *Social anhedonia in the prediction of psychosis proneness. Journal of Abnormal Psychology.*

Phillips, L. (1953). Case history data and prognosis in schizophrenia. *Journal of Nervous and Mental Disease, 117*, 515–525.

Ricks, D. F., & Berry, J. C. (1970). Family and symptom patterns that precede schizophrenia. In M. Roff & D. F. Ricks (Eds.), *Life history research in psychopathology*. Minneapolis: University of Minnesota Press.

Roff, J. D., Knight, R., & Wertheim, E. (1976). Disturbed preschizophrenics: Childhood symptoms in relation to adult outcome. *Journal of Nervous and Mental Disease, 162*, 274–281.

Slater, E., & Cowie, V. (1971). *The genetics of mental disorders*. London & New York: Oxford University Press.

Spitzer, R. L., & Endicott, J. (1977). *Schedule for affective disorders and schizophrenia - Lifetime version (SADS-L)*. New York: New York State Psychiatric Institute.

Spitzer, R. L., Endicott, J., & Robins, E. (1977). *Research diagnostic criteria (RDC) for a selected group of functional disorders*. New York: Biometrics Research, New York State Psychiatric Institute.

Strauss, J. S. (1969). Hallucinations and delusions as points on continua function: Rating scale evidence. *Archives of General Psychiatry, 21*, 581–586.

Watt, N. F. (1972). Longitudinal changes in the social behavior of children hospitalized for schizophrenia as adults. *Journal of Nervous and Mental Disease, 155*, 42–54.

Watt, N. F., & Lubensky, A. W. (1976). Childhood roots of schizophrenia. *Journal of Consulting and Clinical Psychology, 44*, 363–375.

Weissman, M. M., & Paykel, E. S. (1974). Appendix C: Social adjustment scale. From *The depressed woman, a study of social relationships*. Chicago: University of Chicago Press.

Zilboorg, G. (1941). Ambulatory schizophrenias. *Psychiatry, 4*, 149–155.

COMMENTARY

Dr. Joseph Zubin:* I have a lot of admiration for Loren Chapman's approach, especially his ability to apply psychometric approaches to our problems in psychopathology, and his dealing with the question of the general deficit syndrome.

There is one assumption underlying Loren [Chapman's] approach to psychopathology and that is, that you can adopt the usual psychometric methods which have been so successful in intelligence tests and in personality to the problems of psychopathology. This is an admirable assumption, and I suppose if discoveries are made by this method they will certainly be very, very welcome, but I wonder whether we can assume that the data we get in psychopathology obey the linearity, homoscedasticity, and all the other prerequisites that psychometric theory demands from the usual approach to measurement. In dealing with clinical material one should be careful not to accept unquestioningly results expected from clinical hunches, because they are often the basis for self-fulfilling prophecies.

I wonder whether it wouldn't be well for Loren [Chapman] to also consider the possibility of trying to find things that you don't expect. The way to really discover, perhaps, new connections, new possibilities, is to throw away all these requirements of linearity, homoscedasticity, and so on, and apply other kinds of taxonomic methods, clustering methods, and the like, because I always feel that if I get what I expected, I didn't get very much.

* Pittsburgh, Pennsylvania.

Dr. L. J. Chapman: I would differ with Joe [Zubin] on that. I think that any time that a clinician gathers data and compares groups, he is making statistical assumptions, whether or not he states them explicitly. Even a clinical judgment is a measurement and is subject to the laws that statisticians describe. If we ignore the statistical properties of our measures, we won't escape the implications that statistical principles have for our study. We simply will not be aware of them.

I think that, as researchers, we need to attend ever more closely to psychometric features of our measures and to whether we meet such assumptions as linearity, et cetera, because if we don't, we will end up with answers that we believe are valid but are instead statistical artifact.

Dr. Charles Shagass:* We have been looking at brain potentials in overtly sick people for a long time. Some years ago we began a project using Dr. Chapman's perceptual aberration and anhedonia scales, with Dr. Richard Josiassen as the principal investigator. We just had a look at some of the data. The *N*s are relatively small. We started with 300 college students and picked the extremes and compared them with a somatosensory evoked potential selective attention procedure.

I was interested to see that most of the psychopathology reported by Dr. Chapman is coming out in the perceptual aberration group. The one major difference in our data is that the anhedonia group has a very much diminished P300 wave in the selective attention experiment, the results being halfway between those of overt schizophrenics and normals. The perceptual aberration group is quite normal on the selective attention phenomenon, and I just wondered, since you are in touch with probably a number of other people who are making ventures like this, whether you could say something about that.

Dr. Chapman: Yes. Other researchers have reported that same sort of thing: Niels Birbaumer at Tubinger University in Germany, and Bob Simons at the University of Delaware. I am not prepared to discard the Physical Anhedonia Scale, both because of findings such as you report and also because these subjects are socially withdrawn. They qualify for schizotypal personality features. The fact that these subjects don't have marked psychotic-like symptoms or thought disorder should not, I believe; lead us to drop the scale when they do show other features that are consistent with psychosis proneness.

Dr. Marty Harrow†: Loren, I wanted to inquire about whether or not your scales are assessing trait-like features. We've used scales that have some similarity to your anhedonia scale, and we get reasonably high correlations over time. But when we use scales that are similar to the perceptual

* Philadelphia, Pennsylvania.
† Chicago, Illinois.

aberrations scale, and ours is a little different—we call it the Perceptual Experiences Inventory—we didn't get as high correlations over time, suggesting that this feature may not have a trait-like quality to it. Do you have any information on that?

Dr. Chapman: Yes. Among our schizophrenics, high scores on the Perceptual Aberrations Scale are found primarily in the early stages of the disorder. I assume you are speaking of patients.

Dr. Harrow: I was also thinking, though, of your college students. Have you tried them, say, a year or two apart on those kinds of scales?

Dr. Chapman: No. We've examined test–retest stability with a six-week interval, but have not done a long-term study of stability of score. Do you have data of that sort?

Dr. Harrow: We don't have data to provide correlations over time on normals in that area, but we are interested in it, with the worry that the unusual experiences may come and go to a greater extent than the anhedonic kind of quality, but I don't know.

10

Converging Evidence for Vigilance Deficit as a Vulnerability Indicator for Schizophrenic Disorders

KEITH H. NUECHTERLEIN
University of California, Los Angeles

In delineating the symptoms of the disorder that he called dementia praecox, Kraepelin (1913/1919) noted "a disorder of attention, which we very frequently find conspicuously developed in our patients. It is quite common for them to lose both inclination and ability on their own initiative to keep their attention fixed for any length of time" (pp. 5–6). Kraepelin described the patients' difficulties in allocating and maintaining attention over time as "*a certain unsteadiness of attention*; the patients digress, do not stick to the point, let their thoughts wander without voluntary control in the most varied directions" (1913/1919, p. 6). This cognitive-processing abnormality was also among the prominent features described in many other early accounts of the illnesses that we now call schizophrenic disorders, and has remained a central topic of research into the nature of the schizophrenic psychotic period.

The purpose of this chapter is to describe a program of research that seeks to determine whether certain abnormalities in cognitive processing may be present not only in the acute psychotic stages of schizophrenic disorders, but also in persons at risk for these disorders who are not experiencing any psychotic symptomatology. Thus, these studies examine the possibility that some abnormalities in attention and information processing are not only a component of the schizophrenic psychotic state, but are indicators of a vulnerability to developing that state. The results from a variety of laboratory measures of information processing that investigators have recently applied to this question have been examined in detail elsewhere (Nuechterlein & Dawson, 1984a). This description will concentrate on the results of a series of studies in which I and my colleagues have employed measures of vigilance or sustained attention, specifically versions of the Continuous Performance Test (CPT), in an attempt to derive converging evidence for their utility as measures of a vulnerability indicator for schizophrenic disorders.

To converge on the conclusion that certain vigilance tasks may measure a vulnerability factor for schizophrenia, the results of studies that used four different research strategies will be summarized. The first strategy involved the study of children born to schizophrenic mothers, a group known to have a 10% to 15% lifetime risk of schizophrenia as compared to a general population risk of less than 1% (Gottesman & Shields, 1982; Rosenthal, 1970). A second strategy was to examine the vigilance performance of college students who were identified as being schizotypal or psychosis prone based on personality inventory responses. The third strategy reversed the dependent and independent variables in another population by selecting lower socioeconomic status subjects for poor vigilance performance and determining whether they had personality characteristics that are believed to be associated with schizotypy and psychosis proneness. Finally, the fourth strategy examined the stability of the vigilance performance deficit across time within a chronic schizophrenic population to shed light on its possible traitlike quality.

VIGILANCE AMONG CHILDREN OF SCHIZOPHRENIC MOTHERS

The first study (Nuechterlein, 1983) in this program of research involved an assessment of vigilance performance of children at heightened risk for schizophrenic disorder by virtue of having a schizophrenic mother, and was completed as a component of the Minnesota High-Risk Research Project developed by Norman Garmezy. These children, as well as several groups of normal and psychopathological comparison children, were examined on six conditions of a CPT.

Multiple CPT Versions

Although the CPT is often discussed as if it is a single test with standardized parameters, its parameter settings have actually varied substantially across studies. The label CPT has been used to describe a group of related procedures derived from that of Rosvold, Mirsky, Sarason, Bransome, and Beck (1956) in which a subject is asked to monitor a series of briefly presented stimuli (usually letters or numbers) as they are presented individually, with relatively brief, fixed interstimulus intervals over several minutes, and to respond each time that a predesignated target stimulus occurs. The exposure times are typically in the 50–200-msec range, the interstimulus intervals in the 1–1.5-sec range, and the total vigilance period from 5 to 15 min (Kornetsky, 1972; Kornetsky & Orzack, 1978; Rosvold *et al.*, 1956; Sykes, Douglas, & Morgenstern, 1973; Wohlberg & Kornetsky, 1973). The subject's response is usually a button press. The target can be a stimulus on a single presentation (e.g., the letter X) or a sequence of two presentations (e.g., an A followed by an X). The target stimulus occurs with relatively low frequency (target probabilities have ranged from about .10 to .25), as is typical of vigilance tasks (Davies & Parasuraman, 1982).

This initial study (Nuechterlein, 1983) was designed (1) to examine the possibility that children born to a schizophrenic parent show an impairment in vigilance performance, as had been found in a study reported by Erlenmeyer-Kimling and Cornblatt (1978) and Rutschmann, Cornblatt, and Erlenmeyer-Kimling (1977), (2) to relate their new version of the CPT to other CPT adaptations that involved variations in certain stimulus and response dimensions, (3) to examine the role of motivation, and (4) to determine the specificity of the deficit. The CPT version of Erlenmeyer-Kimling, Cornblatt, and Rutschmann involved presentation of slides of playing cards at relatively long (.6 sec) exposures and required children to press a button each time two identical cards occurred on successive trials. This version differed from most conventional CPT versions by employing a relative rather than absolute target, successive matching of the present stimulus to the memory of the preceding stimulus, and two stimulus dimensions (number and suit) rather than one. Thus, the relationship of this CPT adaptation to others needed clarification, as the memory load imposed by vigilance tasks has been found to be an important determinant of their interrelationship (Parasuraman & Davies, 1977).

This study employed six conditions of the CPT: (1) the playing card adaptation of the CPT developed by Erlenmeyer-Kimling, Cornblatt, and Rutschmann; (2) a conventional-numeral CPT that employed a single numeral (5) as the target stimulus and relatively brief exposure durations (40 or 50 msec, depending on the subject's age); (3) a response-reversal CPT that burdened response selection and organization aspects of information processing by requiring the subject to respond to each numeral except the former target numeral; (4) a degraded-stimulus CPT that burdened stimulus encoding and feature-extraction aspects of information processing through blurring of the numerals and superimposing a random pattern of visual noise; (5) a repetition of the degraded-stimulus condition with incentive feedback on correct target detections; and (6) a repetition of the degraded-stimulus condition with incentive feedback on incorrect button presses.

Multiple Comparison Groups

This study involved 24 children of schizophrenic mothers, with index mothers diagnosed by the schizophrenia criteria of Kety, Rosenthal, Wender, and Schulsinger (1968) and Kety, Rosenthal, Wender, Schulsinger, and Jacobsen (1978), as well as two types of normal comparison children and two psychopathological comparison groups. Two normal comparison groups were included in the design to allow for comparison to both a larger, representatively stratified normal sample and a "normal" sample that was individually matched to the children of schizophrenic mothers on sex, age, reading vocabulary and comprehension scores, socioeconomic status, and peer evaluation level. Peer evaluation level was added to the more typical matching variables because it is among the best predictors of global level of adult mental health (Cowen, Pederson, Babigian, Izzo, & Frost, 1973; Roff, 1970). Any vigilance deficits among the children of schizophrenic mothers relative to these sociometrically matched peers might be more specific to vulnerability to schizophrenia than to poor adult mental health in general.

Two psychopathological comparison groups were included in this study to examine further the specificity of any vigilance deficits among the children of schizophrenic mothers. A group of children born to mothers with psychiatric disorders outside the schizophrenia spectrum (Kety *et al.*, 1978; Rosenthal, 1978), most of whom had depressive conditions, was included to examine any generalized effects of maternal psychiatric disorder on children's vigilance performance. In addition, a sample of hyperactive children (without prominent antisocial behavior) was included, to allow an examination of performance in a psychopathological group known for attentional disturbance but without any clearly increased risk for adult schizophrenia (Borland & Heckman, 1976; Mendelson, Johnson, & Stewart, 1971; Stewart, de Blois, & Cummings, 1980; Weiss, Hechtman, Perlman, Hopkins, & Wener, 1979).

Figure 1 presents the mean MMPI profiles of the schizophrenic index mothers and of the index mothers with other psychiatric disorders. Note that the schizophrenic index mothers show their highest elevation on the Schizophrenia scale, followed by the Psychopathic Deviate scale, Paranoia scale, and the Depression scale. This profile type has been associated with schizophrenia in actuarial studies (Lachar, 1968; Marks, Seeman, & Haller, 1974), at least by DSM-II criteria, and is similar to that of the schizophrenic index group of Hanson, Gottesman, and Heston (1976). The profile of the nonpsychotic, psychiatrically disordered index mothers is a very similar in overall elevation level, but includes peak elevations on the Depression, Psychasthenia, and Psychopathic Deviate scales. This profile type has been associated with psychoneurosis (particularly depressive diagnoses) and personality disorders (particularly passive-aggressive personality) in actuarial research (Lachar, 1974; Marks *et al.*, 1974).

Use of Signal-Detection-Theory Indices

Performance on CPTs has traditionally been evaluated by examining errors of omission (missed targets) and errors of commission (responses to nontargets). In this series of studies, signal-detection-theory indices were used as the major dependent variables instead of the traditional raw-error scores

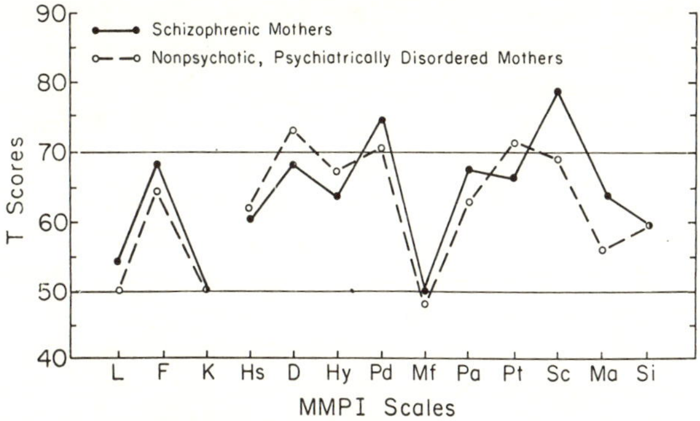

Figure 1. Mean Minnesota Multiphasic Personality Inventory (MMPI) profiles for all index mothers with available test scores ($N = 17$ for schizophrenic mothers; $N = 16$ for nonpsychotic, psychiatrically disordered mothers). (From "Signal detection in vigilance tasks and behavioral attributes among offspring of schizophrenic mothers and hyperactive children" by K. H. Nuechterlein, 1983, *Journal of Abnormal Psychology*, *92*, p. 9. Copyright 1983 by the American Psychological Association. Reprinted by permission.)

because the signal-detection-theory indices allow separation of two hypothesized underlying processes that are not apparent in the raw-error scores. Signal detection theory posits that subjects can be characterized in terms of the accuracy of their discrimination of target (signal) and nontarget (noise) stimuli as well as by their response criterion levels (Davies & Parasuraman, 1982; Green & Swets, 1966; McNicol, 1972). The perceptual evidence that a given stimulus is a signal falls along a dimension, with signal trials forming one distribution and noise trials forming another distribution at a lower level. The trials of the same type form a distribution rather than a single point, even for repeated presentations of the same signal (e.g., a numeral), due to small random fluctuations in the sensory characteristics of the stimulus and in the transmission of the sensory information within the nervous system. The distance between these distributions of perceptual evidence for signal and noise trials for a given subject is an index of signal/noise discrimination, called "sensitivity" in signal detection theory. The sensitivity measure d' refers to the distance between these two distributions in standard deviation units (Green & Swets, 1966).

Subjects also vary on the second variable, response criterion, which corresponds to the amount of perceptual evidence that a person demands before responding that a given stimulus is a signal. On the dimension of perceptual evidence along which the signal and noise distributions fall, the response-criterion cutoff refers to a point beyond which the subject always responds "signal." The response-criterion dimension is independent of the sensitivity dimension. A common measure of response criterion is beta (β), which refers to the ratio of the ordinate of the distribution of perceptual evidence for signal trials to the ordinate for noise trials at the response criterion cutoff point (Green & Swets, 1966; McNicol, 1972).

Although the perceptual-sensitivity and response-criterion indices measure independent underlying processes, differences between subjects in sensitivity and differences in response criterion can have identical effects on one of the raw-error scores considered alone. Thus, more errors of omission by one subject compared to another can be due to either lower sensitivity (poorer signal/noise discrimination) or higher response criterion (greater caution in deciding what to call a signal). More errors of commission can similiarly be due to lower sensitivity or lower response criterion. Thus, one can determine more about the processes that underlie the errors by deriving the signal-detection-theory indices, which consider the joint contributions of the two types of errors in evaluating performance.

Results for Children of Schizophrenic Mothers and Hyperactive Children

A principal components analysis of the signal detection indices d' and β from 5 versions of the CPT and of 14 personality and motivational ratings revealed 5 factors (Nuechterlein, 1983). The d' measure from each CPT version loaded on one factor and the β measure from each version loaded on another factor, suggesting that the two dimensions of perceptual sensitivity and response criterion were common across the five CPT versions. The conventional-numeral CPT did not produce enough errors to derive signal-detection indices reliably and was, therefore, omitted from the principal components analysis, but all versions that involved greater load on processing capacity showed this common performance structure.

The performance of the groups was evaluated by determining whether the children of schizophrenic mothers included an excessive number of cases with extremely poor d' factor scores, as had been hypothesized. The results are shown in Table 1, which presents the percentages of children within each group that obtained extremely low or high factor scores on the d' or β factors, where the 10th and 90th percentiles within the stratified normal comparison group were used as cutoffs to define these extreme scores. The children of schizophrenic mothers were found to include significantly more children with extremely low d' factor scores than the stratified normal comparison children (29% vs. 9%), whereas neither the children of nonpsychotic, psychiatrically disordered mothers nor the hyperactive children showed an excess of low d' scorers (Nuechterlein, 1983). If one subtypes the diagnoses of schizophrenic mothers by narrower diagnostic criteria for schizophrenia, those of the Research Diagnostic Criteria (RDC; Spitzer,

Table 1. Percentages and Frequencies of Children Obtaining Extremely Low or High d' or β Factor Scores

		d'				β			
		Low		High		Low		High	
Group	*N*	%	*F*	%	*F*	%	*F*	%	*F*
Stratified normal children	65	9	6	12	8	8	5	12	8
Children of all schizophrenic mothers[a]	24	29	7**	4	1	4	1	8	2
Children of RDC schizophrenic mothers	13	31	4*	8	1	8	1	8	1
Children of RDC schizoaffective mothers	8	25	2	0	0	0	0	13	1
Children of DSM-III schizotypal personality disorder mothers	3	33	1	0	0	0	0	0	0
Matched comparison children	24	8	2	8	2	4	1	13	3
Children of nonpsychotic, psychiatrically disordered mothers	20	10	2	5	1	0	0	0	0
Matched comparison children	20	10	2	15	3	5	1	10	2
Hyperactive children	14	14	2	0	0	29	4*	0	0
Matched comparison children	14	0	0	0	0	7	1	14	2

Note. RDC = Research Diagnostic Criteria. DSM-III = *Diagnostic and statistical manual of mental disorders* (3rd ed.) (American Psychiatric Association, 1980).

Note. From "Signal detection in vigilance tasks and behavioral attributes among offspring of schizophrenic mothers and hyperactive children" by K. H. Nuechterlein, 1983, *Journal of Abnormal Psychology*, *92*, p. 15. Copyright 1983 by the American Psychological Association. Reprinted by permission.

[a] Diagnoses based on Kety, Rosenthal, Wender, and Schulsinger (1968) schizophrenia criteria.

* $p = .05$, compared to the frequency for the stratified normal group.

** $p = .03$, compared to the frequency for the stratified normal group; $p = .07$, compared to the matched group.

Endicott, & Robins, 1978), the same result holds for the children of these more narrowly defined schizophrenic index mothers. It is noteworthy that the hyperactive children did contain an excessive number of children with extremely low β factor scores compared to the stratified normal children, whereas children of schizophrenic mothers showed no excesses of extreme scores on this performance factor.

In this first study (Nuechterlein, 1983), mean analyses were also completed, and showed essentially parallel results (Table 2). Children of schizophrenic mothers had lower mean d' factor scores than stratified normal comparison children but did not differ on the β factor score. By mean

Table 2. Mean Factor Scores for the Target Groups and Stratified Normal Group (Adjusted for Sex)

Group	Factor				
	d′	β	Task orientation	Emotionality	Fearful inhibition
Stratified normal children	−.01	−.01	.00	.00	−.01
Children of all schizophrenic mothers[a]	−.52*	.03	.04	.33	.10
Children of RDC schizophrenic mothers	−.52*	−.01	−.10	.60	.29
Children of RDC schizoaffective mothers	−.22	.30	.34	−.14	−.22
Children of DSM-III schizotypal personality disorder mothers	−1.36*	−.54	−.13	.39	.11
Children of nonpsychotic, psychiatrically disordered mothers	−.32	−.10	−.30	.10	.46
Hyperactive children	−.35	−.67*	−.70	1.43**	−.67*

Note. RDC = Research Diagnostic Criteria. DSM-III = *Diagnostic and statistical manual of mental disorders* (3rd ed.) (American Psychiatric Association, 1980).

Note. From "Signal detection in vigilance tasks and behavioral attributes among offspring of schizophrenic mothers and hyperactive children" by K. H. Nuechterlein, 1983, *Journal of Abnormal Psychology*, *92*, p. 17. Copyright 1983 by the American Psychological Association. Reprinted by permission.

[a] Diagnoses based on Kety, Rosenthal, Wender, and Schulsinger (1968) schizophrenia criteria.

* $p < .05$, compared to the stratified normal children.

** $p < .01$, compared to the stratified normal children.

analyses, both the children of RDC schizophrenic mothers and the children of DSM-III schizotypal personality disorder mothers showed the hypothesized lower *d′* compared to the stratified normal children. Hyperactive children obtained lower response-criterion-factor scores, but were not significantly lower than the stratified normal comparison group on the perceptual-sensitivity factor. Hyperactive children were also differentiated from the stratified normal children by significantly higher scores on an Emotionality factor and lower scores on a Fearful Inhibition factor based on behavioral ratings.

Analyses that contrasted each target group with its matched comparison group rather than with the stratified comparison group yielded essentially the same results (Nuechterlein, 1983). Thus, the results could not be explained by any of the matching variables, which included sex, age, reading vocabulary or comprehension level, socioeconomic status, or peer evaluation level.

These results suggest that children at risk for schizophrenia by virtue of having a schizophrenic mother show impaired perceptual sensitivity, or signal/noise discrimination, in a vigilance situation, whereas children born to mothers with nonpsychotic disorders outside the schizophrenia spectrum do not. Hyperactive children, who were hypothesized in this first study to have impaired perceptual sensitivity as well as low response-criterion levels, showed only the latter. Low response-criterion levels are consistent with the impulsive cognitive style that some investigators (e.g., Douglas, 1972, 1980) have emphasized as a contributor to the performance of hyperactive children.

It is important to note that we have found that some hyperactive children did show the hypothesized impaired signal/noise discrimination levels during a similar battery of CPT tasks in a second study (O'Dougherty, Nuechterlein, & Drew, 1984), although this deficit was not present to a significant degree at all age levels. In the initial study by Nuechterlein (1983), hyperactive children were selected through the use of factor scores that employed the symptom factors derived by Soli, Nuechterlein, Garmezy, Devine, and Schaefer (1981). Child guidance clinic children were required to have high Hyperactivity factor scores and low Delinquency and Rebelliousness factor scores for inclusion. The presence of learning disability or difficulty was not an aspect of the selection criteria. In the second study by O'Dougherty *et al.* (1984), an elevated score on the hyperactivity index from the revised Conners Teacher Rating Scale (Goyette, Conners, & Ulrich, 1978) was employed as the selection criterion in order to examine a broad hyperactive group comparable to those that have been included in certain previous studies of other research groups. In this second study, marked learning difficulties were often part of the presenting picture and hyperactive children with accompanying antisocial behavior were not excluded. Thus, impaired discrimination of the numeral stimuli in this CPT battery might be linked to the presence of these additional behavioral problems within some hyperactive children (O'Dougherty *et al.*, 1984), particularly learning disability that includes slowed numeral and letter recognition, whereas the hyperactive children in the initial study (Nuechterlein, 1983) were likely to be more purely impulsive. Consistent with the results of the initial study, the hyperactive children in the O'Dougherty *et al.* (1984) study showed a lower response criterion than normal children.

This second study also suggests the possibility that perceptual-sensitivity level during vigilance may be linked to subtle impairment in brain function in at least some instances, because children who had been exposed to chronic oxygen deprivation due to a congenital heart condition were found to have impaired perceptual-sensitivity level, but not motor hyperactivity, in the first several years after corrective surgery (O'Dougherty *et al.*, 1984). Thus, in addition to studies of schizophrenic patients and schizophrenia-prone populations, further research with certain nonschizophrenic populations may shed additional light on whether the processes that cause deficits in perceptual-sensitivity level in such vigilance tasks are similar or different across these groups.

Deficit in Vigilance Level versus Vigilance Decrement over Time

The results presented thus far refer to differences in the overall level of perceptual sensitivity in the vigilance tasks. Decrements in perceptual sensitivity over time within vigilance tasks are viewed as the most meaningful measure of sustained attention, whereas the overall level of vigilance may be determined by separate processes and can be relatively independent of decrement over time (Davies & Parasuraman, 1982; Nuechterlein, Parasuraman, & Jiang, 1983). Thus, using the data from the 11.5-min degraded-stimulus CPT condition, I contrasted children of schizophrenic mothers with the stratified-comparison children in terms of their decrement in performance over time. As shown in Figure 2, the detection of target stimuli (hit rate) did show a tendency to drop more rapidly over time among children of schizophrenic mothers, but this effect was not statistically significant ($p = .08$). More importantly, the perceptual sensitivity (d') did not show a significant differential drop over time for the offspring of schizophrenic mothers (Nuechterlein, 1983). Thus, the deficit in vigilance performance in this first study that may index a vulnerability factor for schizophrenia involves lowering of the overall level of perceptual sensitivity and seems not to be related to any systematic decrement in sustained attention within the task.

Lack of Motivational Basis for the Vigilance Deficit

Another issue that was addressed in the initial study of children of schizophrenic mothers was whether the deficit in vigilance level might be attributable to lower motivation to perform well. Several lines of evidence argue against any simple motivational explanation for the deficit. First, the principal components analysis revealed a behavioral rating factor, Task Orientation, on which several ratings of directed motivation loaded, including ratings of goal orientation, cooperation, and agreeability. This factor was separable from the perceptual-sensitivity (d') factor, and factor scores did not show decreased Task Orientation among children at risk for schizophrenia. Second, signal-detection-theory indices are derived in such a way that motivational influences should be reflected in altered response-criterion levels rather than in changed perceptual sensitivity (Swets & Sewall, 1963), unless the unmotivated subject responds in a wholly random way. Any lowered responding associated with decreased motivation to be engaged in the task

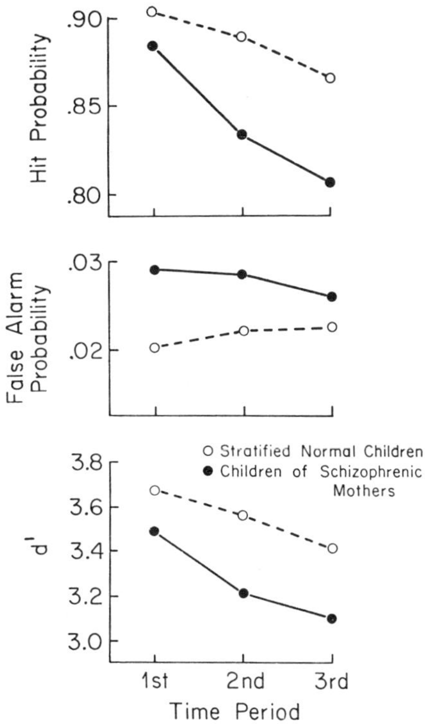

Figure 2. Changes in hit probability, false alarm probability, and *d'* over time periods of the degraded-stimulus continuous performance test for children of schizophrenic mothers and stratified normal children (each time period equals 230 sec). (From "Signal detection in vigilance tasks and behavioral attributes among offspring of schizophrenic mothers and hyperactive children" by K. H. Nuechterlein, 1983, *Journal of Abnormal Psychology*, *92*, p. 21. Copyright 1983 by the American Psychological Association. Reprinted by permission.)

would lead to increased response-criterion levels, which did not characterize the children of schizophrenic mothers. Finally, the children at risk for schizophrenia did not show any differential effect of incentive feedback in the two conditions in which the degraded-stimulus CPT was repeated with auditory feedback on correct or incorrect responses. The perceptual-sensitivity deficit was evident across the three degraded-stimulus CPT conditions rather than disappearing or showing significant lessening under incentive feedback conditions. Thus, the perceptual-sensitivity deficit among children of schizophrenic mothers appears not to be caused by any transient or observable motivational deficiencies.

Specificity of the Deficit to Vigilance Performance

To examine whether the impairments in perceptual-sensitivity level during vigilance represented a cognitive processing anomaly that was specific to this type of task, Nuechterlein, Phipps-Yonas, Driscoll, and Garmezy (1982) examined the pattern of performance across the CPT session, a crossmodal simple-reaction-time session, and a selective-attention session that involved intentional and incidental learning measures. Only the CPT d' factor successfully isolated a disproportionately large poor-scoring subgroup among the children of schizophrenic mothers as compared to the representatively stratified normal children. Neither a Reaction Time factor that indexed slow and variable simple reaction times, an Intentional Learning factor, nor an Incidental Learning factor differentiated such a disproportionately large group of deviant responders. Furthermore, combinations of multiple deviant scores across performance factors and cluster analyses of scores across the major performance factors from these sessions did not improve on the isolation of an excessive number of deviant performers among children of schizophrenic mothers that was achieved by the CPT d' factor alone (Nuechterlein *et al.*, 1982).

Although this pattern of findings suggested that the CPT d' factor was particularly effective at isolating deviant performers among the high-risk group, an underlying factor might be the extent to which the various tasks demanded a high level of moment-to-moment processing capacity or effortful processing (Hasher & Zacks, 1979; Kahneman, 1973; Posner, 1978, 1982). Moderate correlations between the CPT d' factor and the Reaction Time factor ($r = -.39$, $p < .01$) as well as the Intentional Learning factor ($r = .36$, $p < .01$) in the sample as a whole indicated that some common variance was present among performance factors that were likely to involve effortful, focused attention. The Incidental Learning factor, on the other hand, which did not reflect an intentional instructional set, was not significantly correlated with the CPT d' factor ($r = .08$). Nor was the CPT factor significantly associated with a vocabulary score ($r = .16$), which suggests little relationship between the CPT d' factor and general verbal ability level. The CPT conditions that contributed the d' factor were characterized by high stimulus-event rates combined with substantial perceptual-discrimination, short-term memory, or response-organization demands under time pressure. Thus, the CPT d' factor from five CPT versions with relatively high processing loads can be viewed as reflecting performance along an intensity dimension of attentional functioning (Beatty, 1982; Kahneman, 1973) in situations that involve substantial demands on overall processing capacity in addition to any task-specific cognitive operations. Consistent with this emphasis is the finding that the CPT condition with a single, clearly focused target numeral, for which stimulus recognition should demand little or no processing capacity (Posner, 1978; Shiffrin & Schneider, 1977), did not differentiate the children at risk for schizophrenia from the normal comparison groups (Nuechterlein, 1983).

VIGILANCE AMONG YOUNG ADULTS WITH 2–7–8 MMPI PROFILES

The second strategy that was used to determine whether the deficit in perceptual sensitivity during vigilance was related to vulnerability to schizophrenic disorder involved the study of college students who had a 2–7–8 MMPI profile. This profile type, which involves peak elevations on the Depression (2), Psychasthenia (7), and Schizophrenia (8) scales, has been associated with latent schizophrenia, schizotypal, and psychoticlike characteristics (Fujioka & Chapman, 1984; Gilbertstadt & Duker, 1965; Kelley & King, 1979; Peterson, 1954) and later diagnoses of schizophrenia (Peterson, 1954), and was the modal profile type of patients meeting DSM-II criteria for schizotypal personality disorder in a recent study (Edell, 1984). This profile might identify a group at increased risk for psychosis rather than only for schizophrenia, because some studies have suggested that the 2–7–8 profile is associated with affective psychoses (Haier, Rieder, Khouri, & Buchsbaum, 1979; Winters, Weintraub, & Neale, 1981).

Selection of 2–7–8 Group and Two Comparison Groups

To identify a 2–7–8 profile group and comparison subjects, William Edell, Preston West, and I screened with the MMPI-168, a widely used short form of the MMPI, over 1100 college students taking introductory psychology (Nuechterlein, Edell, & West, 1985). Subjects in the 2–7–8 group (N = 16) were required to have elevations on these three scales that were at least 1.5 standard deviations above the MMPI standardization mean (T-score > 65) and could have no other clinical scale with a higher elevation. Subjects who had at least two clinical scales with T-score ≥ 65 and a Schizophrenia scale (8) T-score ≤ 65 were selected for an Other Elevations comparison group (N = 22). A No Elevations comparison group (N = 24) consisted of subjects with no clinical scale more than one standard deviation above the mean (no T-score > 60). Thus, the design compared the performance of a group with schizotypal characteristics with that of (1) a group with profiles at similar overall elevation levels but with lower Schizophrenia scale scores and (2) a group with strictly defined normal MMPI profiles.

Results for MMPI 2–7–8 Young Adults

Subjects were evaluated individually on a degraded-stimulus CPT that paralleled that of the initial study of children born to schizophrenic mothers (Nuechterlein, 1983) but which was adapted for older subjects by increasing the degree of stimulus degradation. This increased stimulus degradation improves the ability of the task to elicit decrements in perceptual sensitivity over time, such that periods of 5–8 min are sufficient to obtain significant sensitivity decrements even with normal young adult subjects (Nuechterlein *et al.*, 1983). The major hypothesis was that subjects in the two comparison groups would not be distinguished by their signal-detection levels during this vigilance task, but that the 2–7–8 group would show significantly poorer signal-detection performance than those groups combined. Consistent with this prediction, subjects in the Other Elevations group, across three conditions of this task that involved presence or absence of simultaneous auditory noise, did not differ in perceptual-sensitivity level from those in the No Elevations group and, in fact, showed no tendency to be lower. Mean overall d' values were 2.28 for the Other Elevations group and 2.15 for the No Elevations group ($p > .50$). The mean overall d' for the 2–7–8 group, on the other hand, was 1.66, which is significantly lower that the level for the combined comparison groups ($p < .03$) (Nuechterlein, Edell, & West, 1985).

The hit rates (target detection rates) showed the same effect, with the 2–7–8, Other Elevation, and No Elevation groups obtaining rates of .60, .76, and .72, respectively. Again, the 2–7–8 group was significantly inferior to the combined comparison groups ($p < .01$), which did not differ from each other ($p > .40$) (Nuechterlein, Edell, & West, 1985). Thus, the significant deficit in signal detection during vigilance performance in this study was found in the group with an MMPI profile associated with schizotypal and psychotic-like characteristics and hypothesized risk for psychosis, but not in subjects either with clearly normal MMPI profiles or with MMPI profiles that suggested similarity to other forms of psychiatric disorder.

Another parallel to the initial study of children born to schizophrenic mothers is that the performance decrement over time within task, although highly significant across all groups, was not significantly greater for the 2–7–8 group than it was for the comparison groups for either perceptual sensitivity (d') or hit rate. The performance of the 2–7–8 group is lower than that of the two comparison groups from the beginning of the vigilance period. Thus, the deficit in performance that is related to the group at hypothesized risk for schizophrenia is again an overall lowering of perceptual sensitivity (signal/noise discrimination) across the periods of performance on this degraded-stimulus CPT.

SCHIZOTYPAL CHARACTERISTICS AMONG SUBJECTS WITH POOR PERCEPTUAL SENSITIVITY DURING VIGILANCE

In a study using a third strategy to examine the possibility that poor perceptual sensitivity during vigilance is related to vulnerability to schizophrenic disorder, I and my colleagues Robert Asarnow and Stephen Marder turned the second strategy upside down. We selected subjects for low perceptual sensitivity (d') during degraded-stimulus CPT performance and examined the possibility that such subjects are characterized by schizotypal traits (Nuechterlein, Asarnow, & Marder, 1985).

Selection of a Socioeconomic High-Risk Sample

To locate a subject pool that was likely to include a greater frequency of persons vulnerable to schizophrenia than the general population, we used subjects from a temporary employment agency who had no personal history of mental disorder but who had relatively low educational level (mean = 12.8 years) and who usually worked in lower-social-class positions. Lower socioeconomic status has been repeatedly associated with a heightened prevalence of schizophrenia (Dohrenwend & Dohrenwend, 1974; Kohn, 1968). Although the reasons for this increased rate of schizophrenia in the lower social classes may include downward drift of predisposed and ill individuals as well as possible triggering of schizophrenic psychosis by the stresses of lower class life (Turner & Wagonfeld, 1967), the increased prevalence of schizophrenia in this segment of society is not in doubt. Thus, this group should provide an increased opportunity to examine the relationship of impaired perceptual sensitivity during the degraded-stimulus CPT to schizotypal personality characteristics.

We tested 50 lower-social-class subjects from a temporary employment agency with the degraded-stimulus CPT with a single target numeral, as part of a larger protocol that included a 4-hour battery of cognitive processing and personality assessment tools (Asarnow, Nuechterlein, & Marder, 1983; Nuechterlein, Asarnow, & Marder, 1985). Subjects with a history of psychiatric disorder, alcohol abuse, or drug abuse were excluded, as were subjects with visual acuity less than 20/30. Subjects were split into two groups based on their score on the overall perceptual sensitivity index, d', during the degraded-stimulus CPT, using the group median as the cutting point.

Characteristics of Subjects with Low versus High Perceptual Sensitivity during the Degraded-Stimulus CPT

The resulting subjects with poor versus good signal/noise discrimination during vigilance were then contrasted on the scales of the MMPI to determine whether the poor-performing group showed evidence of schizotypal characteristics. Indeed, we (Nuechterlein, Asarnow, & Marder, 1985) found that the poor-perceptual-sensitivity group obtained significantly higher scores on the Schizophrenia scale than the good-perceptual-sensitivity group (T-scores = 71.6 vs. 57.7; $p < .01$). Furthermore, the poor-perceptual-sensitivity group did not show higher scores on any other MMPI clinical scale except Psychopathic Deviate (*T*-scores = 71.5 vs. 63.0; $p < .03$), indicating that his group was not simply more psychopathological in general than the remaining subjects. In fact, a stepwise multiple regression analysis using the entire sample identified elevations on the Schizophrenia scale as the best individual MMPI predictor of perceptual-sensitivity level during vigilance, with the only significant remaining predictive variance being contributed by low rather than high scores on the Hysteria scale (Nuechterlein, Asarnow, & Marder, 1985).

Further evidence of an association between poor signal/noise discrimination during the degraded-stimulus CPT and psychosis proneness was found in scores on other recently developed schizotypy and psychosis-proneness scales. The poor perceptual sensitivity group obtained higher scores than the remaining subjects on Chapman, Chapman, and Raulin's (1976) Physical Anhedonia scale ($p \leq .03$), Nielsen and Petersen's (1976) Schizophrenism scale ($p \leq .01$), and Golden and Meehl's (1979) Schizoidia scale ($p \leq .03$). Thus, including the MMPI findings, the subjects with poor perceptual discrimination but without a history of psychiatric disorder showed personality characteristics associated with schizotypy and psychosis proneness across scales from four different sources.

Characteristics of Subjects with Low versus High Brightness Discrimination

To examine the possibility that the association of schizotypy and psychosis proneness with poor perceptual sensitivity in the degraded-stimulus CPT was due to a sensory deficit rather than a deficit in processing features in patterned information, we also split the same group of 50 temporary-employment-agency subjects at the median on their sensitivity (d') in a brightness-discrimination task, to determine whether poor performance on this sensory task was also related to elevated scores on the same personality scales (Nuechterlein, Asarnow, & Marder, 1985). The task involved forced-choice trials in which subjects were asked whether a first or second tachistoscopic flash of light was brighter.

It was striking that subjects who performed poorly on this brightness-discrimination task were not significantly differentiated from those who performed well on any of the schizotypy and psychosis-proneness scales nor on any of the MMPI scales (Nuechterlein, Asarnow, & Marder, 1985). Thus, these data suggest that the deficit that is an indicator of vulnerability to schizophrenic disorders may involve the processing of the features of patterned perceptual information, rather the processing of unpatterned sensory stimuli, because the former is related to personality characteristics associated with schizotypy, whereas the latter is not.

STABILITY OVER TIME OF PERCEPTUAL-SENSITIVITY LEVEL ON THE DEGRADED-STIMULUS CPT

One remaining question is whether the deficit in perceptual sensitivity in the degraded-stimulus CPT is a transient and fluctuating phenomenon or a relatively stable, traitlike characteristic of individuals with schizophrenic disorders or a vulnerability to such disorders. I have recently examined data from a sample of chronic schizophrenic patients, which were collected as part of a larger study in collaboration with Alan Steinberg, Robert P. Liberman, and Charles Wallace, to determine the stability of perceptual sensitivity (d') within the degraded-stimulus CPT over repeated sessions of testing. The patients were diagnosed through a Present State Examination and met the restrictive CATEGO criteria for schizophrenia (Wing, Cooper, & Sartorius, 1974). The numeral stimuli were presented at a degradation level comparable to the high-degradation condition in the Nuechterlein *et al.* (1983) study and used the same 40-msec exposure duration, 1-sec interstimulus interval, and "0" target numeral. For purposes of comparison, a conventional CPT with the same exposure duration, interstimulus interval, and single numeral target, but using clearly focused numerals, was also administered on the same occasions.

Summary data are presented in Table 3. For the degraded-stimulus CPT, both a parametric index of sensitivity, d', and a nonparametric index, $P(\bar{A})$ (also called A'), were calculated (Davies & Parasuraman, 1982; Grier, 1971; Pollack & Norman, 1964). Because the error rates on the conventional single-numeral CPT were extremely low in many cases, only the nonparametric index, $P(\bar{A})$, which makes no assumptions about the underlying signal and noise distributions, was calculated for this version. As shown in Table 3, the test–retest correlations for overall perceptual sensitivity level in the degraded-stimulus CPT indicate that individual differences on this task are fairly stable within chronic schizophrenic patients and are not a transient phenomenon. The parallel correlations for a conventional CPT with a single, clearly focused target numeral (similar to the traditional "X"

Table 3. Stability of Overall Perceptual-Sensitivity Level in the Degraded-Stimulus CPT and a Conventional-Numeral CPT among Chronic Schizophrenic Patients

		Test–retest interval		
CPT version	Sensitivity index	3 months (N = 21)	6 months (N = 20)	12 months (N = 14)
Degraded stimulus	d'	.75	.74	.84
	$P(\bar{A})$	.74	.64	.81
Clear single target	$P(\bar{A})$	.33	.06	.42

version) are substantially lower and indicate relatively low stability of performance on this version.

Thus, perceptual-sensitivity level on the degraded-stimulus CPT, which had been found in the previous studies to be impaired among children of schizophrenic mothers and young adults with 2–7–8 MMPI profiles and also was found to be associated with various schizotypic characteristics on psychometric scales, is a relatively stable characteristic among chronic schizophrenic patients. This reasonable stability over time enhances the argument that perceptual-sensitivity level during this vigilance task is a relatively enduring characteristic that appears to index a vulnerability factor for schizophrenic disorders. In contrast, performance on a conventional CPT with a single, clearly focused target numeral is relatively unstable among chronic schizophrenic patients. As I and Michael Dawson have noted elsewhere (Nuechterlein & Dawson, 1984a), CPT versions with a single, focused target numeral have often failed to detect a significant deficit among children at risk by virtue of being born to a schizophrenic parent (Asarnow, Steffy, MacCrimmon, & Cleghorn, 1977; Cornblatt & Erlenmeyer-Kimling, 1984; Nuechterlein, 1983), even when other CPT versions that make greater demands on processing capacity detect significant deficits in the same samples (Cornblatt & Erlenmeyer-Kimling, 1984; Nuechterlein, 1983). The present evidence that performance on a CPT with a single, focused target is not very stable among chronic schizophrenic patients heightens the contrast in results for these different vigilance tasks. Thus, the evidence for vigilance deficit as an enduring vulnerability indicator for schizophrenic disorder is quite consistent for the more demanding degraded-stimulus CPT, but the cognitive-processing limitations that lead to this deficit are often not evident in performance on CPT versions with a single, focused target stimulus.

CONCLUSIONS AND REMAINING ISSUES

Data from three different subject sampling strategies for examining the relationship between vigilance performance and vulnerability to schizophrenic disorder in nonschizophrenic samples yielded converging evidence that the perceptual-sensitivity level or signal/noise discrimination level in a continuous performance test using briefly presented, degraded stimuli is a promising vulnerability indicator. Children born to schizophrenic mothers and college students with MMPI 2–7–8 profiles showed impaired perceptual sensitivity during this vigilance task, whereas children of nonpsychotic, psychiatrically disordered mothers and college students with other elevated MMPI profiles not including Schizophrenia scale elevations did not differ from normal comparison groups. Among adults without a personal history of mental illness, poor perceptual sensitivity during this vigilance task was associated with elevations on several psychometric measures of schizotypal characteristics and hypothesized psychosis proneness. Furthermore, an examination of chronic schizophrenic patients indicated that perceptual-sensitivity level in this task is relatively stable over a 3- to 12-month interval, suggesting that this task may measure a relatively enduring characteristic rather than a transient deficit.

One important remaining issue concerns the relationships of any changes over occasions in perceptual-sensitivity level during vigilance to changes in psychiatric symptomatology. Although the data from the sample of chronic schizophrenic patients indicated fair stability of performance across occasions, sufficient variance remained to allow substantial relationship to clinical symptomatology as well. To examine this and other vulnerability indicators that may have predictive power for the onset and course of schizophrenic episodes, I and my colleagues in the Mental Health Clinical Research Center for the Study of Schizophrenia at UCLA are currently conducting a longitudinal study of patients who have had a relatively recent onset of schizophrenic disorder. We are examining these patients during their index psychotic period, during clinical remission, and during any psychotic exacerbation or relapse, to determine the extent to which this perceptual-sensitivity deficit during vigilance and other promising vulnerability indicators are related to changes in psychotic symptomatology.

In particular, my colleague Michael Dawson and I seek to separate variables that are "stable vulnerability indicators" from those that are "mediating vulnerability factors" (Nuechterlein & Dawson, 1984b). We use the term *stable vulnerability indicator* to refer to a characteristic that is stably deviant from normal levels, even during symptomatic remission, in schizophrenic patients, and that is independent of symptomatic changes. A *mediating vulnerability factor*, in our terms, refers to a characteristic that is also deviant from normal levels during both psychotic and asymptomatic states, but which covaries with level of symptomatology. We hypothesize that some mediating vulnerability factors may be contributors in causal chains leading to psychotic symptomatology and, therefore, would be expected to show an increased deviation from normal levels simultaneous with or preceding psychotic episodes (Nuechterlein & Dawson, 1984b). In addition to determining whether perceptual sensitivity during the degraded-stimulus CPT and other promising vulnerability indexes are stable vulnerability indicators or mediating vulnerability factors, our ongoing longitudinal study is examining the value of attentional and information-processing vulnerability factors as well as certain psychophysiological abnormalities (Dawson & Nuechterlein, 1984), in combination with stressors such as familial expressed emotion (Vaughn, Snyder, Jones, Freeman, & Falloon, 1984) and discrete life events (Brown & Birley, 1968; Lukoff, Snyder, Ventura, & Nuechterlein, 1984), in predicting the early course of schizophrenic disorders.

Another area that requires further examination is the precise nature of the perceptual-sensitivity deficit in the degraded-stimulus CPT among persons at risk for schizophrenic disorder. We have suggested that this CPT version demands a high level of continuous, capacity-loading, effortful processing, and that this factor distinguishes it from the CPT version with single, clearly focused target numerals that does not detect deficient performance among children at risk for schizophrenia. However, additional comparisons between CPT versions that are carefully matched for overall difficulty level would be very helpful in determining whether specific information-processing operations required by this CPT version, such as the increased emphasis on initial feature extraction processes, contribute to the detection of a vulnerability factor for schizophrenic disorders beyond the increased demand for processing capacity. Such strategies also address the possibility that the psychometric properties of the compared tasks rather than the specific information-processing demands are the determinant of the differential deficit of interest (Chapman & Chapman, 1973, 1978). In collaboration with my colleagues Robert Asarnow and Stephen Marder at UCLA, studies that match CPT versions for difficulty level and psychometric discriminating power are currently underway to examine specific contributions of certain processes and task parameters to differential deficit among schizophrenic patients. These studies should shed additional light on the nature of the perceptual-sensitivity deficit during vigilance that is a promising vulnerability indicator for schizophrenic disorders.

ACKNOWLEDGMENTS

Parts of this research were supported by NIMH Research Grant MH37705, by a grant from the Schizophrenia Research Program of the Scottish Rite, NMJ, U.S.A., and by NIMH Research Grant MH30911, which funds the UCLA Mental Health Clinical Research Center for the Study of Schizophrenia.

REFERENCES

American Psychiatric Association. (1980). *Diagnostic and statistical manual of mental disorders* (3rd ed.). Washington, DC: APA.

Asarnow, R. F., Nuechterlein, K. H., & Marder, S. R. (1983). Span of apprehension, neuropsychological functioning, and indices of psychosis-proneness. *Journal of Nervous and Mental Disease, 171*, 662–669.

Asarnow, R. F., Steffy, R. A., MacCrimmon, D. J., & Cleghorn, J. M. (1977). An attentional assessment of foster children at risk for schizophrenia. *Journal of Abnormal Psychology, 86*, 267–275.

Beatty, J. (1982). Task-evoked pupillary reponses, processing load, and the structure of processing resources. *Psychological Bulletin, 91*, 276–292.

Borland, B. L., & Heckman, H. K. (1976). Hyperactive boys and their brothers: A 25-year follow-up study. *Archives of General Psychiatry, 33*, 669–675.

Brown, G. W., & Birley, J. L. (1968). Crises and life changes and the onset of schizophrenia. *Journal of Health and Social Behavior*, *9*, 203-214.

Chapman, L. J., & Chapman, J. P. (1973). *Disordered thought in schizophrenia*. New York: Appleton-Century-Crofts.

Chapman, L. J., & Chapman, J. P. (1978). The measurement of differential deficit. *Journal of Psychiatric Research*, *14*, 303–311.

Chapman, L. J., Chapman, J. P., & Raulin, M. L. (1976). Scales for physical and social anhedonia. *Journal of Abnormal Psychology*, *85*, 374–382.

Cornblatt, B., & Erlenmeyer-Kimling, L. (1984). Early attentional predictors·of adolescent behavioral disturbances in children at risk for schizophrenia. In N. F. Watt, E. J. Anthony, L. C. Wynne, & J. E. Rolf (Eds.), *Children at risk for schizophrenia: A longitudinal perspective* (pp. 198–211). London & New York: Cambridge University Press.

Cowen, E. L., Pederson, A., Babigian, H., Izzo, L. D., & Frost, M. A. (1973). Long-term follow-up of early detected vulnerable children. *Journal of Consulting and Clinical Psychology*, *41*, 438–446.

Davies, D. R., & Parasuraman, R. (1982). *The psychology of vigilance*. London: Academic Press.

Dawson, M. E., & Nuechterlein, K. H. (1984). Psychophysiological dysfunctions in the developmental course of schizophrenic disorders. *Schizophrenia Bulletin*, *10*, 204–232.

Dohrenwend, B. P. & Dohrenwend, B. S. (1974). Social and cultural influences in psychopathology. *Annual Review of Psychology*, *24*, 417–452.

Douglas, V. I. (1972). Stop, look, and listen: The problem of sustained attention and impulse control in hyperactive and normal children. *Canadian Journal of Behavioral Science*, *4*, 259–282.

Douglas, V. I. (1980). Treatment and training approaches to hyperactivity: Establishing internal or external control. In C. K. Whalen & B. Henker (Eds.), *Hyperactive children: The social ecology of identification and treatment* (pp. 283–317). New York: Academic Press.

Edell, W. S. (1984). *Relationship of borderline syndrome disorders to early schizophrenia on the Minnesota Multiphasic Personality Inventory (MMPI)*. Manuscript submitted for publication.

Erlenmeyer-Kimling, L., & Cornblatt, B. (1978). Attentional measures in a study of children at high-risk for schizophrenia. *Journal of Psychiatric Research*, *14*, 93–98.

Fujioka, T. A. T., & Chapman, L. J. (1984). Comparisons of the 2–7–8 MMPI profile and the Perceptual Aberration-Magical Ideation Scale in identifying hypothetically psychosis-prone college students. *Journal of Consulting and Clinical Psychology*, *52*, 458–467.

Gilberstadt, H., & Duker, J. (1965). *A handbook for clinical and actuarial MMPI interpretation*. Philadelphia: W. B. Saunders.

Golden, R. R., & Meehl, P. E. (1979). Detection of the schizoid taxon with MMPI indicators. *Journal of Abnormal Psychology*, *88*, 217–233.

Gottesman, I. I., & Shields, J. (1982). *Schizophrenia: The epigenetic puzzle*. London & New York: Cambridge University Press.

Goyette, C. H., Conners, C. K., & Ulrich, R. F. (1978). Normative data on revised Conners parent and teacher rating scales. *Journal of Abnormal Child Psychology*, *6*, 221–236.

Green, D. M., & Swets, J. A. (1966). *Signal detection theory and psychophysics*. New York: Wiley.

Grier, J. B. (1971). Nonparametric indexes for sensitivity and bias: Computing formulas. *Psychological Bulletin*, *75*, 424–429.

Haier, R. J., Rieder, R. O., Khouri, P. J., & Buchsbaum, M. S. (1979). Extreme MMPI scores and the Research Diagnostic Criteria: Screening college men for psychopathology. *Archives of General Psychiatry*, *36*, 528–534.

Hanson, D. R., Gottesman, I. I., & Heston, L. L. (1976). Some possible childhood indicators of adult schizophrenia inferred from children of schizophrenics. *British Journal of Psychiatry, 129*, 142–154.

Hasher, L., & Zacks, R. T. (1979). Automatic and effortful processes in memory. *Journal of Experimental Psychology: General, 108*, 356–388.

Kahneman, D. (1973). *Attention and effort.* Englewood Cliffs, NJ: Prentice-Hall.

Kelley, C. K., & King, G. D. (1979). Behavioral correlates of the 2–7–8 MMPI profile type in students at a university mental health center. *Journal of Consulting and Clinical Psychology, 47*, 679–685.

Kety, S. S., Rosenthal, D., Wender, P. H., & Schulsinger, F. (1968). The types and prevalence of mental illness in the biological and adoptive families of adopted schizophrenics. In D. Rosenthal & S. S. Kety (Eds.), *The transmission of schizophrenia* (pp. 345–362). Oxford: Pergamon Press.

Kety, S. S., Rosenthal, D., Wender, P. H., Schulsinger, F., & Jacobsen, B. (1978). The biologic and adoptive families of adoptive individuals who became schizophrenic: Prevalence of mental illness and other characteristics. In L. C. Wynne, R. L. Cromwell, & S. Matthysse (Eds.), *The nature of schizophrenia: New approaches to research and treatment* (pp. 25–37). New York: Wiley.

Kohn, M. L. (1968). Social class and schizophrenia: A critical review. In D. Rosenthal & S. S. Kety (Eds.), *The transmission of schizophrenia* (pp. 155–173). Oxford: Pergamon Press.

Kornetsky, C. (1972). The use of a simple test of attention as a measure of drug effects in schizophrenic patients. *Psychopharmacologia, 24*, 99–106.

Kornetsky, C., & Orzack, M. H. (1978). Physiological and behavioral correlates of attention dysfunction in schizophrenic patients. *Journal of Psychiatric Research, 14*, 69–79.

Kraepelin, E. (1919). *Dementia praecox and paraphrenia* (R. M. Barclay, Trans.). Edinburgh: E. & S. Livingstone. (Original work published 1913)

Lachar, D. (1968). MMPI two-point code-type correlates in a state hospital population. *Journal of Clinical Psychology, 24*, 424–427.

Lachar, D. (1974). *The MMPI: Clinical assessment and automated interpretation.* Los Angeles: Western Psychological Services.

Lukoff, D., Snyder, K., Ventura, J., & Nuechterlein, K. H. (1984). Life events, familial stress, and coping in the developmental course of schizophrenia. *Schizophrenia Bulletin, 10*, 258–292.

Marks, P. A., Seeman, W., & Haller, D. L. (1974). *The actuarial use of the MMPI with adolescents and adults.* London & New York: Oxford University Press.

McNicol, D. (1972). *A primer of signal detection theory.* London: Allen & Unwin.

Mendelson, W., Johnson, N., & Stewart, M. (1971). Hyperactive children as teenagers: A follow-up study. *Journal of Nervous and Mental Disease, 153*, 272–279.

Nielsen, T. C., & Petersen, K. E. (1976). Electrodermal correlates of extraversion, trait anxiety, and schizophrenism. *Scandanavian Journal of Psychology, 17*, 73–80.

Nuechterlein, K. H. (1983). Signal detection in vigilance tasks and behavioral attributes among offspring of schizophrenic mothers and among hyperactive children. *Journal of Abnormal Psychology, 92*, 4–83.

Nuechterlein, K. H., Asarnow, R. F., & Marder, S. R. (1985). *Perceptual sensitivity during vigilance as an indicator of psychosis-proneness.* Manuscript submitted for publication.

Nuechterlein, K. H., & Dawson, M. E. (1984a). Information processing and attentional functioning in the developmental course of schizophrenic disorders. *Schizophrenia Bulletin, 10*, 160–203.

Nuechterlein, K. H., & Dawson, M. E. (1984b). A heuristic vulnerability/stress model of schizophrenic episodes. *Schizophrenia Bulletin, 10*, 300–312.

Nuechterlein, K. H., Edell, W. S., & West, A. P. (1985). *Signal detection during vigilance and span of apprehension in nonpsychotic schizotypal individuals*. Manuscript submitted for publication.

Nuechterlein, K. H., Parasuraman, R., & Jiang, Q. (1983). Visual sustained attention: Image degradation produces rapid sensitivity decrement over time. *Science, 220*, 327–329.

Nuechterlein, K. H., Phipps-Yonas, S., Driscoll, R. M., & Garmezy, N. (1982). The role of different components of attention in children vulnerable to schizophrenia. In M. J. Goldstein (Ed.), *Preventive intervention in schizophrenia: Are we ready?* (DHHS Publication No. ADM 82-1111, pp. 54–77). Washington, DC: U.S. Government Printing Office.

O'Dougherty, M., Nuechterlein, K. H., & Drew, B. (1984). Hyperactive and hypoxic children: Signal detection, sustained attention, and behavior. *Journal of Abnormal Psychology, 93*, 178–191.

Parasuraman, R., & Davies, D. R. (1977). A taxonomic analysis of vigilance performance. In R. R. Mackie (Ed.), *Vigilance: Theory, operational performance, and physiological correlates* (pp. 559–574). New York: Plenum Press.

Peterson, D. R. (1954). The diagnosis of subclinical schizophrenia. *Journal of Consulting Psychology, 18*, 198–200.

Pollack, I., & Norman, D. A. (1964). A non-parametric analysis of recognition experiments. *Psychonomic Science, 1*, 125–126.

Posner, M. I. (1978). *Chronometric explorations of mind*. Hillsdale, NJ: Lawrence Erlbaum Associates.

Posner, M. I. (1982). Cumulative development of attentional theory. *American Psychologist, 37*, 168–179.

Roff, M. (1970). Some life history factors in relation to various types of adult maladjustment. In M. Roff & D. F. Ricks (Eds.), *Life history research in psychopathology* (pp. 265–287). Minneapolis: University of Minnesota Press.

Rosenthal, D. (1970). *Genetic theory and abnormal behavior*. New York: McGraw-Hill.

Rosenthal, D. (1978). The schizophrenia spectrum disorders: Implications for psychiatric diagnosis. In H.S. Akiskal & W. L. Webb (Eds.), *Psychiatric diagnosis: Exploration of biological predictors* (pp. 167–177). New York: Spectrum.

Rosvold, H. E., Mirsky, A., Sarason, I., Bransome, E. D., Jr., & Beck, L. H. (1956). A continuous performance test of brain damage. *Journal of Consulting Psychology, 20*, 343–350.

Rutschmann, J., Cornblatt, B., & Erlenmeyer-Kimling, L. (1977). Sustained attention in children at risk for schizophrenia: Report on a continuous performance test. *Archives of General Psychiatry, 34*, 571–575.

Shiffrin, R. M., & Schneider, W. (1977). Controlled and automatic human information processing. II. Perceptual learning, automatic attending, and a general theory. *Psychological Review, 84*, 127–190.

Soli, S. D., Nuechterlein, K. H., Garmezy, N., Devine, V. T., & Schaefer, S. (1981). A classification system for research in childhood psychopathology. Part I. An empirical approach using factor and cluster analyses and conjunctive decision rules. In B. A. Maher & W. B. Maher (Eds.), *Progress in experimental personality research* (Vol. 10, pp. 115–161). New York: Academic Press.

Spitzer, R. L., Endicott, J., & Robins, E. (1978). *Research diagnostic criteria (RDC) for a selected group of functional disorders* (3rd ed.). New York: Biometric Research.

Stewart, M. A., de Blois, C. S., & Cummings, C. (1980). Psychiatric disorder in the parents of hyperactive boys and those with conduct disorder. *Journal of Child Psychology and Psychiatry, 21*, 283–292.

Swets, J. A., & Sewall, S. T. (1963). Invariance of signal detectability over stages of practice and levels of motivation. *Journal of Experimental Psychology*, *66*, 120–126.

Sykes, D. H., Douglas, V. I., & Morgenstern, G. (1973). Sustained attention in hyperactive children. *Journal of Child Psychology and Psychiatry*, *44*, 267–273.

Turner, R. J., & Wagonfeld, M. O. (1967). Occupational mobility and schizophrenia: An assessment of the social causation and social selection hypotheses. *American Sociological Review*, *32*, 104–113.

Vaughn, C. E., Snyder, K. S., Jones, S., Freeman, W. E., & Falloon, I. R. H. (1984). Family factors in schizophrenic relapse: A California replication of the British research on expressed emotion. *Archives of General Psychiatry*, *41*, 1169–1177.

Weiss, G., Hechtman, L., Perlman, T., Hopkins, J., & Wener, A. (1979). Hyperactives as young adults: A controlled prospective ten-year follow-up of 75 children. *Archives of General Psychiatry*, *36*, 675–681.

Wing, J. K., Cooper, J. E., & Sartorius, N. (1974) *The measurement and classification of psychiatric symptoms*. London & New York: Cambridge University Press.

Winters, K. C., Weintraub, S., & Neale, J. M. (1981). Validity of MMPI codetypes in identifying DSM-III schizophrenics, unipolars, and bipolars. *Journal of Consulting and Clinical Psychology*, *49*, 486–487.

Wohlberg, G. W., & Kornetsky, C. (1973). Sustained attention in remitted schizophrenics. *Archives of General Psychiatry*, *28*, 533–537.

11

Mapping Abnormalities in Language and Cognition

NANCY C. ANDREASEN
University of Iowa

RALPH E. HOFFMAN
Yale University

WILLIAM M. GROVE
University of Iowa

> *Who gives anything to poor Tom? whom the foul fiend hath led through fire and through flame, and through ford and whirlpool, o'er bog and quagmire; that hath laid knives under his pillow, and halters in his pew; set ratsbane by his porridge; made him proud of heart, to ride on a bay trotting-horse over four-inched bridges, to course his own shadow for a traitor. Bless thy five wits! Tom's a-cold,—O, do de, do de, do de. Bless thee from whirlwinds, star-blasting, and taking! Do poor Tom some charity, whom the foul fiend vexes. There could I have him now,—and there,—and there again, and there.*
>
> *King Lear*, III.iv.50–60

In *King Lear*, Edgar is forced to flee for his life because he has been falsely accused by his brother Edmund of conspiring to kill his father. In order to protect his identity after his escape, he feigns madness and pretends to be a "bedlam beggar," a madman from Bethlehem Asylum in London. Experts in "thought disorder" frequently point out that this symptom of schizophrenia is the most difficult for a normal person to feign, and indeed that it is probably impossible for a normal person to sustain for a prolonged period of time the disorganized speech that may occur in schizophrenic patients. Even those of us who have spent most of our careers studying thought disorder and who have observed and collected many examples of it cannot produce long passages of disorganized speech (although of course we may sometimes lack clarity, cogency, or precision—which is a somewhat different matter).

The speech of Poor Tom is, however, an exception to this rule, made possible largely through dramatic license. In his role of Poor Tom, Edgar shows many instances of disorganized speech, as well as the delusions and hallucinations that occur in schizophrenia. All three of these types of schizophrenic symptoms—delusions, hallucinations, and formal thought disorder—are illustrated in the preceding quotation. Although Shakespeare did not have a concept of the disorder "schizophrenia" as it is known in modern times, he clearly had observed people suffering from the disease. When he chose to portray a "typical madman," he therefore gave him symptoms of schizophrenia that would be recognized as classic even today. Indeed, Shakespeare was fascinated with the idea of madness and portrayed it often in his plays, as did many other Renaissance dramatists. Their portrayals indicate that the phenomenology of schizophrenia has remained relatively stable across time and across cultures.

The modern texts of psychopathology that provide extensive descriptions of formal thought disorder include the works of Kraepelin (1913/1919) and Bleuler (1911/1950), both of whom considered it an important symptom of schizophrenia. Kraepelin noted that some patients show a "cessation of the need to express oneself," which corresponds to the diminution in affect and volition: "The patients become monosyllabic, sparing of their words, speak hesitatingly, suddenly become mute, never relate anything on their own initiative, let all answers be laboriously pressed out of them (pp. 55–56)."

He also notes that some patients may produce abundant disorganized speech:

> In states of excitement in place of taciturnity a prodigious *flow of talk* may appear which does not correspond to a need for expression, but usually unburdens itself without any reference to the surroundings. Often it consists of outbursts of filthy abuse, piercing shrieks or screams; a patient whistles tunes all day on a water bottle; many patients carry on monologues or answer voices aloud, often cursing and abusing. . . . Incoherence of the train of thought . . . is usually distinctly noticeable in the conversation of the patients. The most different ideas follow one another with most bewildering want of connection, even when the patients are quiet. (p. 56)

Kraepelin considered formal thought disorder to be one of many important symptoms. His arch-rival, Eugen Bleuler, brought formal thought disorder to the forefront among the various symptoms and considered it to be the most fundamental and important. Until quite recently, Bleuler's work has had more influence on our basic conceptualization of the nature of schizophrenia than has that of Kraepelin. As is well known, Bleuler distinguished between fundamental symptoms, which were present in all cases and did not occur in other illnesses, and accessory symptoms, which were not pathognomonic of the disorder:

> Certain symptoms of schizophrenia are present in every case and at every period of the illness even though, as with every other disease symptom, they must have attained a certain degree of intensity before they can be recognized with any certainty. . . . For example, the peculiar association disturbance is always present, but not each and every aspect of it. . . . Besides these specific or permanent symptoms, we can find a host of other, most accessory manifestations such as delusions, hallucinations, or catatonic symptoms. . . . As far

> we know, the fundamental symptoms are characteristic of schizophrenia, while the accessory symptoms may also appear in other types of illness. (p. 13)

A somewhat loose reading of Bleuler in the United States has given us the Bleulerian "Four A's": association, affect, autism, and ambivalence. A closer reading indicates that he also comments on abnormalities in attention, volition, and activity. Nevertheless, based on a widely accepted (and probably incorrect) understanding of Bleuler, the last several generations of psychologists and psychiatrists have been taught to recognize schizophrenia in terms of the Four A's and to see formal thought disorder as the most important among the fundamental symptoms.

Although recent work has questioned whether formal thought disorder should be considered pathognomonic, nevertheless most investigators interested in understanding the diagnosis and phenomenology of schizophrenia continue to recognize it as a symptom of major importance. Unfortunately, however, research in this area contains considerable conflicting and confused evidence about the nature of schizophrenic thought disorder. Some of the mechanisms that have been proposed to explain the abnormalities in language and cognition include deficits in "association," loss of the abstract attitude, defective concept formation, input dysfunction, overinclusive thinking, disordered attention, disordered family communication, intermittent aphasia, and intermingling and disordered logic (Cameron, 1939; Chaika, 1974; J. Chapman & McGhie, 1962; Cromwell & Dokeckie, 1968; Goldstein, 1944; Harrow, Tucker, & Adler, 1965; Kasanin, 1944; Payne & Friedlander, 1962; Wynne & Singer, 1965). Among these competing explanations, none has emerged as preeminent, and indeed at times the debates among competing theories seem to be primarily of arcane or talmudic scholarly interest, bearing little relationship to the practical questions that the clinicians treating schizophrenic patients must face. Is some type of thought disorder really present in every case? Does it occur only in schizophrenia? How should one interpret the disorganized language manifested by manic patients? What is the course of thought disorder over time? What is its prognostic significance? What is the relationship between disorganized speech and disordered thought? How can one understand that disorder in terms of the neural mechanisms that govern language and cognition?

In an effort to address some of these questions, our research program in language and cognition at the University of Iowa has been pursuing a multiphasic effort for the study of language abnormalities in the major psychoses. This plan has three phases:

Phase I: Clinical description involving definition of terms and determination of the frequency of disorganized language in a broad selection of psychotic patients.

Phase II: Functional mapping of abnormalities in order to determine if specific deficits in linguistic competence occur.

Phase III: Neurological and anatomical mapping in order to determine whether severely disorganized speech can be related to specific brain abnormalities.

PHASE I: THE DEVELOPMENT OF A SCALE TO ASSESS THOUGHT, LANGUAGE, AND COMMUNICATION (TLC)

The first step in this program was to develop a clinical rating scale in order to evaluate "thought disorder." One of the core problems with research on "thought disorder" has been the conceptual entangling of thought and language. Many people who have studied thought disorder have made the simple assumption that thought is reflected in language. Although sometimes acceptable, this assumption is not totally valid. People may have unspoken thoughts or say one thing and think another. Further, thought is probably more than a simple internal representation of spoken language, because otherwise deaf-mutes would be unable to learn to think. Some aspects of cognition, such as listening to music or looking at works of art, clearly have a strong nonverbal component.

Once one recognizes that language and thought cannot be equated, several different strategies are available to deal with this problem. Our own has been to begin by focusing our studies on language behavior. Language behavior is seen as one of several different windows into cognition, and ultimately into the mind or brain. Language behavior is a highly desirable place to begin because it is objective and lends itself readily to empirical study.

Clinical descriptions of "thought disorder" have often used a variety of different terms that in fact refer to various types of language abnormality. Unfortunately, clinicians and researchers have used traditional terms such as "loose associations" or "incoherence" in a relatively precise and nonstandardized way, making communication difficult and research nearly impossible. The first phase of our work thus involved the development of simple but comprehensive definitions of terms or concepts commonly used to describe language abnormalities in the major psychoses. These are contained in the Scale for the Assessment of Thought, Language, and Communication (TLC), a 20-item scale containing definitions and instructions for rating such abnormalities as poverty of speech, poverty of content of speech, tangentiality, derailment (loose associations), and incoherence (Andreasen, 1978, 1979a, 1979b).

The initial results of our work with this scale were quite successful. Although many of the recent standard diagnostic systems such as the RDC or DSM-III have given minimal emphasis to thought disorder because of a concern that it could not be evaluated reliably, we were able to achieve good to excellent reliability using our rating scale. We attribute this good reliability to careful definition of terms and an emphasis on empirical or behavioral observation. The following is a sample definition and example:

Incoherence: A pattern of speech which is essentially incomprehensible at times. The incoherence is due to several different mechanisms, which may sometimes all occur simultaneously. Sometimes portions of coherent sentences may be observed in the midst of a sentence which is incoherent as a whole. Sometimes the disturbance appears to be at the semantic level, so that words are substituted in a phrase or sentence so that the meaning seems to be distorted or destroyed; the word choice may seem totally random or may appear to have some oblique connection with the context. Sometimes "cementing words" (coordinating and subordinating conjunctions such as "and," "although"; adjectival pronouns such as "the," "a," and "an") are deleted.

Incoherence is often accompanied by derailment. It differs from derailment in that in incoherence the abnormality occurs within the level of the sentence or clause, which contains words or phrases that are joined incoherently. The abnormality in derailment involves unclear or confusing connections between larger units, such as sentences or clauses.

This type of language disorder is relatively rare. When it occurs, it tends to be severe or extreme, and mild forms are quite uncommon. It may sound quite similar to a Wernicke's aphasia or jargon aphasia, and in these cases the disorder should only be called incoherence when history and laboratory data exclude the possibility of a known organic etiology and formal testing for aphasia is negative.

Exclusions: Mildly ungrammatical constructions which occur when a person is searching for the right word, phrase, or idea should not be rated as incoherence. (For example, "My father, he, for a long time, well he just started . . . he joined the church and became a, I say he's a Christian now because he used to lie and run around a lot.") Idiomatic usages characteristic of particular regional or ethnic backgrounds, lack of education, or low intelligence should also not be rated as incoherence. ("He ain't got no family." "That there was no good." "The lawn needs mowed." "He took the tools down cellar.")

Interviewer: "Um, what do you think about current political issues like the energy crisis?" *Patient*: "They're destroying too many cattle and oil just to make soap. If we need soap when you can jump into a pool of water, and then when you go to buy your gasoline, m my folks always thought they should, get pop but the best thing to get, is motor oil, and, money. May as well go there and, trade in some, pop caps and, uh, tires, and tractors to grup, car garages, so they can pull cars away from wrecks, is what I believed in. So I didn't go there to get no more pop when my folks said it. I just went there to get a ice cream cone, and some pop, in cans, or we can go over there to get a cigarette. And it was the largest thing you do t to get cigarettes 'cause then you could trade off, what you owned, and go for something new, it w it was sentimental, and that's the only thing I needed was something sentimental, and there wasn't anything else more sentimental than that, except for knick-knacks and most knick-knacks, these cost thirty or forty dollars to get, a good billfold, or a little stand to put on your desk."

Once we had established the reliability of these definitions, we explored the frequency with which these various types of unusual language behavior occurred in patients suffering from schizophrenia, mania, and depression. The results of our first work using this scale are summarized in Table 1.

As this table indicates, several findings are notable. Derailment (or loose associations), argued by Bleuler to be pathognomonic of schizophrenia, is equally common in mania and schizophrenia. Incoherence, or severely disorganized speech, is relatively uncommon but does occur in 16% of both manics and schizophrenics. Some types of thought disorder that are frequently described in textbooks, such as neologisms, echolalia, or blocking, in fact occur very infrequently. Their base rate is too low to give them much diagnostic utility.

Table 1. Reliability and Frequency of Types of Thought-Language-Communication Disorder in Psychiatric Patients

	Reliability (full-scale weighted kappa) (N = 113)	Frequency[a]		
		Manics (N = 32)	Depressives (N = 36)	Schizophrenics (N = 45)
Poverty of speech	.81	6%	22%	29%
Poverty of content of speech	.77	19%	17%	40%
Pressure of speech	.89	72%	6%	27%
Distractible speech	.78	31%	0%	2%
Tangentiality	.58	34%	25%	36%
Derailment	.83	56%	14%	56%
Incoherence	.88	16%	0%	16%
Illogicality	.80	25%	0%	27%
Clanging	.58	9%	0%	0%
Neologisms	.39	3%	0%	2%
Circumstantiality	.74	25%	31%	4%
Loss of goal	.70	44%	17%	44%
Perserveration	.74	34%	6%	24%
Echolalia	.59	3%	0%	4%
Blocking	.79	3%	6%	4%
Global ratings		88%	53%	91%

[a] Based on ratings > 1 on TLC Scale.

Although these results seemed to suggest initially that disorganized speech occurred in all three major psychoses, and therefore that it lacked diagnostic specificity, we were interested in determining whether specific patterns of abnormality might occur. We compared two different patterns in a multivariate analysis of variance. Pattern 1 gave an equal positive weighting to five common types of abnormality usually subsumed under the concept of loose associations: tangentiality, derailment, incoherence, illogicality, and clanging. No significant differences were noted between the manics and schizophrenics. Pattern 2 involved dividing the abnormalities into two groups, positive types of thought disorder and negative types of thought disorder, which were given equal positive and negative weightings. When this was done, the manics and schizophrenics were clearly differentiated, yielding an F-ratio significant at the .05 level. This approach to conceptualizing language or thought abnormalities was also supported by discriminant analysis and factor analysis.

Accordingly, we now conceptualize language and cognitive abnormalities in schizophrenia as being of two main types. One type is negative formal thought disorder, characterized by prominent poverty of speech and poverty of content of speech. Subsequent work has shown that this abnormality is also associated with other negative symptoms. We refer to this type of thought disorder as *alogia*, or absence of the ability to generate speech or ideas. Positive formal thought disorder consists principally of pressured speech, tangentiality, illogicality, derailment, and incoherence. It occurs in both mania and schizophrenia, but more commonly in mania. Among schizophrenic patients, it is modestly correlated with positive symptoms in general, particularly with bizarre behavior (Andreasen, 1982a, 1982b).

We have recently extended this initial work with the TLC in a second sample. The characteristics of this sample are described in Table 2. As this table indicates, in this second study we examined language behavior in a large sample of normals, in addition to studying manics, schizoaffectives, and hebephrenic (disorganized) and paranoid schizophrenics. Patients were defined and classified using the Research Diagnostic Criteria (RDC) (Spitzer, Endicott, & Robins, 1978). As that table indicates, there were some differences between the groups in age, education, and performance on the Shipley–Hartford, but none of these differences is large enough to produce large performance differences on any of the language behaviors under investigation.

The language behavior of these patients was studied in a variety of ways. The overall goal of this second study was to attempt to map language abnormalities in order to examine syntactic, semantic, and discourse aspects of language behavior and to separate perception and processing of language from production or expression. We viewed the TLC as an important clinical method for assessing abnormalities in language production.

Table 2. Demographic and Other Characteristics of Subjects

	Normals (N = 94)		Manics (N = 25)		Schizoaffectives (N = 25)		Hebephrenics (N = 25)		Paranoids (N = 25)	
	X	SD	X	SD	X	SD	$\bar{X}$	SD	$\bar{X}$	SD
Age	28.92	9.13	35.04	14.01	28.16	9.50	26.68	7.41	27.75	6.21
Education, years	14.10	3.42	13.38	2.24	13.50	1.89	12.56	1.66	13.74	2.77
Shipley IQ	115.48	7.71	102.88	11.98	108.00	10.09	95.26	12.28	104.00	9.80
N(%) Female	26	(52)	13	(52)	14	(56)	12	(48)	8	(32)
N(%) Acute					6	(26)	1	(4)	1	(4)
N(%) Good prognosis							3	(12)	8	(32)
Duration of episode, weeks			9.88	9.63	64.48	164.44	246.96	239.55	256.58	262.24
Time in hospital, total weeks			28.46	30.84	41.72	76.27	66.71	160.85	79.71	139.76

Table 3. Frequencies of Thought, Language, and Communication Abnormalities[a] among Diagnostic Groups

	Normals (N = 94)	Manics (N = 25)	Schizoaffectives (N = 25)	Hebephrenics (N = 25)	Paranoids (N = 25)	Chi square[c]	p
Negative FTD							
Poverty of speech	5[b]	4[b]	24[b]	24[b]	36[b]	22.04[b]	.01
Poverty of content	1	8	12	48	8	47.13	.01
Positive FTD							
Pressure of speech	6	88	32	24	16	73.94	.01
Tangentiality	2	4	8	24	16	16.14	.01
Derailment	32	80	56	68	56	24.63	.01
Incoherence	0	24	8	40	20	36.76	.01
Illogicality	0	36	12	48	12	49.39	.01
Other							
Circumstantiality	6	44	16	16	16	21.85	.01
Loss of goal	18	52	20	32	28	12.68	.01
Perseveration	8	44	20	32	16	21.69	.01
Distractible speech	3	20	12	12	0	11.91	.02
Global rating	6	76	60	80	56	81.61	.01

[a] Criterion: Rating > 1.
[b] All values are percentages.
[c] Between patient groups, normals excluded.

TLC data from this second study are summarized in Table 3. As this table indicates, the five samples studied differ significantly from one another on almost all parameters. Interestingly, the normals have a modest amount of abnormal language. Derailment and loss of goal are particularly common. Nevertheless, only 6% of these individuals have a global rating greater than one, indicating that their disturbances were not severe. On the other hand, manics and hebephrenic schizophrenics tend to have a particularly high global rating. Consonant with clinical observation, among the psychiatric patients paranoids have the most normal language behavior. As was shown in the previous study, the schizophrenic patients tend to have a relatively larger amount of negative formal thought disorder, whereas manics in particular have a large amount of positive formal thought disorder. Among the manics, pressure of speech and derailment are especially common, as are circumstantiality, loss of goal, perseveration, and distractible speech.

Because we were interested in both the reliability and the reproducibility of our earlier work, we compared the frequency of TLC abnormalities across the two samples. These results are summarized in Tables 4 and 5. As these

Table 4. Comparison of TLC Abnormalities[a] for Schizophrenics: Initial versus Current

	Initial sample (N = 45)		Current sample (N = 50)			
Variable	N	%	N	%	Chi square[b]	p
Poverty of speech	13	29	15	30	.04	.84
Poverty of content	18	40	14	28	1.53	.22
Pressure of speech	12	27	10	20	.59	.56
Distractible speech	1	2	3	6	—	.35
Tangentiality	16	36	10	20	2.88	.09
Derailment	25	56	31	62	.41	.52
Incoherence	7	16	15	30	2.78	.10
Illogicality	12	27	15	30	.13	.72
Clanging	0	0	2	4	—	.27
Neologisms	1	2	0	0	—	.47
Word approximations	0	0	3	6	—	.14
Circumstantiality	2	4	8	16	3.36	.93
Loss of goal	20	44	15	30	2.12	.15
Perseveration	11	24	12	24	2.41	.12
Echolalia	2	4	0	0	—	.22
Blocking	2	4	0	0	—	.22
Stilted speech	1	2	1	2	—	.77
Ideas of reference	6	13	0	0	—	.01
Global rating	41	91	34	68	7.61	.01

[a] Criterion: rating >1.

[b] Where no statistic is reported, Fisher's exact test was used.

Table 5. Comparison of TLC Abnormalities[a] for Manics: Initial versus Current

Variable	Initial sample (N = 32) N	%	Current sample (N = 25) N	%	Chi square[b]	p
Poverty of speech	2	6	1	4	—	.59
Poverty of content	6	19	2	8	—	.22
Pressure of speech	23	72	22	88	2.20	.14
Distractible speech	10	31	5	20	.92	.33
Tangentiality	11	31	1	4	7.79	.02
Derailment	18	56	20	80	3.56	.06
Incoherence	5	16	6	24	.63	.43
Illogicality	8	25	9	36	.81	.37
Clanging	3	9	1	4	—	.40
Neologisms	1	3	0	0	—	.56
Word approximations	1	3	4	16	—	.11
Circumstantiality	8	25	11	44	2.28	.13
Loss of goal	14	44	13	52	.38	.64
Perseveration	11	34	11	44	.55	.46
Echolalia	1	3	0	0	—	.56
Blocking	1	3	0	0	—	.56
Stilted speech	2	6	4	16	—	.22
Ideas of reference	7	22	1	4	—	.06
Global rating	28	88	19	76	1.28	.74

[a] Criterion: rating >1.

[b] Where no statistic is reported, Fisher's exact test was used.

tables indicate, the rates for almost all types of TLC abnormality are very similar from one sample to the next. This is relatively remarkable because both the patients and the raters were different. The ratings in the first study were done principally by one of us [Nancy C. Andreasen], with the assistance of a research assistant trained in clinical psychology to do the reliability studies. In the replication sample, nearly all ratings were done by two different master's-level clinical psychologists who had been trained in the use of the instrument but had not done ratings in the initial study. These results lead one to conclude that there is relative stability among these types of language abnormality across patient samples. This leads to the conclusion that language abnormalities can probably be rated much more precisely than has been previously thought.

Because we had previously done a discriminant function analysis that was quite useful in classifying patients as manic or schizophrenic, we were interested in determining whether this function would be equally successful in classifying the replication sample. These results are summarized in Table 6. Column 1, "Function from Initial Sample," shows the discriminant function weights derived from the initial sample. When these weights were applied

Table 6. Comparison of Discriminant Functions between Manics and Schizophrenics

Variable	Standardized discriminant weight: Function from initial sample (N = 77)	Function from current sample (N = 75)
Poverty of speech	−.261	—
Poverty of content	−.351	−.457
Pressure of speech	.634	.898
Distractible speech	.422	.685
Detailment	−.406	—
Illogicality	—	−.390
Loss of goal	.223	—
Percent correctly classified	80%[a]	82.7%[b]

[a] Cross-validation performance.
[b] Estimated performance by jackknife.

to the replication sample, 80% of the patients were correctly classified. We also used another newer type of discriminant analysis on the second sample, frequently referred to as the "jack-knife procedure." This procedure yielded a somewhat different set of weights. It too was quite successful in classifying patients, however, correctly classifying nearly 83% of the patients.

We also were able to do follow-up studies on a substantial proportion of these patients six months after the index evaluation. The results of this work are summarized in Table 7. Although the normals were not followed up, their values are shown in this table for purposes of comparison. As this table indicates, the manics tend to normalize rather dramatically on follow-up. The rates of abnormality drop to nearly normal levels. The schizoaffective patients follow a pattern similar to the manics. The paranoids have an intermediate position . Although they have relatively low ratings on almost all subtypes of TLC abnormality, they continue to have a relatively high rate of negative formal thought disorder. The hebephrenics, however, tend to have consistently high ratings and their abnormalities are nearly as severe as they were at the index evaluation.

We were also interested in determining whether type of thought disorder had any prognostic significance. The results of these studies are summarized in Table 8. As this table indicates, negative formal thought disorder is highly correlated with outcome as measured by the Global Assessment Scale (GAS) (Endicott, Spitzer, Fleiss, & Cohen, 1976). It is related both to the GAS rating itself and to the degree of change in the GAS from index evaluation to follow-up evaluation. Thus, although positive formal thought disorder has little prognostic significance, negative formal thought disorder is highly correlated with a poor outcome.

Table 7. Frequencies of Thought, Language, and Communication Abnormalities[a] among Diagnostic Groups: Follow-Up

	Normals (N = 94)	Manics (N = 18)	Schizoaffectives (N = 19)	Hebephrenics (N = 17)	Paranoids (N = 15)	Chi square[c]	p
Negative FTD							
Poverty of speech	5[b]	11[b]	32[b]	29[b]	33[b]	18.53	.01
Poverty of content	1	5	5	55	40	66.23	.01
Positive FTD							
Pressure of speech	6	22	11	12	0	6.48	.17
Tangentiality	2	11	16	53	0	44.08	.01
Derailment	32	33	21	59	33	6.22	.18
Incoherence	0	6	11	11	7	9.70	.05
Illogicality	0	6	5	41	13	39.66	.01
Other							
Circumstantiality	6	11	32	35	0	19.89	.01
Loss of goal	18	28	5	24	0	7.13	.13
Perseveration	8	17	16	41	7	15.31	.01
Distractible speech	3	6	0	0	0	2.22	.69
Global rating	6	33	26	82	33	51.49	.01

[a] Criterion: rating > 1.
[b] All values are percentages.
[c] Between patient groups, normals excluded.

Table 8. Correlation between Index FTD and Outcome as Measured by GAS

	GAS		Change in GAS	
	r	*p*	*r*	*p*
Positive FTD	−.13	.279	−.03	.796
Negative FTD	−.38	.002	−.28	.02

The results of this study suggest that the use of a clinical rating scale in order to characterize types of thought disorder can yield much useful information. Although it is clear that language abnormalities are not pathognomonic of schizophrenia, particular patterns of abnormality can be observed that do have some diagnostic and prognostic significance. In particular, "negative" abnormalities, referred to as *alogia*, tend to be associated with schizophrenia (particularly hebephrenic schizophrenia) and to be associated with a poor outcome in those patients who manifested it at index evaluation.

PHASE II: PSYCHOLINGUISTIC MAPPING OF ABNORMALITIES IN PERCEPTION AND PROCESSING

In addition to the clinical perspective described above, one may also study language abnormalities in schizophrenia using perspectives derived from other disciplines. One of these, aphasiology or neurolinguistics, teaches us that there are several types of language functions that differ in their anatomic mapping in the brain and may be differentially affected by various types of lesions. For example, language perception and processing tends to be located more posteriorly in the brain, whereas language production is located in anterior regions. In attempting to understand language abnormalities in schizophrenia, therefore, it is important to separate input abnormalities from output abnormalities, because of the possibility that these may be differentially produced.

A second perspective is provided by psycholinguistics, or the psychology of language. Psycholinguists frequently divide language into various components that may also be differentially affected. Three components that they frequently discuss are the syntactic component, the semantic component, and the discourse component. These components may be defined as follows:

The syntactic component: Rules governing the ordering of words and the establishment of relationships between them (e.g., subject–verb–object).

The semantic component: Rules governing the interpretation of the meaning of individual words.

The discourse component: Rules governing the manner in which sentences may be combined to construct an idea set or a story.

After completing the initial studies in which we developed the TLC, we began our second, more systematic, study of language abnormalities in schizophrenia, which was designed to explore both input and output and to examine syntactic, semantic, and discourse aspects of language. In this second study, we hypothesized that the schizophrenic is able to perceive and process language normally in terms of both the syntactic and the semantic components. We predicted that the major abnormality would be in language production, rather than perception and processing, and that this abnormality would include primarily semantic and discourse components. We predicted that the abnormalities would be reversible in some patients and irreversible in others, with irreversibility being correlated with greater disorganization at index evaluation. We also suspected that those psychotic patients suffering from affective illness would be more likely to have reversible abnormalities, whereas schizophrenics would more often have irreversible abnormalities.

Our assessment of the syntactic and semantic components of language perception and processing were based on two paradigms developed by psycholinguists to study language functions in normal individuals.

The click task is designed primarily to examine perception and processing of the syntactic components of language. Studies have repeatedly indicated that normal individuals, when listening to sentences containing embedded clicks, tend to report hearing these clicks closer to the syntactical boundaries than the clicks actually occur (Fodor & Bever, 1965; Garrett, Bever, & Fodor, 1966). When this task is used, subjects listen to sentences such as the following:

> *In order to catch* [click] *the train, George rushed furiously to the station.*

In this sentence the syntactical boundary, or end of the clause, occurs after the word *train*. A click may be embedded anywhere in the sentence, but in this example it is embedded in the word *catch*. When asked where they hear the click embedded, normal listeners are likely to report hearing it instead in the word *train* or after the word *train*. This phenomenon occurs even when the sentences are pronounced "flatly" with no clues being provided as to the location of the syntactical boundary through word intonations or pausing. Psycholinguists believe this phenomenon indicates that normal listeners tend to process language as syntactical units. Several studies have used this paradigm to study syntactical processing in schizophrenics and have demonstrated that schizophrenics are, like normals, prone to displace clicks to syntactical boundaries (Carpenter, 1967; Rochester, Harris, & Seeman, 1973). This suggests that schizophrenics are competent in the syntactical processing of language.

The gist task, designed to assess semantic aspects of language perception and processing, also was developed initially in order to study language functions in normal individuals (Bransford & Franks, 1971). This task requires that subjects listen to a series of sentences and later indicate whether they have heard them before. Sample sentences appear in Table 9. During the acquisition phase subjects are never given sentences like the first sentence on the list, which contains four ideas (*the ants are in the kitchen*, *the ants ate the jelly*, *the jelly was sweet*, *the jelly was on the table*). Instead, they are given sentences containing only one idea, two ideas, or three ideas. When later asked if they recognize sentences they have heard previously, normal subjects typically report having heard the longer and more complete sentences containing four ideas, even though they did not actually hear them. This tendency to recognize and group together in memory a set of related concepts is called the "gist effect."

These two tasks, the click task and the gist task, are useful methods for assessing syntactic and semantic aspects of language in schizophrenic patients. In administering these tasks, we introduced a useful innovation developed by Chapman and Chapman (1973), the Matched Task Design.

Table 9. The Semantic Component: The Gist Task

FOUR:	*The ants in the kitchen ate the sweet jelly which was on the table.* (on recognition only)
THREES:	*The ants ate the sweet jelly which was on the table.* (on acquisition only)
	The ants in the kitchen ate the jelly which was on the table. (on acquisition only)
	The ants in the kitchen ate the sweet jelly. (on recognition only)
TWOS:	*The ants in the kitchen ate the jelly.* (on acquisition only)
	The ants ate the sweet jelly. (on both acquisition and recognition)
	The sweet jelly was on the table. (on recognition only)
ONES:	*The ants were in the kitchen.* (on acquisition only)
	The jelly was on the table. (on acquisition only)
	The jelly was sweet. (on recognition only)
	The ants ate the jelly. (on recognition only)

Table 10. Standardized Scores for Click and Control Tasks in Manics, Schizoaffectives, and Schizophrenics

	Click		Digit span control		Difference			
	$\bar{X}$	*SD*	$\bar{X}$	*SD*	$\bar{X}$	*SD*	*t*	*p*
Manics (*N* = 25)	−.31	1.41	−.37	.70	.05	1.59	.16	>.10
Schizoaffectives (*N* = 25)	.32	1.84	−.54*	.80	.97	2.07	2.34	.01
Hebephrenics (*N* = 25)	−.18	1.57	−.70**	.61	.51	1.56	1.63	.06
Paranoids (*N* = 25)	.19	1.73	−.54*	.61	.86	1.26	3.41	.01

Difference from normals: $*p < .05.$
$**p < .01.$

Because the performance of schizophrenic patients on many cognitive tasks is often impaired because of inattentiveness, apathy, or other factors, they typically perform more poorly on most tasks than a matched control group. Chapman and Chapman's innovation involves matching tasks rather than subjects. When an experimental and a control task are matched psychometrically on level of difficulty and internal consistency (as measured by Cronbach's α), other extraneous cognitive factors, such as inattentiveness, are controlled for, and it is possible to determine whether a specific differential deficit in a given area occurs. In our studies of language, the gist task and the click task were treated as experimental tasks and were matched with a digit-span task that served as the control task. Tables 10 and 11 show the results of our investigation. Because these tables report standardized (or *Z*) scores, the scores of the normals are not reported, since by definition they have a mean of 0 and a standard deviation of 1. As Table 10 indicates, the schizoaffectives and the two schizophrenic groups perform considerably worse on the digit-span control task than on the click task. The manics do not differ in their performance on these two tasks, but principally because they perform poorly on both. When the patient groups are compared statistically with the normals, then the schizoaffectives and schizophrenics also differ significantly on the digit-span task. This finding was unexpected. We had hypothesized that all the patients would show normal syntactical processing of language, which they do. We did not expect, however, to find a "reversed differential deficit." That is, the patients were expected to perform at about the same level on the digit-span task as on the click task, just as did the normals. Instead, they performed more poorly. This suggests

Table 11. Gist and Matched Control Task Scores in Manics, Schizoaffectives, and Schizophrenics

Group	Gist		Control		Difference		
	$\bar{X}$	*SD*	$\bar{X}$	*SD*	$\bar{X}$	*SD*	*t*
Manics (*N* = 25)	.84****	1.18	−.62**	.85	1.46	1.47	4.97***
Schizoaffectives (*N* = 25)	.41	1.23	−.57*	1.05	.99	2.07	2.34
Hebephrenics (*N* = 25)	.20	1.28	−1.07***	.70	1.26	1.63	3.79***
Paranoids (*N* = 25)	.06	1.13	−.80***	.87	.73	1.89	1.89

Difference from normals: *$p < .05$.
**$p < .01$.
***$p < .001$.
****$p < .01$, higher than normal.

that these psychotic patients may have a reversed deficit in very short term memory.

The results of the gist task are shown in Table 11. Again, all the patients are able to perform the gist task at normal levels. In fact, they are somewhat better at it than at the click task. As in the comparison between the click and control tasks, however, the patients performed significantly worse on the digit-span control task. Again, they appear to have a reversed differential deficit in very short term memory. This is also evident when control-task scores for the patients are compared to control-task scores for the normals. So, again, we must conclude that these psychotic patients are able to perceive and process semantic aspects of language normally. Instead, they have a differential impairment in their ability to remember random number strings, suggesting a defect in very short term memory.

When we followed up these patients 6 months later, we gave all subjects a psychometrically matched but different version of these tasks. The results of this follow-up evaluation were quite interesting. Just as the language behavior of the manics and schizoaffectives reverted to normal as indicated by performance on the TLC, so too did the performance of manics and schizoaffectives on the tasks just described. In particular, their ability to recall strings of digits improved and normalized, and the reversed-differential deficit disappeared. On the other hand, the schizophrenic patients continued to remain impaired on this test of very short term memory. The hebephrenics tended to remain considerably more impaired than did the paranoids.

Although these studies do not provide an exhaustive mapping of language perception and processing, the results nevertheless seem to provide relatively convincing support that schizophrenics are able to perceive and process language normally. The results of our study of the click task are in conformity with two previous studies (Carpenter, 1976; Rochester *et al.*, 1973). A previous study using the gist task found some indication of impairment in schizophrenics, but it did not apply a rigorous research design similar to our own (Knight & Sims-Knight, 1979). Because of the use of the matched-task design, we have excluded confounding or nuisance variables such as inattention, poor cooperation, or lack of interest and motivation. The finding of a reversed-differential deficit in digit span, while unexpected, is in fact consistent with our studies of discourse. As we shall see in the following section, schizophrenic patients do show significant abnormalities in discourse when it is analyzed psycholinguistically. One explanation for this abnormal discourse might be a deficit in very short term memory, which impairs discourse planning.

PHASE II: PSYCHOLINGUISTIC MAPPING OF ABNORMALITIES IN LANGUAGE PRODUCTION

We have explored abnormalities in schizophrenic language production, or discourse, from three different vantage points. One of them, the clinical vantage point, has already been described in the context of the TLC. The other two vantage points were drawn from psycholinguistics. Both assume that some schizophrenic patients speak language that is unclear and appears abnormal to a person who is listening. Both attempt to account for the heavy burden placed on the listener by exploring the connectedness or interrelationship between words and concepts within the patient's speech.

The first psycholinguistic approach, originally applied to the study of discourse by Rochester and Martin (1979), involves using the analysis of cohesion and retrieval strategies. The methods for measuring cohesion and retrieval strategies are too technical to describe in a relatively brief chapter such as this. One may summarize this approach by stating that it assumes that normal discourse makes sense in part because speakers tie their discourse together through making clear references to ideas or things that have been mentioned earlier and by tying clauses together through a variety of different linguistic techniques. For example, when pronouns such as *it* or *he* are used, they must have a clear earlier reference, either from previous speech or from some other aspect of context, so that the listener can understand what they mean. Otherwise the discourse is confusing. Likewise, transitions and changes of topic must be clearly marked.

When Rochester used these techniques to study the speech of schizophrenic patients, she found those who manifested "thought disorder," as identified by lay raters, to have less coherent discourse than did schizophrenics who were considered to have no evidence of thought disorder. She did not, however, include a nonschizophrenic comparison sample.

We used similar techniques to study the speech of normals, manics, schizoaffectives, and schizophrenics. The details of this analysis are complex and have been described in detail in the work of Rochester and Martin (1979). The results of our work are shown in Tables 12 and 13. Table 12 examines the use of reference in the speech of normal people and psychotic patients. The total items are the number of references appearing in the passage selected for analysis. Participant items refer to either the speaker or the interviewer, whereas nonparticipant items include all other references. Unclear items are those with no clear antecedent references. Cultural items involve a reference to something in the participant's cultural background, whereas situational items refer to something in the current situation. As Table 12 shows, in general there are highly significant differences on most of these variables between normals and the psychotic patients. The psychotic patients do not usually differ among themselves, however, in the reference strategies that they use in their speech. In particular, except for unclear reference, the speech of schizophrenics does not contain any unusual increase in types of reference that distinguish it from the speech of manics or schizoaffectives.

Table 13 shows other indicators of the "connectedness" of discourse. Incomplete clauses are clauses that lack a subject and predicate appropriately tied together. Lexical ties use the same word to tie clauses to one another. Substitution and ellipsis use the deletion of one term and the substitution of another related one to clarify reference. Again, no striking findings emerge. The schizophrenics do speak in incomplete clauses more frequently, and the psychotic patients differ from the normals in the number of lexical ties, with the normals showing more. There are no differences among the groups in substitution and ellipsis. In general, these findings indicate tht psychotic patients as a group show less coherence in their discourse than do normals. When we searched for ways that the patients might differ among themselves, however, the results were far from satisfactory. The psychotic patients tended to have similar types of abnormalities.

Suspecting that these negative results were due to the insensitivity of the method rather than to an actual lack of difference among the psychotic patients, we then applied a second technique to the analysis of psychotic speech (Hoffman, Stopak, & Andreasen, in press). This approach, developed by one of us [Ralph Hoffman], attempts to account for the differences between schizophrenic and manic speech by positing a difference in mechanism. It begins with the assumption, based on psycholinguistic research, that in normal speech, the speaker is working from a "discourse plan" that maps what he is going to say and controls it as he speaks (Deese, 1978). If the discourse lacks a plan or if the speaker changes plan in midstream, then

Table 12. Phoric References in the Discourse of Normals and Psychotic Patients

	Normals (*N* = 25)		Manics (*N* = 23)		Schizo-affectives (*N* = 16)		Schizophrenics (*N* = 24)				
	$\bar{X}$	*SD*	$\bar{X}$	*SD*	$\bar{X}$	*SD*	$\bar{X}$	*SD*	*F*	*p*	Duncan[a]
Total items	71.8	7.1	3.9	9.5	64.7	11.0	63.7	11.4	3.85	.0125	N > M,SA,S
Participant items	38.4	9.1	31.1	13.2	27.7	11.0	29.2	13.2	3.69	.0150	N > M,SA,S
Nonparticipant items	33.4	11.2	33.6	12.5	37.0	10.5	34.5	14.6	.32	.8136	Equal
Unclear items	.2	.4	1.9	1.9	1.1	1.1	2.2	2.4	7.46	.0002	S > SA,N S > N
Cultural items	.5	1.0	1.7	1.8	1.4	1.6	.92	1.3	3.20	.0270	M > N
Situational items	71.2	6.6	60.1	16.0	62.5	10.9	63.2	9.6	4.43	.0062	N > M,SA,S

[a] N = normal; M = manic; SA = schizoaffective; S = schizophrenic.

Table 13. Other Types of Retrieval and Cohesion in the Discourse of Psychotic Patients

	Normals (N = 25)		Manics (N = 23)		Schizo-affectives (N = 16)		Schizo-phrenics (N = 24)				
	$\bar{X}$	*SD*	$\bar{X}$	*SD*	$\bar{X}$	*SD*	$\bar{X}$	*SD*	F	p	Duncan[a]
Incomplete clauses	1.7	2.1	1.3	2.0	1.9	1.4	2.7	2.7	3.37	.0221	S > M,N
Lexical ties	15.6	5.2	9.5	5.5	11.4	5.6	9.9	5.7	6.26	.0008	N > M,SA,S
Substitution and ellipsis	6.4	3.8	5.5	3.2	5.2	3.2	7.8	4.7	2.19	.0941	—

[a] N = normal; M = manic; SA = schizoaffective; S = schizophrenic.

his speech is difficult to follow. Clinically, these patterns would be called *incoherence* or *derailment*.

We theorized that two different mechanisms might account for the abnormalities in manic and schizophrenic speech. The manic, because he tends to be cognitively overactivated, is more likely to develop a plan but to change it midstream, a phenomenon that we call the *structural shift mechanism*. On the other hand, the schizophrenic may have a more primary deficit that makes it difficult for him to generate any type of coherent plan. We call this the *structural breakdown mechanism*.

The psycholinguistic techniques involved in studying these mechanisms are also too complex to describe in detail here and can be examined by studying the work of Hoffman, Kirstein, Stopak, and Cicchetti (1982). Briefly, the techniques involve looking at segments of speech and showing how various clauses within them are tied together conceptually. Discourse "trees" are generated for each conceptual unit. For example, the following unit of discourse might be diagrammed into the type of tree that appears below it:

> Q: *Have you ever been out of New York?*
> A: *No, I've never been nowhere—nowhere . . . if I could go I would go . . . I feel like cashing in my welfare check now and just leaving . . . and I was gonna keep my—my two checks and save them and get an apartment. I wanna save them and just leave.*

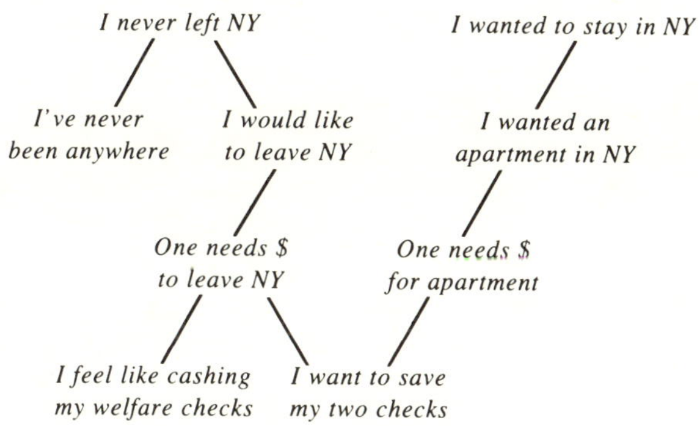

This is an incoherent statement with a relatively disorganized discourse tree because two different ideas related to the basic idea, *I want to save my two checks*, are derived from it.

Using this approach, three different quantitative measures can be developed in order to characterize a person's discourse: the length of utterances,

Table 14. Discourse Trees in Normal, Schizophrenic, and Manic Speech: Predictions

Normals	Manics	Schizophrenics
Short to long utterances	Long utterances	Long utterances
Large subtrees	Large subtrees	Small subtrees
Low deviance	High deviance	High deviance

the size of subtrees, and the degree to which the subtrees show deviance or disorganization. We hypothesized a priori that normals, manics, and schizophrenics would differ on these variables because their speech was informed by different mechanisms. The way they were predicted to differ is summarized in Table 14.

Because the manics are able to generate a discourse plan, they are able to speak long utterances and produce large, complex subtrees. Nevertheless, because their speech is also disorganized due to shifts in topic, they will have a high degree of deviance. On the other hand, schizophrenics may have long or short utterances depending on the degree to which they manifest poverty of speech. Those who do not manifest poverty of speech, however, will have long utterances and yet will have relatively small subtrees because they are unable to generate a complex discourse plan a priori. Nevertheless, even their small subtrees will have a high degree of deviance because of their inability to develop a discourse plan.

The results of this type of analysis are shown in Table 15. As this table indicates, the hypotheses were confirmed. The manics and schizophrenics have much more total deviance than do the normals, with the manics manifesting the most deviance. The manics also tend to have relatively longer utterances than do the schizophrenics and the normals. As predicted, the schizophrenics tend to generate relatively small subtrees in comparison to the manics and normals.

This approach to studying discourse reveals different patterns of abnormality in manic and in schizophrenic patients. It suggests that a different mechanism may underlie the abnormalities in these two patient groups. The language behavior of the manic patients is consistent with a model of cognitive overactivation that leads to over-rapid thoughts, an ability to generate plans quickly, and a tendency to shift quickly from one plan to another. The mechanism producing disorganized speech in schizophrenia is potentially more complex. Clinically, some schizophrenic patients clearly speak very brief but well-formed sentences, which would manifest themselves as short utterances with small but nondeviant discourse trees. On the other hand, in this study, utterance length was approximately the same for schizophrenic patients and normals. This is no doubt in part due to the fact that only

Table 15. Discourse Trees in Normal, Schizophrenic, and Manic Speech: Data

	Normals (N = 40)		Schizophrenics (N = 39)		Manics (N = 24)				
	$\bar{X}$	SD	$\bar{X}$	SD	$\bar{X}$	SD	F Ratio[a]	p	Subsets[b]
Total deviance	1.57	3.69	6.26	8.95	12.29	17.40	20.23	.0001	N/S/M
Utterance length	37.97	14.51	42.5	36.63	65.66	36.41	9,36	.001	S,N/M
Largest subtree	21.52	9.50	18.3	13.3	25.8	12.95	6.47	.002	S/N,M

[a] df = 2,100.

[b] M = manics (N = 24); S = schizophrenics (N = 39); and N = normals (N = 40). Slashes separate groups that are significantly different from each other on the basis of the Duncan multiple range test with alpha set at .05. The group with the lowest score is listed first, and the highest last.

patients with relatively long utterances were selected for inclusion in this psycholinguistic substudy.

The data are clearly consistent with a generalized inability to plan discourse. The neural mechanisms explaining this would be frontal, subcortical, or localized in the left-hemisphere language system. Because the gist and click studies also implicate abnormalities in very short term memory, one also might hypothesize that the structural breakdown in schizophrenic language could be due to defective memory handicapping the patient's ability to form a general discourse plan or to remember it once it has been formulated.

PHASE III: NEUROANATOMICAL MAPPING

The mapping of abnormalities of language function, as defined by psycholinguists, is a valuable descriptive exercise. The ultimate purpose in studying schizophrenic language is to understand how disorganized language reflects impairment in brain function. This may be achieved through neuroanatomical mapping.

Our investigation of this aspect of schizophrenic language abnormalities is still in its preliminary stages. We are using several different techniques in an attempt to understand the underlying neural mechanisms that might explain the linguistic and cognitive abnormalities found in schizophrenia.

One approach involves using the technology of CT scanning in order to search for both focal and diffuse abnormalities. Work with CT scanning has shown that some schizophrenic patients display structural brain abnormalities such as ventricular enlargement. Our current work involves examining density numbers in selected regions of interest, such as the frontal system or the basal ganglia and the thalamus. Limitations in the current technology of CT scanning preclude the examination of specific language areas in the temporal region.

Overall, we think it unlikely that CT scanning will have sufficient power to help us understand the mechanism underlying linguistic and cognitive defects in schizophrenia. NMR and regional cerebral blood flow studies do offer more hope, however. We are just beginning to use NMR and regional blood flow. Our data in this area are as yet very preliminary.

A final approach involves using the aphasias as possible models for language abnormalities in schizophrenia. Like schizophrenic language abnormalities, the types of aphasia are multiple and variable, depending on which components of the language system are affected. In our current work, we are examining the language functions of schizophrenic patients through the use of standard aphasia tests, in order to determine whether characteristic patterns similar to those found in various types of aphasia will emerge.

Preliminary review of this work suggests that schizophrenics clearly show some abnormalities when evaluated by these tests. On the other hand, very few show the classic profiles noted in the typical aphasias, such as Broca's or Wernicke's. Thus, this approach will help us document in more detail the type of language abnormality present, but it also suggests that there is not a simple equivalent between schizophrenic language disorders and the classic aphasias described in neurology.

The future of research in the language of psychotics resides in the study of its neural mechanisms. Developing the technology to study this is the challenge of the future.

ACKNOWLEDGMENT

This research was supported in part by NIMH Grant MH31593, a Scottish Rite Schizophrenia Grant, and The Nelle Ball Foundation

REFERENCES

Andreasen, N. C. (1978). *Scale for the assessment of thought, language, and communication (TLC)*. Iowa City: University of Iowa. (Available from the author on request)

Andreasen, N. C. (1979a). The clinical assessment of thought, language, and communication disorders. I. The definition of terms and evaluation of their reliability. *Archives of General Psychiatry, 36*, 1315–1321.

Andreasen, N. C. (1979b). The clinical assessment of thought, language, and communication disorders. II. Diagnostic significance. *Archives of General Psychiatry, 36*, 1325–1330.

Andreasen, N. C. (1982a). Negative symptoms in schizophrenia: Definition and reliability. *Archives of General Psychiatry, 39*, 784–788.

Andreasen, N. C. (1982b). Negative *versus* positive schizophrenia: Definition and validation. *Archives of General Psychiatry, 39*, 789–794.

Bleuler, E. (1950). *Dementia praecox or the group of schizophrenias* (J. Zinkin, Trans.) New York: International Universities Press. (Original work published 1911)

Bransford, J. D., & Franks, J. J. (1971). The abstraction of linguistic ideas. *Cognitive Psychology, 2*, 331–350.

Cameron, N. (1939). Deterioration and regression in schizophrenic thinking. *Journal of Abnormal Social Psychology, 34*, 265–270.

Carpenter, M. D. (1976). Sensitivity to syntactic structure: Good *versus* poor premorbid schizophrenics. *Journal of Abnormal Psychology, 85*, 41–50.

Chaika, E. (1974). A linguist looks at "schizophrenic" language. *Brain and Language, 1*, 257–276.

Chapman, J., & McGhie, A. (1962). A comparative study of disordered attention in schizophrenia. *Journal of Mental Science, 108*, 487–500.

Chapman, L. J., & Chapman, J. P. (1973). Problems in the measurement of differential deficit. *Psychological Bulletin, 79*, 380–385.

Cromwell, R. L., & Dokeckie, P. R. (1968). Schizophrenic language: A disattention interpretation. In S. Rosenberg & J. H. Koplin (Eds.), *Developments in applied psycholinguistic research*. New York: Macmillan.

Deese, J. (1978). Thought into speech. *American Scientist, 66*, 314–321.

Endicott, J., Spitzer, R. L., Fleiss, J., & Cohen, J. (1976). The Global Assessment Scale: A procedure for measuring overall severity of psychiatric illness. *Archives of General Psychiatry, 33*, 766–771.

Fodor, J. A., & Bever, T. G., (1965). The psychological reality of linguistic segments. *Journal of Verbal Learning and Verbal Behavior, 4*, 414–420.

Garrett, M. F., Bever, T. G., & Fodor, J. A. (1966). The active use of grammar in speech perception. *Psychophysics, 1*, 30–32.

Goldstein, K. (1944). Methodological approach to the study of schizophrenic thought disorder. In J. S. Kasanin (Ed.), *Language and thought in schizophrenia*. Berkeley & Los Angeles: University of California Press.

Harrow, N., Tucker, G. H., & Adler, D. (1965). Concrete and idiosyncratic thinking in acute schizophrenic patients. *Archives of General Psychiatry, 12*, 443–450.

Hoffman, R. E., Kirstein, L., Stopak, S., & Cicchetti, D. (1982). Apprehending schizophrenic discourse: A structural analysis of the listener's task. *Brain and Language, 15*, 207–233.

Hoffman, R. E., Stopak, S., & Andreasen, N. C. (in press). Thought and language abnormalities in schizophrenia and mania: Underlying mechanisms. *Archives of General Psychology*.

Kasanin, J. S. (1944). The disturbance of conceptual thinking in schizophrenia. In J. S. Kasanin (Ed.), *Language and thought in schizophrenia*. Berkeley & Los Angeles: University of California Press.

Knight, R. A., & Sims-Knight, J. E. (1979). Integration of linguistic ideas in schizophrenics. *Journal of Abnormal Psychology, 88*, 191–202.

Kraepelin, E. (1919). *Dementia praecox and paraphrenia* (R. M. Barkley, Trans.). Edinburgh: E & S Livingstone. (Original work published 1913)

Payne, R. W., & Friedlander, D. (1962). A short battery of simple tests for measuring over-inclusive thinking. *Journal of Mental Science, 108*, 362–367.

Rochester, S. R., Harris, J., & Seeman, M. V. (1973). Sentence processing in schizophrenic listeners. *Journal of Abnormal Psychology, 82*, 350–356.

Rochester, S. R., & Martin, J. R. (1979). *Crazy talk: A study of the discourse of schizophrenic patients*. New York: Plenum Press.

Spitzer, R. L., Endicott, J., & Robins, E. (1978). Research diagnostic criteria: Rationale and reliability. *Archives of General Psychiatry, 35*, 773–782.

Wynne, L. C., & Singer, M. T. (1965). Thought disorder and family relations of schizophrenics. *Archives of General Psychiatry, 12*, 187–221.

COMMENTARY

Dr. Robert Rose:* That's very interesting. In the course of your coming to develop this analysis, have you gone back and looked at some of the work of Lyman Wynne and Margaret Thaler Singer in which they talked about a particular kind of concreteness or diffuseness of communication between

* Galveston, Texas.

parents and their schizophrenic children? Have you had a chance to study what they were talking about in that?

Dr. Andreasen: Well, I think what would be interesting, if you could possibly take their language protocols that were generated, would be to apply this kind of analysis to it; they are at a different level of conception. I mean, they are talking about abstract qualities of discourse, and the interesting things is to see if you can then go measure that systematically. Is that what you are saying?

Dr. Rose: Yes. Your approach might further clarify the concepts they were alluding to.

Dr. Samuel Keith:* Just one further question.

Dr. Joseph Zubin†: I'd like to ask the following: Of course, Nancy [Andreasen] writes so much, it is very difficult to keep up with all her findings, and I wonder whether she would be willing to answer this question, even though she may have written about it.

First, is there any connection between the positive thought disorder, negative thought disorder, and positive and negative symptoms? The second question, since the most important aspect of speech in schizophrenia is incomprehensibility, is if there is connection between your general structural analysis and such more simple devices as the cloze technique?

Dr. Andreasen: Yes. Negative thought disorder is related to negative symptoms. Positive thought disorder is related to positive symptoms. So that is relatively easy. To answer the second question, which I guess boils down to a question about the cloze procedure, I find the cloze procedure a relatively simple and extremely gross way of getting at incoherent communication, and as it has been used in the research literature, it has been, I think, more tied to the patience of the people scoring the cloze procedure and their intelligence than it has to actually dissecting anything about schizophrenic or manic discourse. We have done a couple different cloze studies. They've never added up to anything, and I have just never published them.

* Rockville, Maryland.
† Pittsburgh, Pennsylvania.

12

Thought Disorder Specificity in Functional Psychoses

PHILIP S. HOLZMAN, MARGIE R. SOLOVAY,
AND MARTHA E. SHENTON
Harvard University

The intrusion of loose or arbitrarily related associations into the language of psychotic patients has, historically, been regarded as a sine qua non of a schizophrenic condition. Recent evidence, however, suggests that similar thought disorders are present in affective psychoses, and the uniqueness of such intrusions with respect to schizophrenia has therefore been questioned (e. g., Andreasen, 1979; Andreasen & Powers, 1974; Carlson & Goodwin, 1973; Harrow, Grossman, Silverstein, & Meltzer, 1982; Harrow & Quinlan, 1977; Johnston & Holzman, 1979). In addition, disorders of thinking have also been observed in toxic conditions and in some organic brain conditions (e.g., Levine & Finkelstein, 1982; Gerson, Benson, & Frazier, 1977). As a consequence of their presence in different conditions, the mere observation of thought disorder is insufficient for establishing a differential diagnosis among the various psychotic conditions.

The presence of thought disorder in many conditions with diverse etiologies raises the question, "Is thought disorder a nonspecific accompaniment of psychotic behavior, whatever the etiology of that psychosis, just as fever is nonspecific for a variety of systemic conditions; or is there a set of specific disorders of thinking that accompanies specific psychotic conditions?" The answer to this question directs us either to abandon the study of thought disorder as a major avenue to the elucidation of psychotic processes or to take up a more fine-grained analysis of the process–function interrelationships between type of thought disorder and type of psychosis.

In this paper we take the second approach. Evidence is presented that qualitative differences in thought disorders do exist between schizophrenic and manic psychoses. The evidence is based on an exploratory study that requires replication and further exploration before deciding on its usefulness for understanding the pathogenesis and pathophysiology of the functional psychoses.

LANGUAGE OR THOUGHT

Before describing the study, we wish to underscore why we chose to describe the behavioral phenomena under discussion as *thought* disorders rather than as *speech* or *language* disorders. There are, of course, obvious differences among the referents of these three terms and it seems to us important to preface our empirical report with our theoretical argument for considering what seem to be linguistic disorders as essentially disorders of thinking. Indeed, we remain unconvinced that, with respect to psychoses, it is profitable to speak of any language disorder, although we recognize that disagreements about this issue exist in the literature (e.g., Brown, 1973; Chaika, 1974; Fromkin, 1975). We present three arguments for our position.

First, consider the view that language is a medium through which thought is communicated or transmitted. This view is analogous to that proposed by Heider with respect to perception: Colors, slants, constancies of size and shape, for example, are media through which we perceive *things* (Heider, 1959). Thus, when we look directly at a person who is some distance from us we see neither the person's retinal size, nor the changes in shape as a result of orientation shifts, nor the person's various colors. Rather we see the *person* who is recognizable as a friend or a relative or a stranger, whose percept has been mediated by those properties of size, shape, slant, or color. We can, of course, direct our attention to retinal size or skin tone, in which instance those media now become *things* or objects of perception. It is the same with language. In the course of a lifetime we are trained to look through language to the thoughts conveyed by the language. Language, thus, tends to be transparent, although it can be an object for scrutiny, as when a linguist studies various properties of language and usage. Therefore, when we listen to a person speak, psychotic and normal alike, we are apprehending the thoughts of that person, as conveyed by the language.

A second, less theoretical argument for our position takes note of the fact that psychotic patients do not speak a shared language or a shared dialect. There is no such thing as a schizophrenic language. Both schizophrenic persons and nonschizophrenic persons have equal difficulty in understanding the utterances of a schizophrenic patient (Hunt & Walker, 1966).

A third argument for our position observes that language and thought disorders are not only conceptually but empirically separable. There exist thought disorders without the presence of language disorders, and there exist language disorders without thinking disorders. For example, most clinicians have seen patients who display an obvious thinking disorder that is entirely devoid of any language disturbance, as, for example, in cases of pure paranoia. There, the delusional element may be conspicuous in a setting of syntactically and grammatically excellent language. As psychotic people become more disorganized and paranoid constructions are less rigidly organized, language distortions become conspicuous, along with the thinking disorders. On the other hand, there are conditions in which noteworthy language disturbances are patent without any thinking disorder, as in the case of the congenitally deaf. These people, for the most part, are unable to read written English at better than a fifth-grade level, and their spoken speech is peppered with syntactic and grammatical errors. Yet, when they communicate in sign language, their thinking is as well organized as is that of persons with no impaired hearing. Furthermore, one can present a number of examples of disorders of thinking that occur without the mediation of language. The use of noverbal tests such as block designs, digit symbol substitution, maze tracing, for example, yield performance dysfunctions that reflect a thinking disorder in psychotic patients.

Our colleague, Roger W. Brown (1973), has further clarified for us the separability of language and thought, although there are areas of overlap. Professor Brown has called our attention to linguistic factors that are independent of thought. These factors include phonotactics, morphology, and syntactics. *Phonotactics* refers to the sound clusters that are more or less acceptable within a particular language, such as *pr*, *dr*, and *cr*, in English. *Morphology* refers to the rules for linguistic inflection, such as *go*, *going*, *gone*, or *chair*, *chairs*, or *capital*, *capitalize*, in English. *Syntactics* refers to the rules for meaningful word order in a particular language. No studies have shown that psychotic patients violate the tolerance limits of these regularities in these three areas. It seems to us, therefore, that until there is convincing demonstration of a purely linguistic disorder in psychosis, it is more fruitful to regard the verbal productions of psychotic patients as revealing disturbed thought processes. In this paper we will consequently refer to the productions of psychotic patients as reflecting thought disorders.

THE THOUGHT DISORDER INDEX

The assessment of qualitative differences in thought disorder between manic and schizophrenic patients makes use of an instrument, the Thought Disorder Index (TDI), developed by Johnston and Holzman (1979), and revised by the present authors (Solovay, Shenton, Johnston, Gasperetti, & Holzman, submitted for publication). The TDI employs verbal protocols that can be collected independently of clinical diagnostic interviews and of observations of ward behavior. It can also be scored and evaluated blindly with respect to any other identifying information on a particular patient. Although, in principle, any extended verbal protocol can be used as the raw data for the TDI, our laboratory has typically employed verbatim responses to the Rorschach test and to the verbal subscales of the Wechsler Adult Intelligence Scale.

The TDI assesses a range of thought disorder as expressed through verbal samples. The index identifies 22 different categories of thinking disturbances at 4 levels of severity. These categories had been identified previously by Rapaport, Gill, and Schafer (1968), and later presented as an index, called the Delta Index, by Watkins and Stauffacher (1952). The Delta Index was subsequently refined by Johnston and Holzman (1979), and called the Thought Disorder Index (TDI). The categories in the TDI represent a catalog of deviant verbalizations encountered in the course of the psychological testing of psychotic patients. There is no reason to assume that it is an exhaustive catalog, and therefore the TDI can be expected to be revised periodically to reflect the introduction of new categories, probably on the basis of the testing of new patient groups.

Because the TDI includes multiple aspects of thought disorder, it is not tied to a particular theoretical view of "what thought disorder is," that is, whether it represents paralogical reasoning, concrete thinking, or loose associations. The TDI does tag instances of those categories as well as of others. Table 1 presents the categories, scoring levels, and some examples of the kinds of responses scored at those levels.

Table 1. TDI Categories and Levels of Severity with Selected Examples

0.25 LEVEL

1. Inappropriate distance
   - A. Loss or increase of distance (*I'm afraid of what else it could be . . . It scares me to think of what else it could be.*)
   - B. Excessive qualification
   - C. Concreteness (*Some kind of fancy military jet flying up the card.*)
   - D. Overspecificity (*A four-legged lamb.*)
   - E. Syncretistic response (on WAIS—How are wood and alcohol alike? *They both have atoms.*)
2. Flippant response
3. Vagueness (*Nothing but two figures on each side. I don't know what kind of figures. They don't look like animals or people. They just looked like two smears.*)
4. Peculiar verbalizations and responses
   - A. Peculiar expression (*a reverse reflection*)
   - B. Stilted, inappropriate expression (*It's a piece of animation.*)
   - C. Idiosyncratic word usage (*He's all **clowned** up in some kind of suit.*)
5. Word-finding difficulty
6. Clangs
7. Perseverations
8. Incongruous combinations
   - A. Composite response (*a bear with a duck's face*)
   - B. Arbitrary form–color responses (*an orange pelvic bone; green fire*)
   - C. Inappropriate activity response (*a beetle crying*)

(continued)

Table 1. (*Continued*)

0.50 LEVEL

9. Relationship verbalization (an allusion back to an earlier one, *that being the mandibles in the very first picture*)
10. Idiosyncratic symbolism (*the red . . . shows action*)
11. Queer responses
    A. Queer expressions (*inward type of photograph of a flower's reproductive cells*)
    B. Queer imagery (*idealized fire*)
    C. Queer word usage (*pestals on a flower*)
12. Confusion (*some people smoking matches and burning cigarettes*)
13. Looseness (*because it's black, dark, darkness, lovemaking*)
14. Fabulized combinations, impossible or bizarre (*two crows with afros and they're pushing two hearts together*)

0.75 LEVEL

15. Fluidity (*the head of a rocket or the head of a bear or the head of a bird . . . looked like something was becoming something else*)
16. Absurd responses (*This is sticking out there. Remember that's the-uh-cure there. It's our cure, it's called.*)
17. Confabulations
    A. Details in one area generalized to a larger area
    B. Extreme elaboration (*the light bulb is—I think it's man-made. And the pink is down here and it gives energy for the light bulb . . . and the vapors from the pink . . . cause the green and the orange to . . . be there . . .*)
18. Playful confabulation (*an evil witch doing a square dance. . . . She had her dress like this and she was doe-see-doeing.*)
19. Autistic logic (*I see something rather like an appendix. Looked to me totally useless, so then I thought of the appendix.*)

1.0 LEVEL

20. Contamination (*This is definitely a man . . . a man butterfly, a butterfly with a man's face—could be a dark cloud that's dark because it swallows up all . . . uh . . . the dark particles—man butterfly . . . it could be a cloud-like man–butterfly.*)
21. Incoherence (*a duck . . . their disarrangement. They follow out together, they follow one another. The two toes together, meeting one another. They jacked up in back, like spinal cord being broken.*)
22. Neologisms (*That's tevro or neoglyphics.*)

Earlier work has shown that, with training, interscorer reliability for the total TDI is around .90 (Johnston & Holzman, 1979). In that study the TDI was highly elevated for all psychotic patients, which included chronically hospitalized schizophrenics, recently hospitalized schizophrenics, and nonschizophrenic hospitalized psychotic patients. In contrast, nonpsychotic hospitalized psychiatric patients showed less thought disorder than the psychotic patients. The normal control group, while showing some thought disorder, had the lowest TDI total score. Sex differences, ethnicity, social class, and intellectual level do not account for those differences (Haimo & Holzman, 1979).

The TDI has also been used to assess changes in thought disorder in a group of schizophrenic patients undergoing neuroleptic treatment after a drug washout of one to three weeks (Hurt, Holzman, & Davis, 1983). The TDI showed a rapid decrease in thought disorder following the introduction of neuroleptic treatment, and a continual improvement throughout the hospital stay. This pattern of improvement was mirrored by independent clinical assessments on the Brief Psychiatric Rating Scale. Figure 1 displays these data.

These studies evaluated patients with respect to total TDI scores. No diagnostic specificity can be claimed for the total TDI scores because psychotic schizophrenic and manic patients do not significantly differ from each other on total TDI. We report here a first study of qualitative distinctions in thought disorder between manic and schizophrenic patients.

METHOD

Subjects

The pool of subjects from which the study population was drawn consisted of 125 patients at two mental hospitals, one a state hospital for chronic patients and one an active treatment center for more recently hospitalized patients. Each patient was interviewed by one of four diagnosticians who used a standardized instrument that was an amalgam of items from the Present State Examination (Wing, 1970) and the Schedule for Affective Disorders and Schizophrenia—Lifetime Version (SADS-L) (Spitzer & Endicott, 1978). The material from the interview was then combined with information from a standardized chart review to permit classification of the patients on the basis of three diagnostic schemata: the DSM-III (American Psychiatric Association, 1980), St. Louis criteria (Feighner *et al.*, 1972), and the Research Diagnostic Criteria (RDC) (Spitzer, Endicott, & Robins, 1978). For this report we accepted only those patients who met the criteria of all three classification systems for schizophrenia or the equivalents of manic psychosis. These diagnostic procedures were performed independently of the thought-disorder testing, described below.

This process identified 43 schizophrenic and 20 manic patients. Sixty-two patients were excluded from this study; 34 of these 62 patients failed to meet the criteria for all three diagnostic systems, and the remaining 28 cases were classified as "atypical." Our purpose in requiring strict inclusion

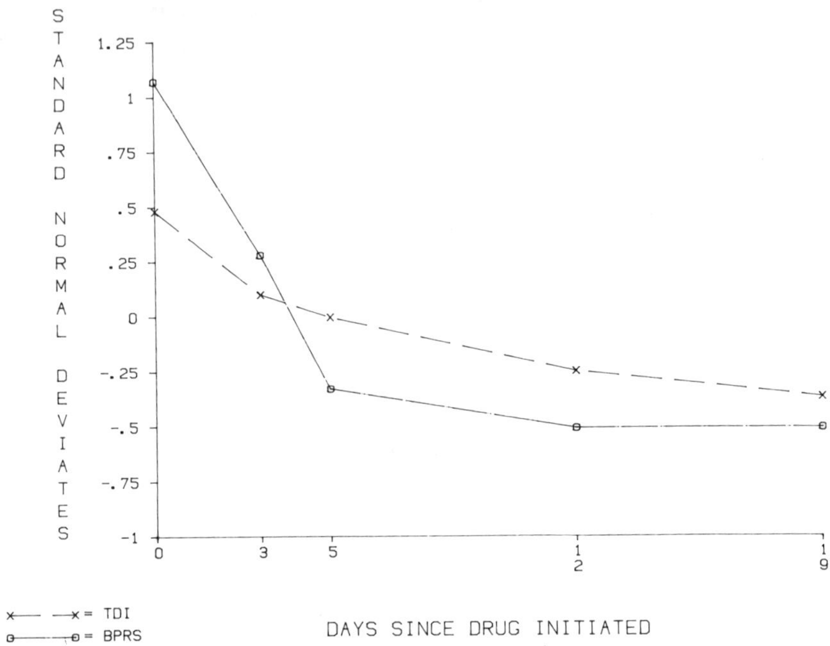

Figure 1. Effects of a neuroleptic drug on thought-disorder level, measured by the TDI total score, and on behavioral symptoms, measured by the Brief Psychiatric Rating Scale total score. Scores are expressed as standard deviation units. Rapid diminution of both thought disorder and behavioral symptoms is shown.

criteria responded to the need to examine groups of schizophrenic and manic patients that were *prototypical* and thereby minimized overlap between the groups. By their "purity," the chosen patient groups avoided biasing by idiosyncratic diagnostic practices of some psychiatrists or of some centers where overdiagnosis of one or another condition may occur. By excluding cases in which there could be a dispute, we believe we maximized the chances of observing whether there are qualitative thought disorder differences between the two psychoses.

In addition to the 63 psychotic patients, we tested 22 normal subjects who were screened for absence of mental illness in themselves and in their first-degree relatives.

Drug Effects

There is no doubt that treatment with antipsychotic medication reduces thought disorder (see, for example, Chapman & Knowles, 1964; Hurt *et al.*, 1983; Orzack *et al.*, 1967; Spohn *et al.*, 1977). The use of drug-free samples is complicated for several reasons, not the least of which is that patients who can be maintained drug-free for the required length of time for a study may represent a sample that is different from those who relapse too quickly to be maintained without drugs. Patients who are admitted to hospitals "drug free" are themselves likely to be atypical (Chapman, 1963). Our solution in this study is clearly a compromise. We tested subjects as close to the beginning of their hospital stay and of their treatment as was possible and thereby we hoped to minimize the ameliorative and masking effects of pharmacological therapy.

All but two schizophrenic subjects were receiving neuroleptic drugs and all manics were being treated with lithium carbonate alone or in combination either with a phenothiazine or a tricyclic.

Table 2 presents the relevant demographic characteristics of the subjects. There were significant group differences in education (manics were better educated), Global Assessment Scale scores (schizophrenics were more disorganized), net hospitalization—the total number of months actually spent in a hospital—(schizophrenics spent more time in the hospital), and length of illness (schizophrenics were ill a longer time).

Procedure

After informed consent had been obtained, all patients and normal controls were administered the Rorschach test in the manner described by Rapaport *et al.* (1968). The inquiry for each card was conducted after the subject had responded to that card; in particular, all strange, idiosyncratic, or deviant

Table 2. Demographic Characteristics of Subjects in the Three Groups: Schizophrenics, Manics, and Normals

	Schizophrenics	*Manics*	*Normals*
N	43	20	22
Sex.			
Male	36	23	8
Female	7	8	14
Mean Age	25.0 ± 5.35	24.1 ± 8.04	20.53 ± 3.16
Education level (in years)	12.7 ± 2.16	14 ± 2.70	13.86 ± 1.83
Socioeconomic class (Hollingshead & Redlich)			
I	13	7	0
II	9	5	2
III	10	4	7
IV	7	3	9
V	4		4
Verbal IQ	103 ± 15	110 ± 15	111 ± 13

verbalizations and responses were probed in the manner described by Johnston and Holzman (1979). All testing sessions were recorded on audio tape and labeled with an identification number, after the subject's name had been removed. These tapes were later transcribed verbatim by an experienced transcriptionist. The typed protocols were then scored for thought disorder by two trained judges, blind to diagnosis, the manner described by Johnston and Holzman (1979).

The TDI takes into account verbal productivity. Verbal productivity was estimated both by counting the number of words spoken by the subject and by tallying the number of Rorschach responses. There were no significant differences in the relationship of these two variables to the total TDI score. We therefore decided to use the number of responses as an estimate of verbal productivity, because this is a more conveniently obtained measure and because it had already been used by Johnston and Holzman (1979). The total scores were therefore divided by the number of responses, and it is to be understood that the total TDI score is the ratio of the sum of weighted scores to the number of responses, multiplied by 100.

The TDI total and category scores are not normally distributed. Therefore, to achieve a closer approximation to a normal distribution, the scores were transformed and then standardized for purposes of statistical analysis. The transformations included negative reciprocals, square root, logarithmic to base 10, and natural logarithmic conversions. Only the category of "neologism" was so skewed that it did not approach normality after transformation: it was therefore dichotomized as "present" or "absent."

RESULTS

The results are presented first in terms of total TDI scores and then in terms of the qualitative distinctions between the subject groups.

Total TDI Scores

As had been the case in the Johnston and Holzman (1979) study, both groups of psychotic patients showed high TDI levels. Although both the manic and schizophrenic groups produced considerably more thought-disordered responses than did the normal control group, the two patient groups did not differ from each other with respect to this global measure. However, both psychotic groups differed significantly from the normal control group. Table 3 presents these data.

Qualitative Distinctions

In order to examine whether these two groups of psychotic patients arrive at their high TDI levels differently—that is, by producing different profiles

Table 3. Total TDI Scores for the Three Subject Groups: Schizophrenics, Manics, and Normals

Subject group	*N*	Mean	*SD*
Schizophrenics	43	34.56	38.77
Manics	20	25.02	16.15
Normals	22	5.95	4.54

of the thought disorder categories—we applied the statistical techniques of factor analysis and discriminant function analysis to the transformed and standardized data. We will present each of these analyses in turn.

FACTOR ANALYTIC EXAMINATION

We explored the usefulness and power of three differently derived sets of factors in the analysis of thought disorder profiles. The first was a set of factors derived from a Principal Components Factor Analysis with Varimax rotation. The second compared the subject groups with respect to factors that had been proposed on an a priori basis. The third examined the separability of the manics and schizophrenics on the basis of a post hoc analysis of TDI category differences between the two diagnostic groups.

Principal-Components Factor Analysis with Varimax Rotation. For the purposes of this analysis, all 97 psychotic subjects were used in order to approximate the desired ratio of subjects to measures. We chose unit weighting over factor loadings in order to minimize sampling fluctuation in what is essentially an exploratory analysis. This analysis yielded six interpretable factors, which reflect recognizable general categories of thought disorder:

1. Idiosyncratic verbalizations
2. Expansive thinking
3. Autistic thinking
4. Fluid thinking
5. Absurdity
6. Confusion

Table 4 shows the composition of these factors with their loadings.

The three groups of subjects were then compared on the extent to which they make use of these six general categories. Figure 2 shows these comparisons. *Expansive thinking* emerges as a clear manic factor, and its composition has a face validity: playful confabulation, incongruous combinations, flippant responses, and fabulized combinations. It is a factor that includes not only expansive thinking but also combinatory ideation. On the remaining five categories, schizophrenic patients produce most of the thought-disordered

Table 4. Factors with Factor Loadings Based on a Principal-Components Factor Analysis with Varimax Rotation

Idiosyncratic Verbalizations	*Fluid Thinking*
Peculiar verbalizations (.827)	Fluidity (.715)
Queer verbalizations (.691)	Contamination (.690)
Expansive Thinking	
Playful confabulations (.834)	*Absurdity*
Incongruous combinations (.602)	Neologism (.863)
Flippant (.576)	Absurdity (.489)
Fabulized combinations (.528)	
Autistic Thinking	*Confusion*
Autistic logic (.789)	Vagueness (.762)
Incoherent (.724)	Confusion (.734)

responses, with the normals and the manics giving only a minimum number of responses that are scorable in these categories.

A Priori Factors. In Johnston and Holzman's (1979) monograph, each thought disorder category was assigned to one of four broad conceptual classifications:

1. Associative looseness
2. Combinatory thinking

Figure 2. Frequencies with which each of the three subject groups (schizophrenics, manics, and normals) produce thought-disordered responses in each of the six empirically derived factors.

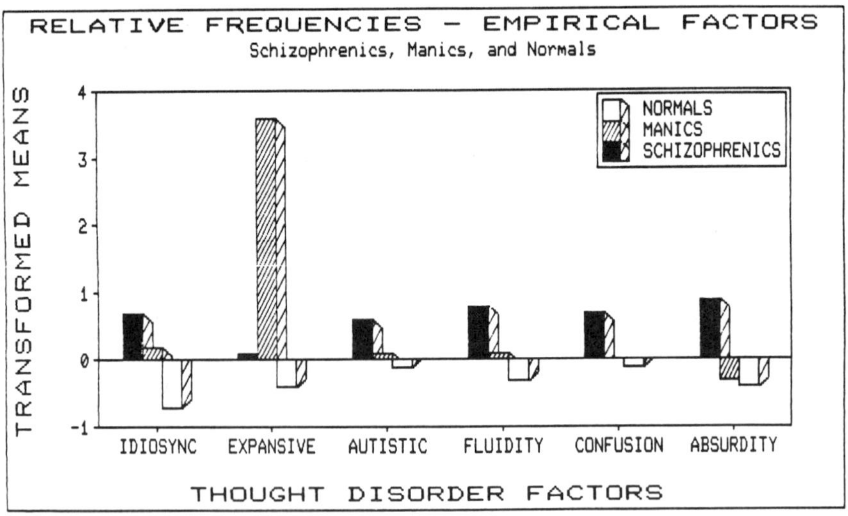

Table 5. Thought Disorder Factors with TDI Categories Based on A Priori Constructions

Associative Looseness	*Disorganization*
Inappropriate distance	Vagueness
Clang	Word-finding difficulty
Perseveration	Confusion
Relationship verbalization	Incoherence
Looseness	
Fluidity	
Combinatory Responses	*Unconventional Verbalizations*
Incongruous combinations	Peculiar verbalizations
Fabulized combinations	Queer verbalizations
Idiosyncratic symbolism	Absurd
Confabulation	Neologisms
Playful confabulation	
Autistic logic	
Contamination	

3. Disorganized thinking
4. Unconventional verbalizations

Table 5 presents the composition of those factors. Associative looseness reflects a tendency for verbalizations to be guided more by internal sets and shifts of set than by the constraints of the task, in this case the appropriate completion of the Rorschach test. Combinatory thinking reflects a tendency to combine percepts, ideas, or images in an incongruous, unrealistic, or inappropriate manner. Disorganized thinking reflects confusion in thinking, perhaps disorganization. Unconventional verbalizations reflect odd word usage which, unlike that of poets and creative writers, is not under voluntary control.

Figure 3 shows the comparison of the three groups of subjects on these a priori factors. There are no differences between the two psychotic groups with respect to the associative looseness factor, suggesting that associative looseness is a general characteristic of psychotic thinking. Strikingly, the manic patients show a significantly greater production of combinatory responses, and the schizophrenic patients show a greater production of disorganized responses and unconventional verbalizations. The alignment is very similar to that obtained by the empirically derived factors.

Post Hoc Factors. Inasmuch as this study is an exploratory analysis rather than a confirmatory one, we attempted to choose those TDI categories that best discriminated the two patient samples. These categories were then grouped according to their conceptual relatedness as five thought disorder factors:

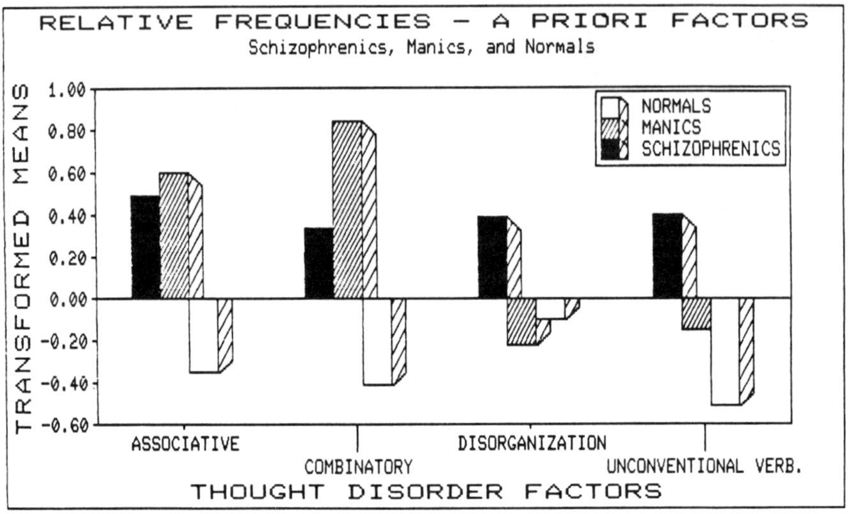

Figure 3. Frequencies with which each of the three subject groups (schizophrenics, manics, and normals) produce thought-disordered responses in each of the four a priori factors.

1. Combinatory thinking
2. Irrelevant intrusions
3. Fluidity of thinking
4. Confused thinking
5. Peculiar verbalizations

Table 6 shows the components of these post hoc factors.

The groups were compared on the basis of this post hoc structure. Figure 4 shows this comparison. It is clear that two manic and three schizophrenic factors distinguish the groups. Combinatory thinking and irrelevant intrusions characterize the manic patients; confused thinking, fluid thinking, and peculiar verbalizations are typical of the schizophrenic patients. Table 6 also shows that eight thought disorder categories of the TDI—called "unspecified categories"—show no power to discriminate the two patient groups, although they are elevated equally in both groups. They therefore seem to represent a general tendency of most psychotic persons, regardless of the type of psychosis, to make use of these categories.

CANONICAL DISCRIMINANT FUNCTION ANALYSIS

We conducted a discriminant function analysis in order to estimate how effectively the set of thought disorder factors separates the manic from the schizophrenic patients. This estimate was accomplished by deriving classification functions that sort subjects into either manic or schizophrenic

Table 6. Post Hoc Factor Structure

Manic factors	Schizophrenic factors
Combinatory Thinking	*Fluid Thinking*
Incongruous combinations	Relationship verbalizations
Fabulized combinations	Fluidity
Playful confabulations	Contaminations
Irrelevant Intrusions	*Confused Thinking*
Flippant responses	Word-finding difficulty
Looseness	Confusion
	Absurdity
	Incoherent
	Neologisms
	Peculiar Verbalizations
	Peculiar

Unspecified categories
Inappropriate distance (excluding flippant)
Vague
Clang
Perseveration
Symbolism
Queer
Confabulation (excluding playful confabulation)
Autistic logic

Figure 4. Frequencies with which each of the three subject groups (schizophrenics, manics and normals) produce thought-disordered responses in each of the five post hoc factors.

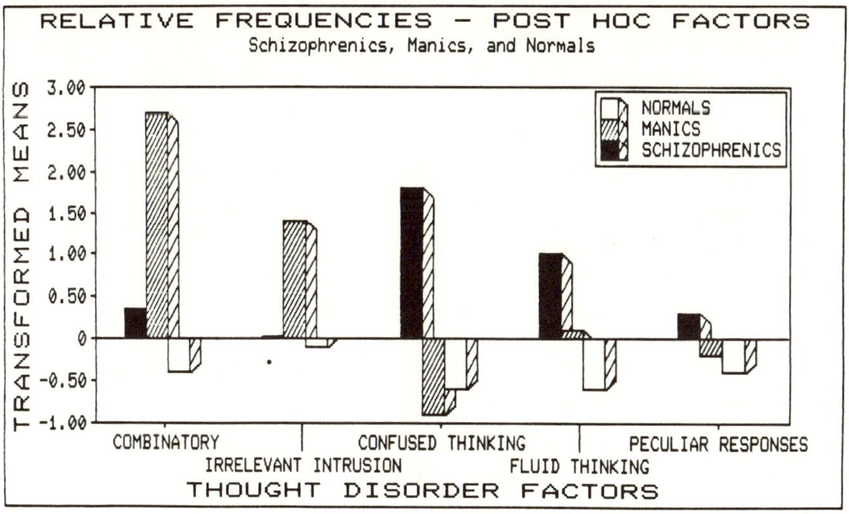

categories on the basis of scores on the thought disorder factors. In order to avoid overestimating the classificatory power that would result from applying classification functions on a sample of subjects that had been derived from that same sample, we randomly divided the sample and derived the functions from one half and applied them to the other half. In order to increase the precision in the now unbiased estimate—precision that was diminished by cutting the sample in half—this technique was repeated several times, and the average of the estimates from each division served as the final unbiased estimate.

When applied to the post hoc factors presented in Table 6 and illustrated in Figure 4, this technique correctly classified 76.5% of the patients, with 82.2% of the schizophrenics and 70.7% of the manics correctly classified. The canonical discriminant function is highly significant ($p < .001$) and correlates .65 ($p < .01$) with the diagnosis of schizophrenia versus mania. In examining the discriminant function, we again see that positive loadings on combinatory thinking and irrelevant intrusions predict mania, and negative loadings on those factors accompany schizophrenia.

The use of the post hoc factors in classifying patients did not overestimate the discriminatory capability of the TDI, because approximately the same results were obtained using the empirically derived factors (see Table 4). There, 75.5% of the subjects were correctly classified, with 80.4% of the schizophrenics and 73.3% of the manics correctly classified. Positive loadings on expansive thinking and negative loadings on idiosyncratic thinking, fluidity, and confusion were predictive of mania; high loadings on those factors characterize schizophrenia.

One additional observation requires mentioning. Schizophrenics tended to produce thought disorder at all levels of severity, from the 0.25 to the 1.0 levels. Manics, on the other hand, did not produce any instance of thought disorder in the most severe (1.0) level.

DISCUSSION

We have presented evidence that manic and schizophrenic psychoses can be distinguished by their distinctive types of thought disorder. The TDI was applied to a group of prototypically "pure" manics and "pure" schizophrenics and has been shown to be sensitive to those differences. On the basis of the data generated by the TDI, manic thought disorder manifests itself as loosely tied together ideas that are easily combined and elaborated to an extravagant degree. One outcome of such a process is irrelevant and incongruous intrusions into social discourse.

Schizophrenic thought disorder, on the other hand, shows very little, if any, of the playful, elaborative, ideationally loose productions of the manics. Rather, fluid thinking, interpenetrations of one idea by another, unstable referents of words, fragmented, and elliptical communications give the impression of inner confusion, which is sometimes not verbalized. The listener, too, may be confused by these communications from the patient.

There is, moreover, a set of thinking disorders that is common to both psychoses. This set includes vagueness, loss of set, and inappropriate distance from the task at hand. Significantly, the normal control group shows evidence of mild thought disorder. Thus, as had been previously reported by Johnston and Holzman (1979), there is continuum of degrees of thought disorder along which people can be arrayed. Most people, however, manifest only mild degrees of thought disorder at some times; fewer people display moderate levels of thought disorder, and as one approaches the higher levels of the continuum, one finds a high prevalence of psychotic people. The transition zones are blurred and inexact, and the mere amount of thought disorder does not distinguish psychotic groups from each other. Indeed, there are a few psychotic persons who produce rather low levels of thought disorder (Johnston & Holzman, 1979). Nevertheless, it appears from the present study that it is principally schizophrenic patients who produce thought disorder at the 1.0 level of severity.

The results reported herein require replication. While awaiting such confirmation or disconfirmation, we can conclude that the TDI is an effective tool which, when employed by trained investigators, can distinguish manic from schizophrenic conditions. This outcome implies two consequences. One concerns the validity of the distinction between mania and schizophrenia, and the second concerns future directions for research in this area.

With respect to the first consequence, that manic and schizophrenic psychoses are two different conditions, the TDI data strongly supports the validity of that distinction. Efforts to elide the distinction between these conditions seem to us to have been based too rigidly on symptom assessments—phenotypic descriptions—that by themselves, in the absence of process variables, can mislead the investigator. The present investigation is consistent with the Kraepelinian distinction between the two major classes of functional psychoses. This, of course, is not to say that mania and schizophrenia are homogeneous disorders. Indeed, the evidence is plentiful that these disorders are heterogeneous, in terms of both their pathogenesis and and their pathophysiology. The present investigation examined the thinking disturbances of indisputable cases of mania and schizophrenia. The task now, in addition to replication, is to examine cases that are not as prototypical and to study cases of so-called atypical psychoses, such as the schizoaffective disorders.

The second consequence of the successful discrimination of manic and schizophrenic thought disorders points to new research directions. We have argued that, in these functional psychoses, language and speech are not impaired, that the capacity to use speech and to use and understand language are unimpaired. The TDI collects instances of impaired language *performance* rather than of language *competence* (cf. Chomsky, 1969). Such impairments of performance reflect the major influences of cognitive factors. For both psychoses it is the cogwheeling, blending, and integrating of thought with language that seems to be dysfunctional. For both psychoses this view would point to pathophysiological investigations that are not confined to speech and language centers of the brain. Yet different processes would be involved in the unbridled combinatory thinking of the manics and in the uncontrolled fluidity and confusion of the schizophrenics. At this juncture, neuropsychological, neuroanatomical, and neuropathological considerations combine with those of psychopathology. This alliance would scrutinize the linkages of concepts, ideas, and images to their sensory aspects, which include their objective referents and their representations in language. These investigations could lead to studies of the inhibitory and disinhibitory control processes involved in the regulation of speech, language, and thought.

REFERENCES

American Psychiatric Association. (1980). *Diagnostic and statistical manual of mental disorders* (3rd ed.). Washington, DC: APA.

Andreasen, N. C. (1979). Clinical assessment of thought, language, and communication disorders. II. Diagnostic significance. *Archives of General Psychiatry, 36*, 1325–1330.

Andreasen, N. C., & Powers, P. (1974). Overinclusive thinking in mania and schizophrenia. *British Journal of Psychiatry, 125*, 452–456.

Brown, R. W. (1973). Schizophrenia, language, and reality. *American Psychologist, 28*, 395–403.

Carlson, G. A., & Goodwin, F. K. (1973). The stages of mania. *Archives of General Psychiatry, 23*, 221–228.

Chaika, E. (1974). A linguist looks at "schizophrenic" language. *Brain and Language, 1*, 257–276.

Chapman, L. J. (1963). The problem of selecting drug-free schizophrenics for research. *Journal of Consulting Psychology, 27*, 540–542.

Chapman, L. J., & Knowles, R. R. (1964). The effects of phenothiazines on disordered thought in schizophrenia. *Journal of Consulting Psychology, 28*, 165–169.

Chomsky, N. (1969). *The acquisition of syntax in children from 5 to 10*. Cambridge, MA: MIT Press.

Endicott, J., Spitzer, R. L., Fleiss, J. F., & Cohen, J. (1976). The global assessment scale: A procedure for measuring overall severity of psychiatric disturbance. *Archives of General Psychiatry, 33*, 768–771.

Feighner, J., Robins, E., Guze, S. B., Woodruff, R., Winokur, G., & Muñoz, R. (1972). Diagnostic criteria for use in psychiatric research. *Archives of General Psychiatry, 26*, 57–58.

Fromkin, V. A. (1975). A linguist looks at "A linguist looks at 'schizophrenic' language." *Brain and Language, 2*, 498–503.

Gerson, S. N., Benson, D. F., & Frazier, S. H. (1977). Diagnosis: Schizophrenia versus posterior aphasia. *American Journal of Psychiatry, 134*, 966–969.

Haimo, S., & Holzman, P. S. (1979). Thought disorder in schizophrenics and normal controls: Social class and race differences. *Journal of Consulting and Clinical Psychology, 47*, 963–967.

Harrow, M., Grossman, L., Silverstein, M., & Meltzer, H. (1982). Thought pathology in manic and schizophrenic patients: Its occurrence at hospital admission and seven weeks later. *Archives of General Psychiatry, 39*, 665–671.

Harrow, M., & Quinlan, D. (1977). Is disordered thinking unique to schizophrenia? *Archives of General Psychiatry, 34*, 15–21.

Heider, F. (1959). On perception, event structure, and the psychological environment. *Psychological issues* (No. 3). New York: International Universities Press.

Hunt, W. A., & Walker, R. E. (1966). Schizophrenics' judgments of schizophrenic test responses. *Journal of Clinical Psychology, 22*, 118–120.

Hurt, S. W., Holzman, P. S., & Davis, J. M. (1983). Thought disorder: The measurement of its changes. *Archives of General Psychiatry, 40*, 1281–1285.

Johnston, M. H., & Holzman, P. S. (1979). *Assessing schizophrenic thinking*. San Francisco: Jossey-Bass.

Levine, D. N., & Finkelstein, S. (1982). Delayed psychosis after right hemisphere parietal stroke or trauma: Relation to epilepsy. *Neurology, 32*, 267–273.

Orzack, M. H., Kornetsky, C., & Freeman, H. (1967). The effects of daily administration of carphenazine on attention in the schizophrenic patient. *Psychopharmacologia* (Berlin), *11*, 31–38.

Rapaport, D., Gill, M. M., & Schafer, R. (1968). In R. Holt (Ed.), *Diagnostic psychological testing*. New York: International Universities Press. (Original work published 1946)

Solovay, M., Shenton, M., Johnston, M. H., Gasperetti, C., & Holzman, P. S. *The Thought Disorder Index revised*. Submitted for publication.

Spitzer, R. L., & Endicott, J. (1978). *Schedule for affective disorders and schizophrenia - Lifetime version*. New York: Biometrics Research, New York State Psychiatric Institute.

Spitzer, R. L., Endicott, J., & Robins, E. (1978). Research diagnostic criteria: Rationale and reliability. *Archives of General Psychiatry, 35*, 773–782.

Spohn, H. E., Lacoursiere, R. B., Thompson, K., & Coyne, L. (1977). Phenothiazine effects on psychological and psychophysiological dysfunction in chronic schizophrenia. *Archives of General Psychiatry, 34*, 633–644.

Watkins, J. G., & Stauffacher, J. C. (1952). An index of pathological thinking in the Rorschach. *Journal of Projective Techniques, 16*, 276–286.

Wing, J. K. (1970). A standard form of psychiatric present state examination (PSE) and a method for standardising the classification of symptoms. In S. H. Hare & J. K. Wing (Eds.), *Psychiatric Epidemiology*, London: Oxford University Press.

General Discussion

Dr. Samuel Keith:* I would like to compliment today's presenters. I have been very much impressed by the clarity, the creativity and the integrative nature of their papers. I have not always felt this way about the area of attention, perception, and cognition, and when Dr. Alpert first asked me to chair this session, I had a déjà vu to my entrance to the NIMH some ten years ago when I was asked to prepare a review of this field, and about two-thirds of the way through this review, which fortunately never saw the light of day, I become so overwhelmed that even applying Dr. Andreasen's suggestions of serial analysis or even global analysis to it still failed understanding.

What I was struck by was that it seemed to me that no matter how complex the data turned out to be, a theory could be generated that could explain it, and somehow I found that a little bit like the argument between the proponent and the opponent of the death penalty, where the proponent said, "You know, if you execute somebody, he'll never kill another person," to which the opponent said, "But suppose you execute an innocent man?" To which the proponent then responded, "Still works." I think the field has indeed progressed beyond the "still works" potential, and I think the people who presented in this session are indeed responsible. The careful, incisive criticism of the methodologies that was put forth by the Chapmans in the mid-1970s, the scholarly consolidation of many of the areas in written work by Dr. Nuechterlein, and the application of intuitive and clinical relevance to research instrumentation and interpretation by Dr. Andreasen, and finally, the integrating and synthesizing translation of the potentially exciting new findings into a relevant framework for cognitive research by Dr. Holzman, I think has brought this field enormously forward.

Today's presentations represent an excellent sampling, of the current work being done in the field, but we should not forget where the field has been, and in turning this program back to the people you actually came to hear, I would like to ask them where it is going and how, perhaps, it can be integrated with some of the other discussions that we have heard. So in

* Rockville, Maryland.

responding to questions, I'd like for them to consider the future direction of the field, and now I would like to open the floor to general discussion questions.

Dr. Gerald Rosenbaum:* I had a question for Phil Holzman. Considering all of the effort and clinical skill that goes into the use of the TDI (and it is a very thoughtful instrument), it was a little disappointing to me to see how much the TDI index improved with the neuroleptic treatment. Particularly because many of us think of indices of thought disorder as very fundamental to schizophrenia, and we have been looking for markers of schizophrenia. Hence, it was kind of disappointing to see that the thought disorder score was reduced so much with neuroleptic treatment. Now, since Dr. Holzman has done such a clever job in his presentation of separating out the manic component of thought disorder from the schizophrenic component by variables such as amount of associative flow, some empirical factors, and some post hoc factors, I wonder if applying that same analysis to the data you have on the neuroleptic treatment research would result in less drop in the thought disorder index, if you pulled out the manic component.

Dr. Philip S. Holzman†: Yes, I think you raise a very good point. There is another slide, which I did not show, from Steve Hurt's data. That slide shows that even though there is a remarkable drop in the thought disorder index as a result of these neuroleptic treatments, the thought disorder index does not descend to the levels of the normal nonpsychotic, population. It remains elevated, not by terribly much, but it is statistically significantly elevated above normal levels. It would seem to me, therefore, that the thought disorder index reflects two processes: it reflects a state variable and a trait variable, and it is as yet, hard to tease them out separately. When somebody is acutely psychotic the Thought Disorder Index probably is inflated, thus reflecting state variables.

When there is a remission or a settling down of the acute psychosis, there is still an elevation of thought disorder, which may indicate the enduring, state, aspects of this process.

Dr. Rosenbaum: I'm wondering whether the state component might not be this manic component you have pulled out.

Dr. Holzman: I would tend to doubt that, but we haven't done that kind of study. What you are asking for is a study that applies these factors to patients in remission, and we don't have that information.

Dr. Rosenbaum: Thank you.

Dr. Ann Hardesty‡: When I was in graduate school, of course Rapaport *et al.*'s book was biblical, and liturgy was very much similar to some of the thought, the sort of variables you've listed, and I was delighted to see

* Detroit, Michigan.

† Cambridge, Massachusetts.

‡ New York, New York.

the way you've handled them and some of the results. More particularly, the answers from patients that you demonstrated show how clearly a Rorschach can pull out this kind of material—and you've classified it. I think that's nice.

My question to you is twofold: One is the same one that the previous questioner asked: since a lot of us who have been involved in quantitative measurement have looked at follow-ups in drug studies and have found thought disorders, most of them intractable to haloperidol, including haloperidol intervention, I was surprised at the results.

Second, I was wondering, since delusional material and the kind of Rorschach answers that you used were very verbal with very much output, if haloperidol may indeed reduce the verbal output and reduce the indices of thought disorders.

Dr. Holzman: To take the last one first, Dr. Hardesty, there is a way of controlling the TDI for verbal output. The unit thought disorder here is longer than the word and shorter than the response. So something in between those two events has to be used as a divisor, that is, one must divide the total amount of thought disorder by verbal output. As a matter of fact, verbal output seems to make no difference in acutely disturbed patients or recently hospitalized patients. It makes a lot of difference in the chronic, so-called process schizophrenic, where there is a paucity of verbal productivity. If you control for verbal productivity by dividing by the number of Rorschach responses, which seems to me better than by the number of words, then you do get a very reliable index of the amount of thinking disorder. A chronic schizophrenic can produce one clear neologism in five responses, and the patient won't give you any more. But one neologism will give you a very high thought disorder index once verbal productivity is taken into account, oddly enough.

Dr. Nancy C. Andreasen:* Listening to the questions, one of the problems I think we have in talking about thought disorder is treating it globally. Why does the thought disorder go up or down? In fact, what Phil [Holzman] has been doing, what I have been doing, has been trying to dissect apart kinds of thought disorder, and I really think we have to orient our thinking more that way—what kind of thought disorder responds to neuroleptics, what doesn't respond—and tease those things apart. Otherwise, we are just going to keep on with this muddle—we expect it to be a state, we expect it to be a trait, we expect it to respond or not to respond. So what I am trying to do—to characterize more specifically the kinds of thought disorder, language, abnormality, or whatever.

* Iowa City, Iowa.

Dr. Solomon C. Goldberg:* My question is mainly to Phil Holzman. There is other evidence on the basis of clinically judged thought disorder, in an article by Kendler and Hayes, showing that thought disorder occurs mainly in patients who have a positive family history for schizophrenia—that is, in those patients with a higher genetic loading. Keith Nuechterlein pointed out two studies on the CPT, showing that it too is associated with positive family history. It would appear that these two variables—thought disorder and CPT—may be associated with a higher genetic loading. I wonder if you had any opportunity to see what the relationship is between thought disorder and family history for schizophrenia. Second, I wonder whether there's any association between CPT and thought disorder.

Dr. Holzman: Excuse me, Sol. The two variables being what? The genetic loading and the thought disorder?

Dr. Goldberg: Yes, but also add the CPT. I'm wondering if you had any opportunity to look at that or whether anyone knows of any relationship between CPT and thought disorder and genetic loading for schizophrenia.

Dr. Holzman: I can tell you about CPT and eye tracking. There's no relationship there. But I can't tell you about CPT and thought disorder. I can tell you about families, but I cannot address the issue of whether there is a positive relationship between so-called genetic loading and the amount of thought disorder or the quality of thought disorder in the patients. I don't know the answer to that. I think it would be very difficult for us, perhaps impossible, to address that question with the sample that we have, because at McLean Hospital we have a very small number of parents with a positive history of schizophrenia, not because there is generally, a small number of parents with schizophrenia, but because of the kinds of samples that McLean Hospital draws. They tend to draw people from the middle classes and the upper middle classes who are relatively well put together to begin with. So they have screened out those people who can address the issue that you raise. I would say it's a dandy question, but our data can't address it.

Dr. Keith H. Nuechterlein†: Could I make a comment on that? I'm happy to say that we have collected the data to answer your first question. We have collected data on two different versions of the CPT and on Dr. Holzman's thought disorder index. We haven't analyzed it yet, but we should be able to address that issue soon.

Dr. Goldberg: So it is unproven. I had another question about your factor analysis and whether there is any difference in the factors in the way they respond to drugs?

* Richmond, Virginia.

† Los Angeles, California.

Dr. Holzman: I don't know. This is brand new, and that's certainly something that has to be done. We have not analyzed how these factors respond to neuroleptic treatment.

*Dr. Nina Schooler**: This is for Phil Holzman also. First, I just want to offer an interpretation of your finding of a correlation between the GAS score and your thought disorder index. It might be simply that, to the clinicians who are rating, who are making a global assessment, the kinds of things that you are picking up in the thought disorder index may seem to them to be particularly pathognomonic of schizophrenia. That may be why you find a significant correlation for that population and not for the others. A propos of that, I was wondering if you applied the index to any other verbal corpus other than the Rorschach and whether it does work. You mentioned early on that it was equally applicable.

Dr. Holzman: I am very pleased to have that interpretation, that we are dealing with a contaminated variable. It's terrible to be dealing with variables that may not be independent, but I guess that's the way the cookie has crumbled. Nevertheless, the TDI does make explicit what may be implicit in the BPRS & GAS ratings. Yes, we are using the thought disorder index with another kind of discourse. We are studying, in collaboration with Drs. Kety, Kinney, Jacobsen, and Schulsinger, the Danish adoption sample. For a variety of reasons, we were forbidden to administer the Rorschach test to the Danish adoption sample. Instead, we have a collection of answers to a number of questions such as "What was the most exciting thing that happened to you?" and "What do you think about birth control?" There were 10 questions like that, and we have Danish translators, bilingual and quite good, who are going over these protocols with us in order to see what is there, and I can tell you that in some of the protocols there is a lot of thought disorder that you can score in exactly the same way as the Rorschach. I was surprised, because I had been a little worried about it, but we've been scoring them for about a year now, and you can do it.

Dr. Jeff Mattes†: I have a question for Dr. Nuechterlein. Of course, one of the difficulties with the theory that schizophrenics have attentional problems, which you try to address, is that hyperactive children have attentional problems, now called attention deficit disorder. Your results with hyperactive children varied somewhat from study to study. You are using the CPT, which is typically a test for attention problems. Although you've modified it somewhat, I wasn't clear whether your conclusion is that the deficit you found in schizophrenics is not an attentional difficulty, or whether it's something other than attentions that you're measuring with your modified CPT?

* Bethesda, Maryland.
† Belle Meade, New Jersey.

Dr. Nuechterlein: I think the difficulty that you're talking about has a lot to do with the definition of attention and the amorphous quality of the concept. Actually, based on data that I didn't have a chance to present, we still believe that the nature of the deficit in hyperactive children is likely to be somewhat different than that in schizophrenic individuals and in persons at risk for schizophrenia. As I pointed out, the consistency across our two studies with hyperactive children involves the response criterion index. Hyperactive children set the cutting score for responding lower than normal children, but children at risk for schizophrenia use normal response criterion levels. The signal/noise discrimination index, also called perceptual sensitivity, in one study did not show significant overall deficit among the hyperactive children; in another it did at some age levels and not at others. Signal/noise discrimination was impaired among children at risk for schizophrenia.

My sense of this (we've written about this issue in the *Schizophrenia Bulletin*, 1984, Vol. 10, Issue 2) is that if you examine the deficit across tasks in subjects at risk for schizophrenia, the deficit appears to be related to the momentary processing load of the task. That concept is a little difficult to explain very briefly, but processing load involves a very specific meaning of the word attention, in which the key element is the extent to which a task can be performed without interfering with other simultaneous cognitive processing.

I would argue that the data from a number of tasks right now suggest that high processing load might be a common factor. The total amount of possible shared processing, which may reflect the total amount of available processing capacity in the terms of some modern cognitive theorists, may be decreased in schizophrenia. The total pool of processing capacity might be normal, but the allocation to specific task-relevant stimuli is decreased.

I think that it is likely that hyperactivity is characterized by a somewhat different deficit that doesn't have as much to do with momentary processing load. However, I really can't tell you at this moment exactly how to characterize that difference, except for the observation that the response criterion cut-off is lowered among hyperactive children.

Dr. Marty Harrow:* I want to point out a discrepancy between Nancy [Andreasen's] and Phil [Holzman's] data. Nancy noted how the schizophrenics stay high in thought disorder over time, at least for some period, whereas the manic go down. Now, when Phil presented Steve Hurt's dissertation from his research program, basically thought disorder went down with phenothiazine and with treatment. With our data, we also find that schizophrenics seem to go down in thought disorder over time, although many of them

* Chicago, Illinois.

don't reach normal levels, and there is still a certain percentage flagrantly thought disordered after the acute phase. I was wondering, Nancy, if you were using a more chronic sample or you had any thoughts about it.

Dr. Andreasen: I doubt that I have a more chronic sample, because I don't know your patients that well, but I think our three groups are probably relatively similar. These are people who come into the hospital for a period of time and go back to the community, some of them returning to work and functioning and some of them not.

What I showed was that in a subset of schizophrenics, the hebephrenics, the thought disorder didn't go down, and in particular, it was a kind of thought disorder, a negative thought disorder, that didn't diminish, and that's why I think it is important that we look at both kinds of schizophrenia and kinds of thought disorder, so that we know what it is that we are actually saying, not globally that schizophrenics do or don't improve or thought disorder does or doesn't improve, but what can we predict about this kind of schizophrenic with this kind of language or thinking abnormality.

Dr. Holzman: There are some additional data. Carla Solomon did a test–retest study in which she examined patients from the state hospital, the very chronic patients, and McLean patients. I think there was about a 6- to 9-month interval between test and retest. She found that in the McLean schizophrenics, thought disorder did go down, but in the chronically hospitalized state hospital patients, there was no significant change over those months.

So it's possible that if global thought disorder stays up, that you are dealing with the more intractible trait-related disorders or something like that.

SECTION FOUR

OTHER ASPECTS OF PHENOMENOLOGY

13

The Signs and Symptoms of Schizophrenia

MURRAY ALPERT
New York University Medical Center

We set a difficult task for ourselves when we attempt to define schizophrenia solely in terms of behavioral signs and symptoms. It might be useful to compare this problem with the situation at the end of the last century in regard to the diagnosis of neurosyphilis. Here, a definitive diagnosis could be made in postmortem tissue. I have heard, but have not been able to locate the reference, that when Wassermann's serological procedure was introduced in 1906 there was a sharp decrease in the frequency of the diagnosis of late syphilis, to about one-half of the rate of the previous year. Although the serology is vulnerable to false negatives, it appears that some patients, perhaps a significant portion, were misdiagnosed when diagnosis was based solely on clinical signs and symptoms.

Today it is felt that late syphilis is not difficult to diagnose from its clinical features, although no one would be willing to forego the available laboratory procedures. In contrast with syphilis, in schizophrenia a postmortem examination is not helpful. To characterize the disorder we are totally dependent on clinical signs and symptoms. It is sobering to consider how often patients are misdiagnosed.

In Appendix F of DSM-III (American Psychiatric Association, 1980), Williams and Spitzer have provided an estimate of the interrater reliability of field-trial tests of the new, criterion-based approach to diagnosis. In regard to the schizophrenic disorders, kappas of .81 are reported for each of two trials. The overall kappa for diagnoses on axis I was about .7. Affective disorders did not fare better than did schizophrenia.

An imperfect reliability of measurement sets a limit on the validity of measurement. Guidelines for the minimally acceptable interrater reliability for the evaluation of nominal categories are not hard and fast, but .81 is not overly reassuring. It seems inevitable that many patients are misclassified. With the most optimistic view, many of the patients included in the studies reported at this meeting as schizophrenic would not have been included in this category if we had a serological test for this disorder. However, compared with the clinical exigencies, researchers frequently have the luxury of discarding doubtful cases, when they know they are doubtful.

Some of our difficulty in identifying markers and traits for schizophrenia may be related to the likelihood that our study populations are heterogeneous for the condition. Efforts to improve diagnostic precision would seem of the highest priority and DSM-III is a response to such concerns. But questions about diagnosis tend to be referred to committees, and the committees have sought consensus rather than attempting to develop empirical approaches. This is not to belittle the accomplishments of DSM-III. The task was enormous, with extensive economic and social implications. However, it seems that greater emphasis could have been placed on efforts to develop objective measures in areas where they are clinically important and technologically feasible.

For example, central to decisions as to whether a patient is showing signs of mania or retarded depression or Type 2 schizophrenia is the patient's speech rate. But speech rates are never measured. An internist who reported bradycardia without noting the pulse rate, or fever without reporting the temperature, would not be viewed favorably. To my knowledge, no clinician has ever reported the rate of speech of a patient described as showing disturbance in speech productivity. The operations for making such measurements are straightforward and the explanation of the lack of interest in this direction seems most directly attributable to a charismatic view of psychiatric diagnosis.

There is a pervasive feeling in psychiatry that clinically important phenomena reside primarily in the intrapsychic experience of our patients, and that access to this experience depends on subjective report. In regard to the functional psychoses, this is not so. Most of the phenomena that are important in the evaluation of schizophrenic patients reside in the signs, not the symptoms, of the disorder. This may be seen, for example, in one of the most used of the clinical rating instruments, the Brief Psychiatric Rating Scale (BPRS) (Overall & Gorham, 1962). We train raters to use this scale and, in order to improve rating reliability, have developed operations for specifying the phenomena referred to by the various scales.

Table 1 contains the behavioral referent system that we use. Only 5 of the 18 scales are symptoms in the usual sense that they are evaluated solely through the subjective report and complaint of the patient. It might be argued that even the 5 exceptions may be construed as showing some "sign-like" quality, for example, the arbitrary separation of anxiety and tension, or the shading off between sign and symptom for depression. I will return to the issue of hallucinations subsequently, but note at this point that some clinicians feel that they can detect hallucinations in patients who deny that they are present.

The point of my emphasis on the prevalence of signs in the characterization of schizophrenia refers to that distinction between signs and symptoms

Table 1. Behavioral Referents for the Brief Psychiatric Rating Scale

Scales	1	2	3	4	5
1. Somatic Concern	X				
2. Anxiety	X				
3. Emotional Withdrawal			X	X	X
4. Conceptual Disorganization		X	X		
5. Guilt Feelings	X				
6. Tension				X	X
7. Mannerisms and Posturing				X	X
8. Grandiosity		X	X		
9. Depressive Mood	X	X	X	X	
10. Hostility		X	X		
11. Suspiciousness		X	X		
12. Hallucinatory Behavior	X	X			
13. Motor Retardation				X	X
14. Uncooperativeness		X	X		
15. Unusual Thought Content		X	X		
16. Blunted Affect			X	X	X
17. Excitement			X	X	X
18. Disorientation		X	X		

1 = Symptom based on subjective report and complaint
2 = Based on content, but not purely subjective or purely complaint
3 = Based on relation between what is said and manner of speaking or responsiveness to question
4 = Based on infra-content talking behavior
5 = Based on posture, movements, facies, appearance

that contrasts their objective and subjective origin. Signs are objective, observable and, at least potentially, are accessible to measurement. Where there has been an attempt at measurement in psychopathology it has been directed largely at observationally inaccessible phenomena such as through the use of word association tests, reaction times, or evoked potentials. An exception may be seen in the measurement of intelligence. The many rating scales and forms in use are, largely, convenient instruments for quasi-quantitative and comprehensive recording of the clinician's impressions.

This is not to deny that the clinician's impressions are a rich and efficient system for processing a very complex data set. My argument is that measurement of the behaviors that are the signs of the disorder will improve diagnostic precision and, potentially, understanding of their underlying processes.

There is a second source of difficulty in the development of a systematic approach to the study of the phenomena of schizophrenia, and that is a tacit assumption that the signs of the disorder reflect phenomena that are discontinuous with those seen in normals. This "discontinuity" hypothesis has discouraged investigators from using available behavioral science techniques in the study of the behavioral signs of schizophrenia; to relate hallucinations to perceptual mechanisms, for example, or to study thought disorder as a cognitive variant. There have been some exceptions to this, of course, as in the psycholinguistic approach to thought disorder, but these studies appear more as exceptions that prove the rule.

In our labs we have been trying to measure disturbances in feeling, and view the use of acoustic measures of voice as a reasonable analogy to study of fever with a thermometer, albeit a fairly complex thermometer. In our first studies we found that clinicians could judge disturbances in mood and affect from an audio recording of an interview about as well as they could from a face-to-face contact (Alpert, Hekimian, & Frosch, 1966). The clinically relevant information that is present visually appears to be redundant with the fairly complete set of cues relevant to disturbed feelings encoded in the acoustic energy recordable on an audio cassette. We were interested in the observation that our raters could judge depression, pressure of speech, and flat affect even from segments of interviews where the patient was not discussing personally significant events. This suggested that the information was encoded in the manner of talking rather than what was said.

In other studies we found that it was useful to distinguish between affects, moods, and emotions (Alpert, 1982). Affects appear to be encoded in voice through patterns of emphasis, utilizing stress, inflection, and timing to highlight salient words. Flat affect appears as a failure to vary stress, pitch, and rhythm in ways that help the listener appreciate the differential values of the different words being said. It may be fair, if a little extreme, to suggest that affects are to talking as associated movements are to walking. This definition should include facial and gestural activity as well as voice.

This is not to suggest that flat affect necessarily reflects a lesion of the basal ganglia. Although patients with Parkinson's disease show the stigmata of flat affect (Alpert & Rush, 1983), there are also cortical lesions that disturb the expression and perception of feelings. Ross and Mesulam (1979) have speculated that mechanisms underlying prosodic aspects of production and perception of speech are distributed across structures of the "minor" hemisphere in a manner analogous to the organization of the "phasias" on the "major" hemisphere.

In a study of flat affect that Mayer (1983) did for her doctoral dissertation, a cohort of 48 RDC chronic schizophrenics, half in hospital continuously for at least 18 months, the other half out of hospital continuously for at least 3 years, were evaluated. All were on neuroleptic medication. The patients were examined on a number of measures in an attempt to identify predictors of global ratings on Andreasen's scale for rating flat affect (1979a).

Using a multiple-regression model, we were able to show that the following measures independently contributed significant efficiency to the prediction: a measure of extrapyramidal disturbance using a modification of the Simpson–Angus Scale (Simpson & Angus, 1970); a measure of retarded depression based on our pause-duration measure from the acoustic analysis of the patient's voice (Alpert, 1982); and a measure of right-hemisphere dysfunction using the Benton, Van Allen, Hamsher, and Levin (1978) test of face recognition.

A number of issues are raised by these observations, assuming that they can be replicated. The behavioral signs of flat affect, manifest in immobile face and lack of gestures, can be a reflection of the retardation seen in depression or a product of neuroleptic side effects as well as an aspect of schizophrenia. One of the items in the Andreasen scale, that concerning slowed speech, probably adds to confounding the differentiation of flat affect and depression. We have not found that flat-affect schizophrenics talk slowly. They do not speak very much and they tend to speak softly, as do patients with Parkinson's disease (Alpert & Rush, 1983). Clinicians may confuse slowed speech with poverty of speech, and measurement of the speech rate and voice level would be useful here. Slowed speech (really increase pause time) should be reserved for the evaluation of retarded depression.

Incidently, we do not find that disturbed eye contact, another of the items in Andreasen's scale, is related to flat affect in schizophrenia, nor is it defective in Parkinsonian patients (Alpert & Rush, 1983). It may be that restricting flat affect to associated aspects of communication would help to purify the measure clinically, although multiple brain mechanisms could still be implicated.

Differentiating depression from flat affect is both important and difficult. The glossary of DSM-III (American Psychiatric Association, 1980) advises us that "affect is to mood as weather is to climate" (p. 353), which is the sort of definition that helps those who are helped by that sort of definition. A clinical approach to this differential is suggested by a study by Levin, Hall, Knight, and Alpert (in press) in which vocal and verbal aspects of expression of positive and negative feelings were evaluated in a small sample of schizophrenics, depressives, and controls. The results could be interpreted as suggesting that the depressives were defective in the vocal expression of positive but not negative feelings, whereas the schizophrenics failed to produce vocal samples that could be reliably identified in either the positive or negative direction. It may be useful, when attempting to differentiate flat affect from a mood disorder, to examine the patient while discussing both sad and glad events.

Our evidence (Alpert & Anderson, 1977), suggesting that affects are language-related behaviors, is provocative because it appears, then, that all of the cardinal signs of schizophrenia implicate a defect in language processing. Few would object to the suggestion that some sort of a disturbance in language function is implicated in thought disorder. The role of language in schizophrenic auditory hallucinations has not often been stressed. Bear in mind that these are *always* verbal hallucinations in which the patients hear people talking to them. I will attempt to show later in this chapter that schizophrenic hallucinations have other important language-related characteristics.

At this point we emphasize that disturbances in aspects of language function are implicated in flat affect, thought disorder, and hallucinations. This convergence on language may help guide the search for pathophysiological processes in schizophrenia toward language-integrating mechanisms. Aspects of minor-hemisphere language processing are suggested by flat affect and auditory hallucinations, and an argument could be developed for such a contribution to certain aspects of disordered thought. Some investigators have guided their search for disturbed brain function through analysis of dopaminergic tracts or study of limbic structures, based on the premise that schizophrenia is an emotional disorder or that there is an underlying hyperdopaminergia (Alpert & Friedhoff, 1980). It was Bleuler (1911/1950) who first emphasized the central role of language processing in schizophrenia, and our study of the psychopathology of schizophrenia would suggest that brain scientists attend to minor-hemisphere language areas.

Returning to our discussion of hallucinations, we investigated the characteristics of hallucinations as we manipulated suggestion and arousal. Subjects were in a sound-isolated room, wore headphones that had an acoustic seal, and heard varying levels of white noise. They were interrogated every 5 minutes as to what they had heard. We were confident that they could not actually hear anything from outside the room. One group was of schizophrenics who had never reported hallucinations. There were two groups of hallucinating schizophrenics in this study, one in a high and the other in a low suggestion-to-hallucinate condition, and, also, a group of alcoholics who had hallucinated on the current admission.

The nonhallucinating schizophrenics reported hearing things in our experimental situation, but never intelligible words. They heard footsteps, or hammering, perhaps even a voice. We rated the reported hallucinations on a scale in which 1 was assigned to an unidentifiable sound, 2 to an identifiable sound but not a voice, 3 to an unintelligible voice, 4 to words that were intelligible but not personally meaningful; 5 to a personally significant message; and 6 to occasions in which subject conversed with the hallucinated voice.

Four of the 10 nonhallucinating schizophrenics reported non-object-bound perceptions, but none received a score above 2 on the scale. The two groups with clinical hallucinations had verbal hallucinations. Suggestion increased the frequency but not the score on the scale with which we measured the verbal elaborateness of the messages. For the schizophrenics, hallucinations tended to occur more frequently at the moderate levels of white noise. In fact, the hallucinated schizophenics were very sensitive to the higher level of white noise. Significantly more of this group said that they could not tolerate the noise and requested to withdraw from the experiment, compared to the alcoholic and nonhallucinated schizophrenic groups. The alcoholic group hallucinated more frequently as the white noise became louder, suggesting to us that the hallucinogenic mechanism might overlap with their disturbance in arousal.

As part of this series of studies we also made an audio recording of a series of brief phrases. We varied the intelligibility of the phrases by adjusting a low-pass filter so that some of the phrases could be understood at less than a 10% rate, some at about 50%, and the others at about a 90% rate. Thus, intelligibility could be varied independently of the signal-to-noise ratio of the phrases. The subject's task was simply to report what was heard.

Hallucinating schizophrenics differed from nonhallucinators in the nature of the errors they made while performing this task and, also, in the confidence with which their errors were offered. The hallucinators produced errors that were more semantically constrained. They were coherent phrases that tended to be quite remote from the stimulus phrase. And they were inappropriately confident that they were right when they were wrong. The errors of the nonhallucinators had a different quality. They tended to preserve fragments of the stimulus phrase, and their confidence was more closely correlated with their accuracy.

In an interesting extension of this work, Bash used the tape with a group of 30 malingerers (Bash & Alpert, 1980). These were subjects remanded to the forensic service at Bellevue for pretrial examination who complained of hearing voices. The impression of the forensic psychiatrists, arrived at independently of our procedures, was that these subjects were not hallucinating. They were compared with another group, also 30 subjects, who complained of hearing voices and who were felt to be schizophrenic and hallucinating. Although there were 4 false positives and 4 false negatives, the groups could be separated on the basis of this measure with a phi coefficient of .73, rejecting the null hypothesis that the two groups had the same response style at a probability less than .0001. Even hallucinations, which on the BPRS are considered a symptom and rated on the basis of the patient's subjective report, may be accessible to objective measurement procedures.

Thus, instead of viewing hallucinations as de novo phenomena or as a visitation, they can be examined within the context of auditory verbal processing. In an opportune study done at a military hospital, Johnson and Miller (1965) contrasted a group of hallucinators with one of nonhallucinators on the Army General Classification Test scores that were obtained when their patients were first inducted into the army, and before they developed schizophrenia. The groups were found to be different before they became ill, with those who eventually developed hallucinations showing a relative impairment on verbal scores. Two observations seem apt. First, the results suggest that personality variables, which appear to be unrelated to the disease process, may contribute to the development of signs and symptoms of schizophrenia. Second, the findings support the impression that there is a language-related locus for the genesis of hallucinations.

Similar arguments could be made in the complex area of thought disorder. In her scale to assess thought, language, and communication disorders, Andreasen (1979b) has attempted to define and systematize the evaluation of this group of disorders. As we inspect this scale we find a heterogeneous list of phenomena. For example, speaking too little or too much are both included. Easily losing the thread of a theme or sticking too persistently to a theme are also variations of disordered thought. Word salad, alogia, and derailment seem so different from one another that it is not clear how they can be alternate manifestations of the same process. What seems disturbed is, as Andreasen suggests by the title of her scale, communication.

In an ingenious study, Cohen, Nachmani, and Rosenberg (1974) developed experimental control of a communication network by asking subjects to describe stimuli of controlled similarity, thus controlling task difficulty. Schizophrenics were as competent as controls when decoding the descriptions, but proved defective when encoding. Schizophrenics were equally as puzzled as controls when trying to decode the transmissions of other schizophrenics. They could not even decode their own faulty transmissions.

Thus, the difficulty appears to reside somewhere in the encoding process. The schizophrenic, when encoding information, seems unable to appreciate the task of the listener, while able to function well when in the listener's role. When encodings are impoverished or pressured, when the thematic relations between one sentence and the next are too loose or too tight, the transfer of information is impaired. When this occurs in a clinical interview this disturbance in information flow is seen as a thought disorder.

Disorders of thought are generally divided into two parts, one in which the thoughts are unusual, overvalued, or delusional and another in which the formal structure of language is disturbed. The communication network paradigm that is the basis for Cohen and Camhi's experimental model focuses on the autistic aspects of thought disorder. It ignores the fact that for some schizophrenics the problem is not so much a lack of empathy with the audience as a lack of anything to say. It is not clear whether this alogia is a disturbance of language, thought, or communication.

We have been examining bilingual schizophrenics (Marcos & Alpert, 1980) to see how the thought disorder translates. Proficient bilinguals are of two types: the compound, who learned both languages in the context of the home, and the coordinate, who learned the two languages at different times and places. The coordinate bilingual has dual independent language systems. If the compound bilingual shows similar patterns of thought disorder in the two languages whereas the coordinate shows differences, the results might be seen as evidence for a locus of the disorder in language function rather than in the area of thought.

This observation invites a comment on an issue of considerable current vogue. At this meeting and in the literature many workers are busily sorting out positive and negative symptoms and relating them to presumably orthogonal disease processes. The negative symptoms are thought to be related to brain changes (Crow, 1980), the positive to hyperdopaminergia. The positive symptoms are "active," "productive," the negative symptoms "passive," "asocial." The separation between the two clusters is on an intuitive basis, although new statistical approaches (Lewine, Fogg, & Meltzer, 1983) may begin to permit some empirical tests.

We have discussed our discontent with the hyperdopaminergia model of schizophrenia (Alpert & Friedhoff, 1980) and we will not review that argument here. If the deficit state reflected in Parkinson's disease (Alpert & Rush, 1983) has anything to tell us about Type II schizophrenia, then a role for dopamine seems immanent. Why does no one wonder why Type I and Type II schizophrenia so frequently coexist? Aside from violating parsimony, the two-disease hypothesis appears to ignore biological and clinical interconnections between the two conditions.

We have considered the contribution of nondisease factors to the development of individual signs and symptoms of schizophrenia. Hallucinators differ from nonhallucinators before they develop schizophrenia. Knight, Roff, Barrnett, and Moss (1979) have shown that aspects of the deficit cluster can be identified in the primary-school records of schizophrenics perhaps a decade prior to the onset of the disorder. It is striking that the course of the disorder that eventually developed was predictable from the cluster of deficit symptoms that were detectable in the primary-school records. I don't know of similar predictors of thought disorder from measures collected prior to the development of schizophrenia, but as far as I am aware, this issue has not been pursued. Anyone who has had the humbling experience of correcting a transcription of their public comments must come away with the conviction that there is a high rate of disordered expression in nonclinical populations.

We sometimes fail to appreciate the importance of social contingencies in the maintenance, if not the origin, of the signs and symptoms of schizophrenia. I was interviewing a schizophrenic patient some time ago, trying to understand the process by which his hallucinations had stopped. They seemed to have faded away, first during the day, then during quiet times. As I pursued the issue he was reluctant to go into detail, and seemed dysphoric. I commented that he seemed sad when he discussed the voices and he said, "At least they were company." He missed them. If the consequences of the behavioral signs and symptoms are reinforcing, the signs may be perpetuated through mechanisms that differ from those involved in their origin. We have reported a study in which the frequency of hallucinations could be decreased through negative reinforcement (Anderson & Alpert, 1974) and Slade has reported a series of such studies (Slade, 1973, 1974).

In line with this observation, we studied schizophrenic hallucinators and nonhallucinators on a series of cognitive tasks in Bellevue Hospital, where we found that about half of the schizophrenics hallucinated. The study paradigm is a convenient one because both the experimental and the control groups share the assigned patient role, both are on neuroleptics, etc., and the study can be carried out with only modest intervention in the usual course of treatment of these patients. When my collaborator moved to the Veterans Administration (VA), we attempted to continue the studies there. We found plenty of hallucinating schizophrenics, but we could not find nonhallucinators.

We could not attribute the prevalance of hallucinations in the VA schizophrenic cohort to the obvious factors, such as the sex or the age of the subjects; nor did alcohol or substance abuse seem to be the likely factors. The admitting services at both facilities were staffed by the same group of psychiatric residents who were equally motivated at both facilities to discourage unnecessary admissions. One likely possibility is that the symptoms are responding to different contingency systems. In Bellevue, when the patient hallucinates they raise the dose. At the VA they raise the compensation.

I began this chapter by noting how dependent we are, in the study of schizophrenia, on the patient's clinical presentation. I lamented this dependence and suggested that it might be moderated if greater effort were directed toward the development of objective approaches to the assessment of the signs of the schizophrenic disorder. Such work might lead to a clearer separation between similar signs, such as the separation between flat affect and retarded depression. It might also lead to identification of different underlying mechanisms, such as the not-intuitively-obvious observation that flat affect is associated with difficulty on a neuropsychological task that estimates right-hemisphere function, whereas depression shows an inverse association with the same task. We have also pointed to the importance of further study of the relations between the signs of schizophrenia within the context of nondisease-related aspects of cognition, perception, and feelings. We must always, of course, contemplate our next grant renewal.

ACKNOWLEDGMENT

This work was supported in part by MH-37952 and MH-35976.

REFERENCES

Alpert, M. (1982). Encoding of feelings in voice. In P. J. Clayton & J. E. Barrett (Eds.) *Treatment of depression: Old controversies and new approaches*, (pp. 217–228). New York: Raven Press.

Alpert, M., & Anderson, L. T. (1977). Imagery mediation of vocal emphasis in flat affect. *Archives of General Psychiatry*, *34*, 208–212.

Alpert, M., & Friedhoff, A. J. (1980). An un-dopamine hypothesis of schizophrenia. *Schizophrenia Bulletin*, *6*, 387–390.

Alpert, M., Hekimian, L. J., & Frosch, W. A. (1966). Evaluation of treatment with recorded interviews. *American Journal of Psychiatry*, *122*, 1258–1264.

Alpert, M., & Rush, M. (1983). Comparison of affects in Parkinson's disease and schizophrenia. *Psychopharmacology Bulletin*, *19*, 118–120.

American Psychiatric Association. (1980). *Diagnostic and statistical manual of mental disorders* (3rd ed., pp. 261–281). Washington, DC: APA.

Anderson, L. T., & Alpert, M. (1974). Operant analysis of hallucination frequency in a hospitalized schizophrenic. *Journal of Behavioral Therapy and Experimental Psychiatry*, *5*, 13–18.

Andreasen, N. C. (1979a). Affective flattening and the criteria of schizophrenia. *American Journal of Psychiatry*, *136*, 944–947.

Andreasen, N. C. (1979b). The clinical assessment of thought, language, and communication disorders. II. Diagnostic significance. *Archives of General Psychiatry*, *36*, 1325–1330.

Andreasen, N. C. (1981). *Scale for the assessment of negative symptoms*. Iowa City: Department of Psychiatry, University of Iowa College of Medicine.

Bash, I. Y., & Alpert, M. (1980). The determination of malingering. *Annals of the New York Academy of Sciences*, *327*, 86–99.

Benton, A. L., Van Allen, M. W., Hamsher, K. de S., & Levin, H. S. (1978). The test of facial recognition, form SL, Manual. Iowa City: Benton Laboratory of Neuropsychology, Division of Behavioral Neurology, University of Iowa.

Bleuler, E. (1950). *Dementia praecox, or the group of schizophrenias* (J. Zinkin, Trans.). New York: International Universities Press. (Original work published 1911)

Cohen, B. D., Nachmani, G., & Rosenberg, S. (1974). Referent communication in acute schizophrenia. *Journal of Abnormal Psychology*, *83*, 1–19.

Crow, T. J. (1980). Molecular pathology of schizophrenia: More than one disease process? *British Medical Journal*, *12*, 16–68.

Johnson, R. L., & Miller, M. D. (1965). Auditory hallucinations and intellectual deficit. *Journal of Psychiatric Research*, *3*, 37–41.

Knight, R. A., Roff, J. D., Barnett, J., & Moss, J. L. (1979). Concurrent and predictive validity of thought-disorder and affectivity: A 22-year follow-up of acute schizophrenics. *Journal of Abnormal Psychology*, *88*, 1–12.

Levin, S., Hall, J. A., Knight, R. A., & Alpert, M. (in press). Verbal and nonverbal expression of affect in speech of schizophrenic and affect disorder patients. *Journal of Abnormal Psychology*.

Lewine, R. R. J., Fogg, L., & Meltzer, H. Y. (1983). Assessment of negative and positive symptoms in schizophrenia. *Schizophrenia Bulletin*, *9*, 368–382.

Marcos, L., & Alpert, M. (1980). Bilingualism: Implications for the evaluation of psychopathology. In R. Reiber (Ed.), *Applied linguistics and mental health* (pp. 129–138) New York: Plenum Press.

Mayer, M. (1983, October). *The relation between right hemisphere cognitive processing and flat affect in a schizophrenic population*. Doctoral Dissertation, Department of Psychology at New York University's Graduate School of Arts & Science.

Overall, J. E., & Gorham, D. R. (1962). The brief psychiatric rating scale. *Psychological Reports*, *10*, 799–812.

Ross, E.D., & Mesulam, M. M. (1979). Dominant language functions of the right hemisphere? Prosody and emotional gesturing. *Archives of Neurology* (*Chicago*), *36*, 144–148.

Simpson, G., & Angus, J. (1970). A rating scale for extrapyramidal effects. *Acta Psychiatrica Scandinavica*, Supplementum *212*, 11–19.

Slade, P. D. (1973). The psychological investigation and treatment of auditory hallucinations: A second case report. *British Journal of Medical Psychology*, *46*, 293.

Slade, P. D. (1974). The external control of auditory hallucinations: An information theory analysis. *British Journal of Social and Clinical Psychology*, *13*, 73–79.

COMMENTARY

Dr. Alpert: I've been invited to take a few questions if there are some that are pressing in the audience. Yes?

Dr. Arnold J. Friedhoff:* I may be prejudiced, but I think that was a brilliant talk. I think Murray has delivered a message that is long overdue—that clinical psychiatry can move into the modern age, that we don't have to wait for the development of new technology to begin measuring things, and I congratulate him on conveying that message so effectively.

Dr. Alpert: Thank you, Arnold.

* New York, New York.

14

Clinical Definition of Negative Symptoms as a Reflection of Theory and Methodology

RICHARD J. LEWINE
Illinois State Psychiatric Institute and
University of Chicago Pritzker School of Medicine

ALISON A. SOMMERS
Illinois State Psychiatric Institute

INTRODUCTION

As pointed out by both Andreasen and Holzman (Chapters 11 and 12 in this volume), the study of schizophrenic phenomenology requires attention to delineated subcategories that presumably reflect underlying processes. In this chapter, we examine a specific aspect of negative symptoms, namely the conceptualization of "loss," and its theoretical contexts. In so doing we hope to demonstrate that the search for underlying processes must be preceded by careful articulation of theory.

The impetus for this chapter derives, in part, from our experiences in the implementation of a construct validation study of negative symptoms in schizophrenia. We have undertaken a systematic comparison of three currently available empirical scales for the assessment of negative symptoms: Scale for the Assessment of Negative Symptoms (SANS; Andreasen, 1981), Scale for Emotional Blunting (SEB; Abrams & Taylor, 1978), and Scales for the Assessment of Negative and Positive Symptoms based on the SADS-C (Lewine, Fogg, & Meltzer, 1983). In the process of training raters in the various methods we have encountered ambiguities, the sources of which have implications for the empirical study of schizophrenia in general. We have been forced to clarify item definition, identify anchors for judgments, and examine critically the theoretical contexts within which the different scales have been developed. Although the empirical study of negative symptoms is clearly approaching bandwagon proportions (as is evident in other chapters in this volume), as assessed by current empirical scales they represent considerable conceptual confusion, despite what at first blush appears to be at least operational clarity.

Some of this confusion regarding the definition and measurement of negative symptoms, as well as their differentiation from other similar syndromes, is due to the failure to articulate covert but omnipresent theory. Once we begin to articulate theory we quickly find a conflict having its roots in a Kraepelinian versus a Bleulerian conceptualization of schizophrenia. Additional confusion is created by unnecessary ambiguities in assessment that allow considerable individual freedom to raters in making their judgments and thereby lead to greater likelihood of rater bias. Finally, there is some ambiguity that is an inherent aspect of trying to measure something that is by definition not present.

NEGATIVE SYMPTOMS

Put most simply, negative symptoms represent the absence of normal functioning and are presumably specific to schizophrenia, although the latter is more implied than explicitly stated (Andreasen, Olsen, Dennert, & Smith, 1982; Strauss, Carpenter, & Bartko, 1974). For purposes of discussion, symptoms and signs can be arbitrarily divided into four domains: affect-arousal, physical, perception-cognition, and interpersonal. Table 1 summarizes various negative symptoms and signs based on a selected review of the literature (Abrams & Taylor, 1978; Andreasen, 1981; Astrup, 1979; Bleuler, 1978; Carpenter, Heinreichs, & Haulon, 1981; Crow, 1980; Fish, 1962, 1964; Haase, 1980; Huber, Gross, Schuttler, & Linz, 1980; Mackay, 1980; McGlashan, 1982); the items are ordered by our impression of their status as negative symptoms, with the most commonly cited ones in uppercase letters and the least-cited negative symptoms in lowercase letters.

The range of items listed under the rubric of negative symptom is rather wide. There are several items that are almost universally accepted as negative, such as blunted affect, loss of drive, and poverty of content of speech. Others, such as inappropriate affect, are included on all current empirical scales for the assessment of negative symptoms, but are more controversial in nature. Yet other symptoms, such as anxiety, sleep disturbance, and hypochondriasis, are only infrequently mentioned and are more commonly associated with affective syndromes.

A close examination of the published work in this area suggests the existence of two different literatures, an empirically oriented negative-symptom literature (Andreasen *et al.*, 1982; Crow, 1980; Lewine *et al.*, 1983) and a clinically oriented, deficit-state literature that emphasizes the characterological consequences of psychopathology (Astrup, 1979; Huber *et al.*, 1980; McGlashan, 1982). The misleading use of the terms negative

Table 1. Negative and Deficit-State Symptoms in Schizophrenia

AFFECT–AROUSAL	PERCEPTION–COGNITION
LOSS OF DRIVE, WILL BLUNTED ANHEDONIA EMPTY	POVERTY OF SPEECH BLOCKING POVERTY OF CONTENT CONSTRICTION OF IDEATIONAL FIELD
Inappropriate Fatigue	Impaired attention Impaired intellectual functioning Weakness of judgment
anxiety irritability subdepressive moods	incoherence compulsion to reflection hypochondriasis
PHYSICAL	**INTERPERSONAL**
RETARDED MOVEMENT DECREASED SPONTANEOUS MOVEMENT SLOWED SPEECH	WITHDRAWAL ACTIVE SECLUSION LOSS OF EMPATHY
Physical exhaustion Asthenia	
vegetative/sensorial disturbance hypersensitivity to noise sleep disturbance	

symptoms and deficit state as synonymous further muddies the conceptual waters, a point to which we shall return at the conclusion of this chapter.

The point we wish to emphasize here is that the lack of a clear, consensual boundary for the negative-symptom syndrome ultimately results in rating scales that vary in item composition (or operational definition) and hence in the constructs they attempt to assess; that they are all called *negative-symptom scales* does not eliminate this difference.

Despite this state of affairs, a lively controversy has arisen regarding the etiology and treatment of negative symptoms, especially in contradistinction to positive symptoms. Do negative and positive symptoms represent different aspects of the same process (Mackay, 1980) or do they represent different processes (Strauss *et al.*, 1974)? Do negative symptoms respond to medication (Meltzer, Chapter 7 in this volume) or not (Crow, 1980)? Are negative symptoms associated with enlarged ventricles, low platelet monoamine oxidase, or both? The ultimate answers to these questions require explication of the theoretical positions underlying the measurement of negative symptoms; in the absence of this, empirical findings are likely to be contradictory and difficult to interpret. What then are these theories?

KRAEPELIN

Kraepelin (1919/1971) stated quite explicitly that the loss of will (or the destruction of the individual's "inner psychic unity") was the "*real fundamental disorder* in dementia praecox" (p. 221, emphasis in original). Rather than address the thorny issue of "will," we can turn to Kraepelin's own partial operationalization of the concept as "the singular indifference of the patients towards their former emotional relations, the extinction of affection for relatives and friends, of satisfaction in their work and vocation, in recreation and pleasures. . . ." (p. 33). Today, the same phenomenon would be called *blunted affect:* literally nothing seems to matter to the patient and he gives every indication that he could tolerate any change in the environment without experiencing either dysphoria or pleasure. We can assume that the indifference and extinction of affection are permanent on the basis of Kraepelin's language (e.g. the "annihilation" rather than the "diminution" of will and affect) and on the fact that in his final text he discussed only nonrecovered cases.

A second feature of a Kraepelinian perspective on schizophrenia is the assumption of an underlying neurological dysfunction. Kraepelin listed many neurological signs, such as sluggish pupillary response, hyperresponsive reflexes, disequilibrium, tremors, aphasia, and nystagmus as occurring in dementia praecox. He even went so far as to suggest that this disease was due to a permanent loss of nerve tissue, probably in the frontal and temporal lobes. A Kraepelinian orientation, then, would lead us to emphasize the extinction or permanent loss of will as reflected in loss of affective ties and indifference to all aspects of functioning. This would require a longitudinal framework in which to assess deterioration without recovery.

BLEULER

In contrast to Kraepelin, who pointed to the loss of will or drive, Bleuler (1911/1950) emphasized the loss of *direction*; all the normal drives, affects, and intellectual functioning continue to exist, even if very difficult to demonstrate, but in the absence of clear goal orientation. If we think of the schizophrenic as analogous to a car, then for Kraepelin it is without an engine, whereas for Bleuler it lacks a driver. A striking example of how we would expect loss of goal orientation to be manifested clinically was provided by Andreasen (Chapter 11 in this volume) in her description of the schizophrenic's failure to generate organized discourse trees. Based on what would now be considered a naive associationist psychology, Bleuler quite clearly stated that schizophrenia was first and foremost a cognitive disorder and, more specifically, that a predisposition to cognitive loosening underlay every case of schizophrenia. This fundamental cognitive deficit interferes with the schizophrenic's ability to marshall his psychological and intellectual resources for the purpose of reaching well-defined goals.

In sharp opposition to Kraepelin, Bleuler believed that "there can be no doubt at all that the psyche's capacity to produce affects has not disappeared in schizophrenia" (1911/1950, p. 47). When blunting did appear, it was thought to be secondary to the cognitive disorder. Similarly, Bleuler argued that what characterized schizophrenia was neither uniform intellectual deterioration nor absolute inability to work, but rather an excessive variability of performance. Within a short period the schizophrenic might at one time be capable of successfully completing complex intellectual tasks while at other times not; work history might yield evidence not only of poor work performance, but also of a marked discrepancy between education/training and job status.

Bleuler exhibited considerable ambivalance of his own when addressing the etiology of schizophrenia. His most impassioned arguments were those for the importance of psychological factors, namely the loss of goal orientation or loosening of associational structures. In short, what is lost in schizophrenia is a presumed higher order cognitive function which results in variable performance, not necessarily a loss which is permanent.

ITEM SELECTION AS THEORY

Consider blunted affect, poverty of speech, inappropriate affect, and poverty of content of speech, four symptoms commonly accepted as negative symptoms and included in current empirical scales for their assessment. The first two (blunted affect and poverty of speech) easily fall under a Kraepelinian rubric of *extinction of function,* more specifically the extinction of affect and the extinction of speech. There is, in each case, an easily observed absolute loss of product, an absence of behavior. (We are assuming here, as did Kraepelin, that the absence of performance reflects loss of capacity.)

Inappropriate affect and poverty of content of speech reflect the loss of a presumed higher level of integration, a concept more Bleulerian and psychological in nature, as argued previously. In both of these negative symptoms there is adequate raw material (affect and speech), but a deficit in higher levels of integration that facilitate social communication. In the case of inappropriate affect, the integration of thought and affect is missing, whereas in poverty of content of speech, integration of cognitive functioning is missing as reflected in loss of meaning.

Two very different types of phenomena are included in a single construct, adversely affecting our efforts to validate the "negative-symptom" syndrome. Adopting for heuristic purposes the "Kraepelinian" versus "Bleulerian" distinction, we would expect symptoms such as blunted affect and poverty of speech to be associated with signs of permanent structural change such as cortical atrophy (as suggested in part by Crow, 1980), whereas symptoms such as inappropriate affect and poverty of content of speech might be expected to be associated with state-dependent process variables. Inclusion of both types of negative symptoms in a single additive scale confounds these theoretical predictions. Put simply, there is inherent in the current conceptualization of "negative symptoms" a confounding of a loss of quantity and a loss of quality, a distinction that ultimately may be arbitrary but which for immediate research purposes has many implications.

Having once accepted that the "loss" in negative schizophrenic symptoms may represent either quantity or quality, it then becomes difficult to defend the separation between negative thought disorder (e.g., poverty of content, alogia) and positive thought disorder (e.g., loosening of associations, incoherence). All schizophrenic thought disorder is characterized by poor *quality,* and thus would qualify as a negative symptom. Conversely, if we want to restrict negative symptoms to those that represent a quantitative loss of functioning, then current scales would have to delete symptom items to reflect this decision. In any event, careful consideration of what is meant by *loss* must necessarily result in a new generation of negative-symptom scales.

There is a resemblance between the view spelled out here and Crow's (1980) distinction between Type I and Type II syndromes. Type I is associated with positive symptoms (which include thought disorder), acute onset, good neuroleptic response, and a putative increase in dopamine receptors, whereas Type II is characterized by negative symptoms (affective blunting, poverty of speech, and loss of volition), chronic disorder, poor neuroleptic response, and presumed cell loss or structural changes in the brain. The Type II syndrome is clearly meant to reflect what we have labelled a quantitative loss and is consistent with a Kraepelinian perspective. The Type I syndrome, however, includes all thought disorder, one aspect of which is poverty of content of speech (a commonly accepted negative symptom) and, by inference, inappropriate affect. To the extent that such symptoms account for the responsiveness of negative symptoms to treatment, there is no discrepancy in empirical findings, but rather a difference in the label used for the symptoms. That is, there may well be general agreement that neuroleptics reduce poverty of content of speech, but disagreement about whether to call this a positive or a negative symptom. At this stage, argument about the "facts" of negative-symptom treatment may reflect semantic and theoretical confusion far more than differences in empirical findings.

IMPLICATIONS FOR RESEARCH

Some of these distinctions (Bleulerian vs. Kraepelinian theory, quantitative vs. qualitative loss, and structural vs. process dysfunctions) are necessarily arbitrary and in some respects ultimately false. It is recognized, for example, that there would be considerable overlap between the lists of negative symptoms generated by Bleuler and by Kraepelin. Furthermore, the truth value of any given theory is not at issue here; that is a matter for later empirical testing. Finally, we do not believe there is a single best way to conceptualize negative symptoms, but rather, that it is the process of comparing carefully defined and measured constructs that will lead to meaningful answers.

We suggest first of all that clear theoretical perspectives be adopted. There are at least two heuristics whose roots lie in Krapelinian and Bleulerian psychiatry, respectively, to which we could turn. However, a simple oath of loyalty to one or another is not sufficient; the appropriate measures must be employed, the logical predictions of adopting one theory over another must be spelled out, and when possible theories must be pitted against one another. Consider for example how we might address some of the issues raised in this chapter:

1. Create separate "negative symptom" scales to reflect quantitative and qualitative loss. Items such as poverty of speech, blunted affect, and loss of interest would be included on one scale, whereas items such as poverty of content of speech, loosening of associations, and inappropriate affect would appear on the other. Systematic comparison of such scales would generate theoretically meaningful results.

2. Selection of mathematical parameters for analysis can also follow from theory. For example, if our Kraepelinian theory predicts quantitative loss, then we might examine mean scores, whereas a Bleulerian theory that predicts variability might be better served by an examination of standard deviation or variance, a suggestion made 20 years ago by Wishner (1964).

3. Quantification of criterion variables would follow in similar fashion. Absolute work history is of importance within a Kraepelinian context, whereas the discrepancy between education and job status is of importance to a Bleulerian view. In studying the relationship between "negative symptoms" and work history, therefore, we would want to employ both an absolute measure of work functioning (such as that found in the Hollingshead–Redlich two-factor index of social competence) and a relative measure (such as the difference between education level and current job status).

4. If we had two types of negative-symptom scales (reflecting quantitative and qualitative loss), we would expect them to be differentially related to other clinical variables in a way predicted by the theories from

which they emerge. Kraepelinian negative symptoms should correlate more highly with signs of neurological disorder than should Beulerian negative symptoms, a hypothesis for which some evidence already exists (Crow, 1980).

Consideration of theories of psychopathology and of assessment also suggests that we engage in "testing the limits" in the assessment of negative symptoms. It has been argued that negative-type symptoms as assessed in the typical hospital setting are not a fundamental part of the disease process but rather a response to an unstimulating environment. It would be useful, therefore, to actually manipulate the social environment in an attempt to eliminate these types of symptoms. Put another way, unless we specifically attempt to test a patient's capability, we cannot know to what extent negative symptoms are a reflection of environmental contingencies. Distractor and high-versus-low incentive paradigms provide excellent models for such assessment of negative symptoms (Garmezy, 1974; Harvey, Winters, Weintraub, & Neale, 1981; Oltmanns, 1978).

A related need is the assessment of negative symptoms across situations and across domains. Current assessment procedures for negative symptoms assume consistency across situations and domains of assessment. A recent patient in our own study received the highest rating we have yet given on Abrams and Taylor's (1978) Scale for Emotional Blunting, yet was reported by ward staff to exhibit considerable enthusiasm, energy, and normal psychomotor behavior whenever she received a telephone call. In a psychiatric interview she would be called blunted, but clearly exhibited different behavior in a different setting. Negative-symptom scales such as Abrams and Taylor's and Lewine *et al.* (1983) will necessarily be restricted in comparison to scales that provide a broader range of situation sampling (such as the SANS).

An overlooked aspect of negative-symptom assessment (and, indeed, much clinical assessment in general) is the fact that the assessment interview is an interpersonal situation, one that by definition varies from interviewer to interviewer. It is clear from personality research that differences in interviewers can exert a powerful influence on the interviewee's behavior (Endler & Magnusson, 1976). Recall also that some have defined the deficit syndrome as the "expected minus the observed" (Carpenter, Chapter 3 in this volume), requiring someone to do the expecting, in his study "someone" being the clinicians. Therefore, individual differences among clinicians as to what is expected could have considerable impact on deficit-syndrome scores. Given that the assessment of negative symptoms requires the interviewer to provide emotional stimuli via his own affect in determining, for example, the patient's affective responsivity, it follows that negative-symptom scores are influenced by the genuineness and intensity of the interviewer's "pull" for affect. Although it might be argued that such individual differences in interviewers ought to be minimal compared to the gross distortions of cognition, affect, and behavior in psychopathology and should have little impact on the assessment of negative symptoms, we would urge that interviewer characteristics (including basic sociodemographic features at the very least) be regularly entered into negative-symptom analyses until it is demonstrated for a particular rating team that such differences do not matter. Ideally, ratings of the interviewer's affect and characteristics as a social stimulus would also be assessed and included in the data analyses.

Some of the ambiguity about the nature of negative symptoms lies in what has to date been the often-synonymous use of the terms *negative symptom* and *defect state*. We would suggest that the two are not the same but, rather, are related in the following way:

1. *Defect, end, or terminal states refer to pervasive changes in the personality.* A judgment of defect state implies consideration of the individual's global psychosocial competence, including social relationships, work performance, self-care, management of personal affairs, community role, etc. It is implicitly a molar, normative judgment of overall functioning that is the long-term outcome of unremitting negative symptoms in interaction with the social environment. As such, additional extraindividual factors may have a part in its determination (e.g., family support, labelling, reward contingencies within the welfare system, and employment opportunities). Negative symptoms are molecular psychiatric symptoms and signs. The concept of the defect state is a higher order construct than that of negative symptoms and is embedded in a richer, more multidimensional nomological net than the lower-order signs and symptoms.

2. *Defect states are longitudinal in nature, whereas negative symptoms are cross-sectional.* As emphasized by many clinicians, defect states represent a progressive deterioration in functioning, the assessment of which requires a developmental context. Negative symptoms may be assessed at any given point in time, with minimal reference to temporal change. Furthermore, defect states have been commonly believed to be immutable, although some clinicians have suggested that end states fluctuate. Nevertheless, we can expect that defect-state schizophrenics, having undergone extensive personality change and deterioration in functioning, will only rarely return to their full level of premorbid functioning.

Although negative symptoms have been described as chronic and inflexible (especially in contrast to positive symptoms), there is evidence that negative symptoms do respond to treatment albeit to a lesser degree and/or less rapidly than do positive ones. Although we believe that the malleability of both defect states and negative symptoms is open to empirical investigation, we would suggest that any single negative symptom implies far less about chronicity or inflexibility than the more global concept of defect state.

3. *Both positive and negative symptoms may be present in defect states.* Sometimes it is the reduction in affective responsivity to the positive symptom

that characterizes the defect state; at other times the positive symptoms themselves change. Fish (1962), for example, has described how the content of hallucinatory voices often becomes stereotyped in chronic defect states.

4. *Defect states and negative symptoms stand in a hierarchical, non-reflexive relationship to one another.* That is, a defect state always implies the presence of negative symptoms, but negative symptoms do not necessarily imply a defect state.

CONCLUSION

The empirical interest in negative symptoms is to be viewed with considerable enthusiasm by those who have argued over the years that the fundamental, complex aspects of schizophrenia reflected in negative symptoms have been overlooked because it has been easier to study positive symptoms (Kety, 1980). Because negative symptoms force us to operationalize concepts such as *will,* and to measure things (that are noteworthy by virtue of their absence) not easily translated into the language of empirical research, we must be especially careful to be as precise as possible. The worst possible outcome of our efforts to study negative symptoms empirically would be to forsake the complex for the simple, leaving us no closer to understanding the core process of schizophrenia than we are now.

ACKNOWLEDGMENT

Preparation of this chapter was supported in part by grants MH37898-01 and MH30095, both from the National Institute of Mental Health.

REFERENCES

Abrams, R., & Taylor, M. (1978). A rating scale for emotional blunting. *American Journal of Psychiatry, 135*, 226–229.

Andreasen, N. (1981). *Scale for the assessment of negative symptoms (SANS).* Iowa City: University of Iowa College of Medicine.

Andreasen, N., Olsen, S., Dennert, J., & Smith, M. (1982). Ventricular enlargement in schizophrenia: Relationship to positive and negative symptoms. *Archives of General Psychiatry, 139*, 297–302.

Astrup, C. (1979). *The chronic schizophrenias.* New York: Columbia University Press.

Bleuler, E. (1950). *Dementia praecox or the group of schizophrenias* (J. Zinkin, Trans.). New York: International Universities Press. (Original work published 1911)

Bleuler, M. (1978). *The schizophrenic disorders. Long-term patient and family studies* (S. Clemens, Trans.). New Haven, CT: Yale University Press.

Carpenter, W. T., Heinrichs, D. W., & Haulon, T. (1981). Methodologic standards for treatment outcome research in schizophrenia. *American Journal of Psychiatry, 138*, 465–471.

Crow, T. (1980). Molecular pathology of schizophrenia: More than one disease process? *British Medical Journal, 280,* 66–68.

Endler, N., & Magnusson, D. (1976). Toward an interactional psychology of personality. *Psychological Bulletin, 83,* 956–974.

Fish, F. (1962). *Schizophrenia.* Bristol: John Wright and Sons, Ltd.

Fish, F. (1964). A guide to the Leonhard classification of chronic schizophrenia. A followup study. *Psychiatric Quarterly, 38,* 1–13.

Garmezy, N. (1974). Children at risk: The search for the antecedents of schizophrenia. Part II. Ongoing research programs, issues, and intervention. *Schizophrenia Bulletin, 1,* 14–90.

Haase, H. (1980). Follow-up treatment and aftercare of discharged schizophrenic patients. *Schizophrenic Bulletin, 6,* 619-626.

Harvey, P., Winters, K., Weintraub, S., & Neale, J. (1981). Distractibility in children vulnerable to psychopathology. *Journal of Abnormal Psychology, 90,* 298–304.

Huber, G., Gross, G., Schuttler, R., & Linz, M. (1980). S. Clemens (Trans.). Longitudinal studies of schizophrenic patients. *Schizophrenia Bulletin, 6,* 592–605.

Kety, S. S. (1980). The syndrome of schizophrenia. Unresolved questions and opportunities for research. *British Journal of Psychiatry, 136,* 421–436.

Kraepelin, E. (1971). *Dementia praecox and paraphrenia.* (R. Barclay Trans.). Huntington, NY: Krieger Publishing. (Originally published 1919)

Lewine, R., Fogg, L., & Meltzer, H. (1983). Assessment of negative and positive symptoms in schizophrenia. *Schizophrenia Bulletin, 9,* 368–376.

Mackay, A. (1980). Positive and negative schizophrenic symptoms and the role of dopamine. *British Journal of Psychiatry, 137,* 379–383.

McGlashan, T. (1982). Aphanasis: The syndrome of pseudo-depression in chronic schizophrenia. *Schizophrenia Bulletin, 8,* 118–134.

Oltmanns, T. (1978). Selective attention in schizophrenic and manic psychoses. *Journal of Abnormal Psychology, 87,* 212–225.

Strauss, J. S., Carpenter, W. T., & Bartko, J. (1974). The diagnosis and understanding of schizophrenia. Part III. Speculations on the processes that underlie schizophrenic symptoms and signs. *Schizophrenia Bulletin, 11,* 61–69.

Wishner, J. (1964, August). *Efficiency in schizophrenia.* Paper presented at the Symposium on Clinical Psychology and Experimental Psychopathology, International Congress of Applied Psychology.

COMMENTARY

Dr. Joseph Zubin:* There was a rather interesting contrast between the beginning of the talk we have just heard and the end, and I want to call attention to that. In a sense, what I'm going to say really might have better come from you [Dr. Lewine] than me, because what I'm going to say, even though I've lived during the period when Kraepelin was still alive and Bleuler was still alive, is that I now feel very much in doubt as to whether

* Pittsburgh, Pennsylvania.

what they were saying about negative symptoms really is part of schizophrenia. You have picked up the cudgels for them, even though perhaps you might have been in better position to be negative about them because of the fact you were not their contemporary.

Positive symptoms and negative symptoms have been described by Rue Cromwell in a rather interesting way. He says, positive symptoms are things that patients *do* but normals *don't,* and negative symptoms are things that normals *do,* namely they interact and they have motivation and they have will, but patients *don't* do those things. So we have an interesting contrast between Cromwell's view and the established view. I would really like to challenge you on the following:

I accept positive symptoms as reflecting the episode of schizophrenia. I reject negative symptoms as having anything to do with schizophrenia! They are either a continuation of the premorbid personality or they are the impact of having had an episode, in other words, a side effect, an artifact, arising from the fact that the individual has suffered an episode and has undergone all the troubles resulting from being labeled as schizophrenic just as you were describing toward the end of the talk. Therefore, I believe that our search for negative symptoms as being part of the disorder is entirely unwarranted. You'd have to demonstrate that these negative symptoms don't occur in nonschizophrenics under conditions of deprivation in long prison terms and other types of isolation and that they don't occur in schizophrenics who are in an affluent nonnoxious niche and therefore don't depend upon having to get jobs and don't feel denigrated and rejected.

In other words, the burden of proof upon you is to demonstrate that the negative symptoms are really part of the disorder, rather than a side effect and not an indigenous part of the disorder itself.

Dr. Lewine: First, I think that we should be looking at psychiatric symptoms in the affluent, and in various and sundry populations that don't generally get labeled as psychopathological. As Nancy Andreasen, I think it was, suggested this morning, I think we would be rather surprised to find a fair amount of thought disorder in a "normal" population. I don't see that as evidence against the existence of psychopathology but rather that some people with psychopathology can exist outside of the mental health system.

Second, there occur many positive symptoms in nonschizophrenics, but we haven't been called upon to prove that those symptoms are not related to schizophrenia—for example, bereaved people hearing voices, auditory hallucinations in other sorts of psychopathology—though, as suggested by Murray Alpert just a little while ago, there may in fact be some differentiation between them.

Third, however, and I think from my point of view this is the most important part, in some respects I am quite willing to concede the point. It may be that what I am talking about here is personality. It may be longstanding. It may be chronic. In some respects, ultimately, that may not be the critical question but rather, can be begin to identify subcategories as urged by Holzman? Can we begin to trace longitudinally specific functions in an individual? Can we begin to examine functions that look like schizophrenia, that look like depression, whatever, that are identified as risk factors? I think that Dr. [Raymond] Knight will be talking about that.

There is evidence suggesting that some of these processes are longitudinal, more trait-like in nature; whether one wants to call them *personality* or *psychopathology* ultimately may not be the issue. Finally, we have the logical impasse that has been pointed out by Hansen, Gottesman, and Meehl, that once we have any behavioral indicator, we simply can't get away from the fact that we may have the first signs of a disease process that has already begun.

15

Affectivity in Schizophrenia

RAYMOND A. KNIGHT
Brandeis University

JAMES D. ROFF
Eastern Michigan University

THE PREDICTIVE AND DISCRIMINANT VALIDITY OF AFFECTIVE DEFICITS

Although both thought and affect disturbances have traditionally been described as primary or fundamental symptoms of schizophrenia (Bleuler, 1911/1950; Kraepelin, 1913/1919), recent efforts to specify the criteria for differentiating schizophrenia from other psychopathologies have focused almost exclusively on various manifestations of thought disorder. For instance, Schneider's (1959) First Rank Symptoms do not include any consideration of affective deficits. Both Spitzer, Endicott, and Robins (1978) and Feighner *et al.* (1972) clearly enumerate the thought-disorder symptoms necessary for a diagnosis of schizophrenia. For affect, they require only that the schizophrenic lack periods of depressive or manic symptoms that would suffice to qualify him for an affective-disorder diagnosis. The New Haven Schizophrenia Index (NHSI) (Astrachan *et al.*, 1972) contains many thought-disorder symptoms, but allocates only one item for inappropriate affect. DSM-III, following this trend, relegates consideration of affectivity to the weak position of one of multiple conditional moderators of formal thought disorder or to one of many prodromal or residual symptoms.

This emphasis on measures of thought disorder and relative neglect of assessments of affectivity as diagnostic discriminators for schizophrenia persists despite contrary evidence from two crucial domains, discriminant and predictive validity. In the 18 descriptive studies reviewed by Pope and Lipinski (1978) it was found that between 20% and 50% of well-defined cases of manic–depressive illness (MDI) manifested "schizophrenic" thought-disorder symptoms. In contrast, in these same studies, "flatness of affect" was not reported as present in any MDI cases. The data on prognosis coincide with these discriminant-validity results. Early studies of the predictive validity of thought-disorder symptoms yielded at best contradictory results (Zubin *et al.*, 1961). More recent studies (e.g., Astrup, Fossum, & Holmboe, 1962; Astrup & Noreik, 1966; Harrow, Bromet, & Quinlan, 1974; Jansson, 1968; Knight, Roff, Barrnett, & Moss, 1979; Stephens, 1978; Stephens, Astrup, & Mangrum, 1966; Strauss & Carpenter, 1972) have consistently found that such thought-disorder symptoms lack prognostic utility. Indeed, both the Langfeldt (1937) and Schneider (1959) thought-disorder symptoms, widely touted to identify "true schizophrenia," have had their prognostic significance tested in 2- and 5-year follow-up studies (Hawk, Carpenter, & Strauss, 1975; Strauss & Carpenter, 1974) and have been found to lack predictive validity. In contrast, affective deficits have consistently been found to predict poorer outcome among schizophrenics (e.g., Astrup & Noreik, 1966; Carpenter, Bartko, Strauss, & Hawk, 1978; Knight *et al.*, 1979; Langfeldt, 1969). Although the relation of positive affective symptoms to favorable outcome among schizophrenics has not always been found (e.g., Carpenter *et al.*, 1978; Gift, Strauss, Kokes, Harder, & Ritzler, 1980), the majority of studies have yielded positive results (e.g., Astrup & Noreik, 1966; Huber, Gross, Schüttler, & Linz, 1980; Kant, 1937; Langfeldt, 1937; Levenstein, Klein, & Pollack, 1966; Odegaard, 1964).

The predictive primacy of affectivity and the temporal instability of thought disorder are clearly demonstrated in two follow-up studies that we have conducted. In the first study we followed up the child guidance records of "disturbed preschizophrenics" through armed service records and Veterans Administration Claim files (cf. Knight & Roff, 1983, for a more complete discription of this study). The patients in this sample had experienced their first psychotic break during young adulthood while in the armed service. We generated a path model that included assessments of this sample at three periods—childhood (average age = 10.9), young adulthood (average age = 21.7), and middle adulthood (average age = 43.7).

Ratings and analyses were done independently for each time period. A principal-components analysis of the childhood data yielded four factors from which factor scorres were derived: neurosis, low IQ–poor school achievement, schizoid syndrome, and unsocialized aggression. We have described these factors elsewhere (Roff, Knight, & Wertheim, 1976). Separate principal-components analyses with oblique rotation[1] were calculated for the young adult (armed service records) and middle adult (Veterans Claim files) periods. The former produced three theoretically cohesive factors that accounted for 56.4% of the variance, and the latter yielded four cohesive

1. Both oblique and varimax rotations resulted in essentially the same factor structure. We created scales from the oblique solution because we did not wish to restrict artificially the hypothesized correlations between affectivity and thought disorder.

factors that accounted for 79.2% of the variance. These factors are presented in Tables 1 and 2.

For the young and middle adult periods we created Likert scales for each factor by standardizing each variable, inverting variables with negative loadings, and summing all those variables that had loadings at least .45 on each factor. In instances where a variable loaded at least .45 on two factors, it was included only on the factor on which it had the greater loading. The single exception to this rule was the middle adult Thought Disorder Judgment. It had a slightly greater loading on the Affect Deficit/Social Incompetence factor (.74), but was included on the Thought Disorder Scale because it

Table 1. Final Young Adulthood Item-Groups Entered into the Path Analysis

Item groups	Variables	Loadings	Percent of variance	Cronbach alpha
Thought Disorder			24.2	.85
	New Haven Schizophrenia Index[a]	.92		
	Thought Disorder Symptom Scale[b]	.88		
	Paranoia[c]	.77		
	Conceptual Disorganization[c]	.71		
	Disorientation[c]	.65		
	Aggression Scale[d]	.57		
Affect Deficit/Social Incompetence			19.6	.78
	Affect Deficit Clinical Judgment[b]	.84		
	Service Performance[b]	−.69		
	Prehospital Time in Service[b]	−.57		
	Marital Status[e]	−.56		
	Service Social Adjustment[b]	−.49		
	Affect Deficit Scale[b]	.46		
Discipline Problems			12.6	.74
	Discipline Problems[b]	.75		
	Depression Scale[f]	−.79		
	Neurosis Scale[g]	−.67		

[a] Astrachan *et al.* (1972).

[b] Knight, Roff, Barrnett, and Moss (1979).

[c] Hautaluoma (1971).

[d] The Aggression Scale includes the sum of 0–1 ratings of physical aggression, verbal aggression, rebelliousness, and temper tantrums.

[e] For Marital Status 1 = single, 2 = widowed, divorced, or separated, and 3 = married or remarried.

[f] The Depression Scale includes the sum of 0–1 ratings of depression, guilt and/or shame, self-harm or suicide attempts, and inferiority feelings.

[g] The Neurosis Scale includes the sum of 0–1 ratings of anxiety, compulsions or obsessions, fears (phobias), worrying, vague somatic complaints, and hypochondriasis.

Table 2. Final Middle Adulthood Item-Groups Entered into the Path Analysis

Thought Disorder			48.5	.94
	New Haven Schizophrenia Index[a]	.93		
	Paranoia[b]	.91		
	Disorientation[b]	.87		
	Conceptual Disorganization[b]	.84		
	Thought Disorder Symptom Scale[c]	.73		
	Thought Disorder Clinical Judgment[c]	.68		
Depression/Anxiety			15.5	.67
	Neurosis Scale[d]	.89		
	Depression Scale[e]	.81		
Affect Deficit/Social Incompetence			8.0	.85
	Affect Deficit Clinical Judgment[c]	.81		
	Marital Status[f]	−.80		
	Affect Deficit Symptom Scale[c]	.77		
	Bizarre Behavior[g]	.65		
	Employment History[h]	−.65		
Aggression			7.2	—
	Aggression Scale[i]	.90		

[a] Astrachan *et al.* (1972).

[b] Hautaluoma (1971).

[c] Knight, Roff, Barrnett, and Moss (1979).

[d] The Neurosis Scale includes the sum of 0–1 ratings of anxiety, compulsions or obsession, fears (phobias), worrying, vague somatic complaints, and hypochondriasis.

[e] The Depression Scale includes the sum of 0–1 ratings of depression, guilt and/or shame, self-harm or suicide attempts, and inferiority feelings.

[f] For Marital Status 1 = single, 2 = widowed, divorced, or separated, and 3 = married or remarried.

[g] The Bizarre Behavior Scale includes the sum of 0–1 ratings of bizarre behavior (rocking, mannerisms, etc.), bizarre behavior (general conduct), smearing feces, unusual idiosyncratic language, mutism, and autistic thinking.

[h] For Employment History 1 = unemployed, 2 = marginal or unsteady employment, and 3 = full-time employment.

[i] The Aggression Scale includes the sum of 0–1 ratings of physical aggression, verbal aggression, rebelliousness, and temper tantrums.

was theoretically more consistent with this scale. Tables 1 and 2 present the final list of variables included in each scale, the factor loadings of these variables, the percent of variance accounted for by each factor, and the Cronbach α's of the final scales.

These three sets of scales were used to compute the path analysis presented in Figure 1. Path analysis is a family of statistical methods that allows one to assess the strength of causal links, when the direction of these links has been set a priori (cf. Kim & Kohout, 1975). We applied the simplest of path models, based on simultaneous multiple regressions. The

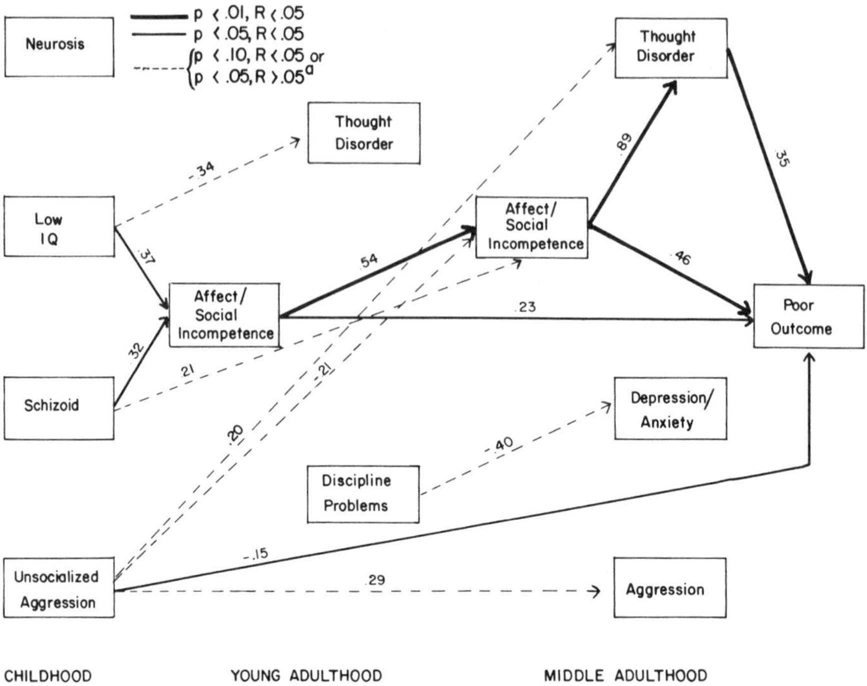

Figure 1. Path-analysis diagram of the childhood factors, young- and middle-adult factor scales, and consensus outcome for the Child Guidance Study. Solid lines indicate that the standardized beta contributed significant variance ($p < .05$ or $< .01$) to an overall R that was also significant ($p < .05$). Dashed lines indicate either that the standardized beta approached significance ($p < .10$), when the overall R was significant, or that the standardized beta was significant ($p < .05$), but the overall R was not ($p < .05$).

causal assumptions that generated our model included developmental progression (earlier events were hypothesized to cause later events), the causal primacy of affectivity in relation to thought disorder within a single assessment time (derived from our earlier cross-lagged panel analyses [Knight *et al.*, 1979]), and, within a single time set, the independence of all relations other than between affect deficit and thought disorder. We made this last assumption because we had no a priori theoretical or empirical justification to specify the causal directions among other variables. A posteriori, this seems to have been a reasonable assumption, because there was only one significant, unspecified zero-order correlation within a time set (between thought disorder and aggression in the middle adult period [$r_{(49)} = .48, p < .001$]).

This path analysis clearly illustrates both the temporal stability and predictive validity of an affective deficit, and its interrelation with social competence. Its manifestation in young adulthood was predicted by both the low-IQ factor and the schizoid syndrome of childhood. It showed substantial consistency through middle adulthood and was related to a poor global outcome. In contrast, young adult thought disorder was only related in this sample to a higher childhood IQ. It showed no temporal stability and was completely unrelated to outcome. It is also noteworthy that in this sample, aggression showed some temporal stability from childhood to middle adulthood. Moreover, the childhood unsocialized aggression factor was tentatively related to greater middle adult thought disorder and less affective deficit, and predcited better outcome.

We wanted to replicate some of these findings on a more representative sample of schizophrenics, one that did not, as did our original sample, require contact with a child guidance clinic prior to their first psychotic break. Thus, we undertook a second study, a 7-year follow-up of a group of young, psychiatric in-patients admitted to the Veterans Hospital in St. Cloud, Minnesota, between 1970 and 1971.

At initial assessment, our sample of veterans was young ($\bar{X}$ age = 27.34, *SD* = 5.4) and had experienced relatively little cumulative hospitalization ($\bar{X}$ total hospitalization = 5.57 months, *SD* = 7.62). During the initial evaluation, these patients were administered a battery of standardized tests, were rated on a standard assessment of ward behavior (Psychotic Inpatient Profile), were given a choice-reaction-time task, were interviewed about both their social and their employment history, and were administered a standard social competence questionnaire (General Information Questionnaire [DeWolfe, 1968]). From the interview and questionnaire we derived Phillips (1953) social competence scores and Zigler and Phillips (1961) ratings of employment and occupation. In addition, independent judgments of affectivity and thought disorder were made from abstracted clinical records according to the same criteria we used in our previous follow-up study (Knight *et al.*, 1979). Finally, using clinical file abstracts that included mental status and social work reports, ward notes, and testing data, two clinical psychologists (R. K. and J. R.) independently diagnosed 110 of the 132 patients according to DSM-II criteria.

Follow-up data were collected by a thorough search of VA medical records and VA claim files. Indications of hospitalizations or imprisonments outside of the VA system were checked and appropriate record sources accessed. We were able to find sufficient follow-up data to rate 126 of the 132 patients in the initial sample on at least a portion of the outcome measures.

A group of six research assistants was trained to rate the follow-up data. They had access to and rated only the extensive clinical file data written on patients between 1972 and 1978. Two assistants first independently rated a file and recorded their ratings for reliability assessment. They then met to resolve any discrepancies by a consensus procedure. Inability to reach an agreement on a discrepant judgment was coded as a missing datum in the consensus database.

These assistants were divided into two groups. The two assistants who had had the most extensive experience with clinical files were trained to make diagnostic and clinical judgments and to rate consensus outcome. In this chapter we will be concerned only with their consensus global outcome rating described in Table 3. The other four assistants were trained to make social-competence and work-history judgments, to compile data on hospitalizations, and to assess patients on a symptom checklist. Each rater coded approximately the same number of files and was paired for the consensus procedure approximately an equal number of times with each other rater. The symptom checklist and social-competence judgments were coded independently and combined by the consensus procedure. The hospitalization

Table 3. Selected Outcome Measures for the 7-Year Follow-Up Study of Young, Acute Psychiatric Inpatients

Variable	Description	Interrater reliability
Consensus Outcome	(1) Recovered (2) Neurotic, characterological symptoms (3) Nonschizophrenic psychosis (4) Paranoid/hostile, questionable schizophrenia (5) Schizoid (flat affect with minimal thought disorder) (6) Process schizophrenia (with periods of remission) (7) Process schizophrenia (deteriorated)	.78
Hospitalization	*Number* of admissions between 1972 and 1978 Total cumulative *months* between 1972 and 1978	
Social Relationships/ Contacts	(1) Sociable and outgoing (2) Good social contact (3) Some social contact (4) Avoided social contact	.59
Social Relationships/ Depth	(1) Married or cohabiting (2) Some close friends (3) Some casual friends (4) No friends	.86
Highest Job	Warner, Meeker, and Eells's (1949) 7-point scale (1) Professional to (7) Odd-job man, janitor	
Steadiness of Employment	(1) Steady and progressive (2) Steady (3) Erratic (4) Nonexisting	

and work ratings were made by a single assistant and checked for errors by the independent ratings of a second assistant. Table 3 presents a description of their ratings and interrater reliabilities, where appropriate.

The outcome symptoms were analyzed by choosing all those consensed symptom ratings (cf. Roff, 1981) that had both at least .70 Spearman–Brown interrater reliability[2] and at least 10% prevalence in the sample. We computed a principal-components analysis with rotation to varimax on the 30 symptoms that reached these criteria. This analysis yielded 5 theoretically consistent factors that accounted for 63.6% of the variance. Table 4 presents a summary of the symptom loadings on each factor.

A symptom scale was created for each factor by summing the consensed ratings of all symptoms that loaded .40 or more on a factor. If a symptom loaded .40 or more on two factors, it was included only on the factor on which it had the greater loading.[3] Table 4 presents both the Cronbach α's and interrater reliabilities for these final symptom scales. The former were computed on the consensus ratings, and the latter were calculated by summing the independent preconsensus ratings for each rater and correlating these sums.

Tables 5 and 6 present the correlations of the clinical judgments of thought disorder and affective deficit, and several measures of social competence—the Phillips scale (Farina, Garmezy, & Barry, 1963; Farina, Garmezy, Zalusky, & Becker, 1962; Phillips, 1953); the Ullmann–Giovannoni scale (Ullmann & Giovannoni, 1964); and the occupation and employment subscales of the Zigler–Phillips (1961) scale—with two sets of outcome measures. Table 5 focuses on the number and total cumulative months of hospitalization between 1972 and 1978, outcome measures of the number of social contacts and depth of relationships during this period, and follow-up assessments of work history. Table 6 presents the correlations with our outcome-symptom scales and the global-consensus outcome. The 49 subjects analyzed in both of these tables were selected to approximate the diagnostic composition of our original child-guidance sample—they included all patients who had ward diagnoses of schizophrenia and were diagnosed by one of us as schizophrenic in 1970–1971, with the alternative diagnosis always an affective or paranoid psychosis. Thus, like the child-guidance sample, they constituted a broadly defined group of schizophrenics.

2. A single exception was made for illogical thinking which had a consensed reliability of only .60. It was included because of some evidence suggesting that it is a discriminator between Schizophrenia and Major Depressive Disorder (Andreasen, 1979).

3. The single exception to this general rule was flat or blunted affect, which had a greater loading on the first factor (.70). Since in our previous study (Knight *et al.*, 1979), flat affect consistently covaried with the symptoms of the current fifth factor and not with the symptoms of the current first factor, we decided to include it on the fifth factor scale only.

Table 4. Principal-Components Factor Item-Groups for the Outcome Analyses of the Symptom Checklist in the 7-Year Follow-Up Study

Item-Groups	Variables	Loadings	Percent of variance	Cronbach alpha	Interrater reliability
Thought Disorder			40.4	.91	.95
	Tangential Thinking	.77			
	Loose Associations	.76			
	Incoherence	.68			
	Inappropriate Affect	.68			
	Crazy Thinking	.66			
	Delusions	.63			
	Paranoid Thinking	.60			
	Concreteness	.56			
	Attention Problems	.54			
	Hallucinations-Auditory	.47			
Aggression			9.1	.87	.90
	Physical Aggression	.87			
	Verbal Aggression	.78			
	Temper Tantrums	.76			
	Inappropriate Behavior	.66			
	Rebelliousness	.65			
	Hyperactivity	.52			
	Impulsivity	.51			
Depression/Anxiety			6.0	.84	.93
	Depression	.77			
	Suicidal Ideation	.72			
	Anxiety	.69			
	Sleep Disturbances	.65			
	Inferiority Feelings	.61			
Loneliness/Frightful			4.3	.70	.90
	Loneliness	.78			
	Daydreaming	.64			
	Frightful	.62			
Withdrawal/Affect Deficit			3.8	.80	.89
	Poor Social Relations	.72			
	Withdrawal/Seclusion	.67			
	Flat or Blunted Affect	.42			

The results presented in Tables 5 and 6 are very clear. Affect deficit predicted multiple aspects of outcome, including months of hospitalization, depth of interpersonal relationships, the highest job level achieved, steadiness of employment, three of the five outcome-symptom scales (depression, loneliness, and withdrawal), and global outcome. Thought disorder predicted only the outcome thought-symptom scale. Measures of social and work competence predicted only aspects of outcome social and work adaptation.

Table 5. Correlations of 1970–1971 Clinical Judgments and Social-Competence Measures with Outcome Measures of Hospitalization, Social Relationships, and Employment for the 7-Year Follow-Up

	Hospitalization		Social relationships		Employment	
	Number	Months	Contact	Depth	Highest Job	Steadiness
Clinical Judgments						
Affect deficit	.24	.30*[a]	.27	.46**	.30*	.40**
Thought disorder	.28	.24	.17	.19	.03	.14
Social Competence						
Phillips	.10	.24	.09	.48***	.44**	.16
U–G Scale[b]	−.16	.13	−.24	.18	.37*	.35*
Zigler–Phillips Work						
Occupation	−.14	−.26	−.25	−.35*	−.40*	−.32
Employment	−.03	−.04	−.24	−.03	−.55***	−.32
Age						
Onset	−.19	−.26	.04	.05	.06	.06

[a] Because of missing data, different absolute levels of correlations are significant at different levels (*N* = approximately 49).

[b] U–G = Ullmann–Giovannoni (1964) Scale.

* $p < .05$ (two-tailed).

** $p < .01$ (two-tailed.

*** $p < .001$ (two-tailed).

Thus, thought disorder and social competence seem to be semi-independent domains of functioning (Strauss, Bartko, & Carpenter, 1981), showing continuity over time, but at best only weakly linked to other domains within a particular time frame. In contrast, the affect-deficit judgment predicted a wide range of outcome domains and was the only variable among those presented to predict global outcome.

When we further restricted the sample and analyzed only the 31 cases on whom there was unanimous agreement about the diagnosis of schizophrenia, the affective-deficit judgment still predicted months of hospitalization ($r_{(28)} = .36, p < .05$), depth of social relationships ($r_{(27)} = .50, p < .01$), highest job level ($r_{(27)} = .40, p < .05$), steadiness of work ($r_{(24)} = .58, p < .01$), and global outcome ($r_{(27)} = .57, p < .001$). It lost only its ability to discriminate among outcome symptoms.

THE RELIABILITY PROBLEM

The consistency of the relation of an affective deficit to poor outcome among schizophrenics would seem sufficient to earn measures of such a

Table 6. Correlations of 1970–1971 Clinical Judgments and Social-Competence Measures with Outcome-Symptom Scales and Global-Consensus Outcome for the 7-Year Follow-Up

	Symptom scales					Global-consensus outcome
	Thought Disorder	Aggression	Depression/ Anxiety	Loneliness/ Frightful	Withdrawal/ Affect Def.	
Clinical Judgments						
Affect Deficit	.24	.24	.34*[a]	.31*	.42**	.42**
Thought Disorder	.32*	.12	.13	.23	.21	.26
Social Competence						
Phillips	−.03	−.04	−.04	.14	.24	.24
U–G Scale[b]	−.00	−.03	−.14	.03	.10	.21
Zigler–Phillips Work						
Occupation	−.06	−.02	.08	−.09	−.15	−.19
Employment	.02	−.01	.17	.13	−.14	−.06
Age						
Onset	−.18	−.10	−.06	−.27	−.04	−.28

[a] Because of missing data, different absolute levels of correlations are significant at different levels ($N =$ approximately 49).

[b] U–G = Ullmann–Giovannoni (1964) Scale.

* $p < .05$ (two-tailed).

** $p < .01$ (two-tailed).

deficit a secure place in both the diagnostic assessment and clinical investigation of schizophrenia. Yet, as we have noted, it has been virtually excluded from diagnostic criteria and, compared to the number of studies on thought disorder, the research aimed at understanding both the nature of the affective deficit and its role in schizophrenia has been meager. The long history of difficulty in reliably assessing affectivity (e.g., Alpert, Hekimian, & Frosch, 1966; Astrup & Noreik, 1966; Endicott *et al.*, 1982; Feighner *et al.*, 1972; Harris & Metcalfe, 1956; Schwartz, Grinker, Harrow, & Holzman, 1978) might account for this relative neglect. Indeed, as can be seen in Table 7, the reliabilities of the affect judgments in our two follow-up studies have not always been impressive, despite the predictive validity of these judgments. An analysis of the discrepancies in our judgments revealed that our greatest problem involved discriminating between flat or blunted affect and

Table 7. Interrater Reliabilities for the Affective-Deficit Judgments for the Two Follow-Up Studies

	Young adulthood	Middle adulthood
Child Guidance Study	.66	.87
7-Year follow-up	.47	.71

depression. Difficulty with such a differentiation has been a common problem (e.g., Andreasen, 1979; Harrow, Grinker, Holzman, & Kayton, 1977). A recent attempt (Lewine, Fogg, & Meltzer, 1983) to derive a negative-symptom scale empirically, using a latent-trait model to cluster the symptoms of carefully defined schizophrenics, illustrates an interpretive problem that arises from this difficulty of discriminating depression and flat affect. The negative-symptom scale they derived included symptoms of both "depressed appearance" and "blunted affect." It is difficult to determine from this scale and from the additional analysis the authors did to explore this unexpected covariation whether there is some real relation between depression and negative symptoms, or if the loading of "depressed appearance" on this scale simply represents the failure of clinicians to differentiate depression and flat affect adequately.

Several investigators have attempted to address the problems of reliably assessing affective deficits by creating rationally derived scales that specify the criteria for affective flattening (e.g., Abrams & Taylor, 1978; Andreasen, 1979, 1982). Two somewhat similar procedures have been followed in developing such scales. Abrams and Taylor's (1978) method for constructing the Scale for Emotional Blunting (SEB) illustrates the first approach. They combed the classical clinical literature, amassed and organized descriptive phrases relating to emotional blunting, chose prototypic exemplars of each class, and assigned numerical values to assess the presence and severity of each descriptive statement. The summation of ratings on these statements constitutes a patient's global affective score. Following a slightly different procedure, Andreasen (1979) first generated a series of "observable phenomena" by describing the behavioral criteria that clinicians seemed to use in judging affective deficits. These criteria were specified and a numerical scale assessing presence and severity was assigned. Once again, a global assessment of affect could be produced by summing the ratings of individual phenomena.

Although these and similarly constructed scales have had the important effect of encouraging research on affectivity in schizophrenia, two problems limit their usefulness. First, many of the proposed criteria lack behavioral and criterion specificity. When other investigators use such scales, they are required to generate their own behavioral referents and norms if adequate reliability is to be attained. For instance, Boeringa and Castellani (1982) in their study of the SEB reported in their Method section, "We initially examined and rated a number of patients openly with the SEB, then discussed each SEB item until we reached agreement on its meaning and how it was manifested" (p. 1132). The necessity of such procedures has serious negative consequences because they produce assessments that vary across research sites and they can result in inflated estimates of reliability as investigators at particular institutions settle on their own idiosyncratic, but easily agreed upon manifestations of such constructs as "incongruous mood."

The second problem with the extant summative scales centers on the inadequacies of the source from which they originated—clinical experience. To illustrate these deficiencies we will briefly review in the next section selected research on four of the behavioral domains that have been employed in the summative affect-deficit scales. As we will see, the empirical research on the discriminant validity of some of the observables chosen to characterize flat affect clearly indicates that, even if we provided precise descriptions and quantified norms for these behaviors, they would not adequately differentiate flat affect from depression. Thus, clinical experience was inaccurate about the specificity of these behaviors. We will suggest an alternative solution to this discrimination problem, generated from an integration of the empirical findings.

BEHAVIORAL STUDIES OF AFFECTIVITY INDICATORS

Gestures

Andreasen (1979) clearly specified two categories of gestures that were included on her affective-flattening scale (AFS)—decreased spontaneous movement and paucity of expressive gestures. Although gestures were not directly specified as criteria in the SEB, aberrations in the quantity of gestures could contribute to SEB judgments of "constricted affect," "unvarying affect," and "lacks spontaneity."

The typology and meaning of gestures and individual differences in gesture patterns has been one of the focuses of the programmatic research of Ekman and Friesen (e.g., 1972, 1974) on emotional expression. Two of their empirically validated categories, illustrators and adaptors, are relevant to our discussion of flat affect. Illustrators are gestures that bear a temporal relationship to the course of speech and serve to elaborate upon or illustrate what is being said. Adaptors are gestures that serve to cope with bodily needs, and are hypothesized to occur in response to tension or anxiety. As part of their program S. A. Kiritz (1971, reported in Ekman & Friesen, 1974) analyzed the gestures of 31 female psychiatric patients (9 psychotic depressives, 7 neurotic depressives, and 15 schizophrenics) who were filmed at both admission and discharge. He also obtained independent ratings by three experienced clinicians of Overall and Gorham's (1962) Brief Psychiatric Rating Scale (BPRS). Although for the entire sample the BPRS scale of *blunted affect* was significantly negatively correlated with illustrating at admission and discharge, the scale of *depressive mood* was also negatively correlated with illustrating. Moreover, the psychotically depressed patients showed significantly fewer illustrators than schizophrenics at admission.

In another study of nonverbal communicative behavior of schizophrenics, Grand, Freedman, Steingart, and Buchwald (1975) analyzed the gestures of two groups of "chronic" schizophrenics. They used the Hospital Proneness Scale (Freedman, Rosen, Engelhardt, & Margolis, 1967) to differentiate their sample into "prone" and "nonprone" subtypes. Patients categorized as prone were characterized as socially isolated, nonbelligerent schizophrenics with an impoverished form of cognitive functioning. The nonprone schizophrenics showed greater social effectiveness, were more overtly oppositional, and evidenced more adaptive cognitive functioning. Thus, the prone patients are descriptively similar on a number of dimensions to our affectively deficient schizophrenics and the nonprone types share many features with paranoid, positive-affect schizophrenics. Grand *et al.* assessed two gesture types that closely approximated Ekman and Friesen's categories. Their "object-focused movements," closely resembling illustrators, were "communicative acts closely linked to the rhythm and content of speech . . . [that] qualify, punctuate, illustrate, or depict some verbalized or partially unverbalized aspect of thought" (p. 294). "Bodily-focused activity," descriptively similar to adaptors, were defined as "apparently unrelated to speech and invariably involv[ing] more or less continuous self-stimulation" (p. 294). Grand *et al.* found that their schizophrenic subtypes were equivalent in the frequency of illustrator-like gestures, but prone schizophrenics engaged in significantly more continuous bodily focused adaptor-like gestures.

Knight, Levin, and Miklowitz (1984) studied the patterns of schizophrenics' gestures during the telling of stories with different emotional content. During a videotaped interview they had patients tell stories about themselves that were happy, sad, or angry. The content of these stories was transcribed, purged of obvious references to the intended nature of the emotion, and rated by college students ignorant of the source of the stories. Trained research assistants ignorant of patient diagnosis and story content rated voiceless videotapes on the frequency and duration of illustrating and adaptive gestures. The sample for this study consisted of 31 psychiatric inpatients and 8 normal controls. The psychiatric patients, who were rather heterogeneous with respect to age and chronicity ($\bar{X}$ age = 35.0, *SD* = 12.3; $\bar{X}$ total hospitalization = 2.8 years, *SD* = 3.8) included 24 patients who met the Research Diagnostic Criteria (RDC) (Spitzer *et al.*, 1978) for schizophrenia. Eight of these 24, whom we will refer to as "negative-affect schizophrenics," were judged from a detailed examination of their extensive clinical files to have a modal history of flat or inappropriate affectivity. The remaining 16 "positive-affect schizophrenics" manifested irritable, hostile, emotionally unstable, or depressive affectivity. The 7 nonschizophrenic patients in this sample met the RDC for major depressive disorder.

The emotional-content ratings of all patient groups' stories did not differ from the ratings of normals' stories. All groups produced stories that were rated as highest on the intended emotion. In contrast, the patterns of gestures that accompanied these stories differed radically. Figure 2 presents the percent of time each group was engaged in each gesture type while

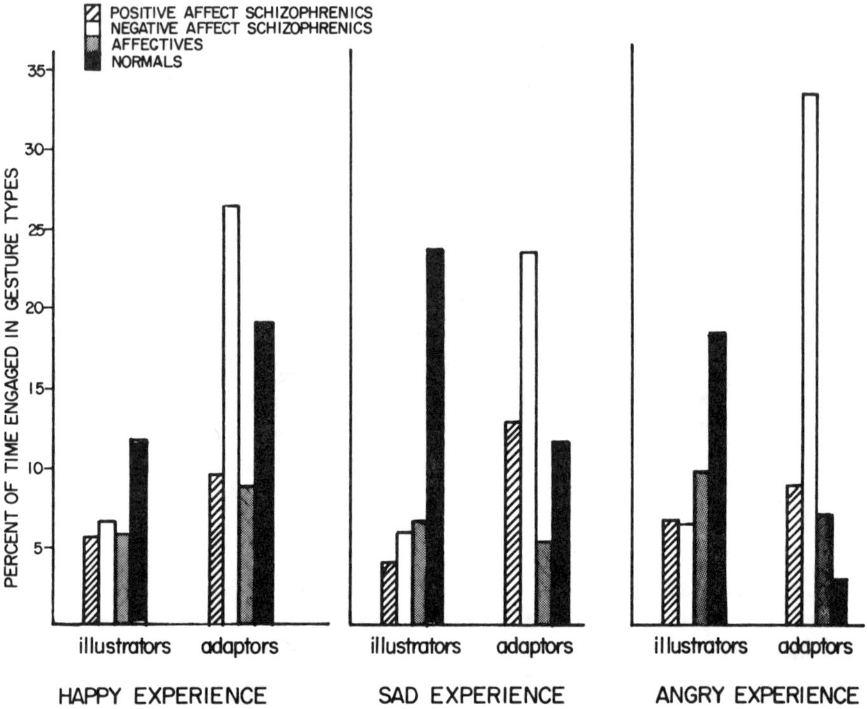

Figure 2. The percent of time each diagnostic group was engaged in illustrators and adaptors while telling about happy, sad, and angry experiences.

telling about happy, sad, and angry experiences. Four results are noteworthy. First, Grand *et al.*'s finding that prone schizophrenics produced more adaptors was replicated. Negative-affect schizophrenics, who were similar to Grand *et al.*'s prone schizophrenics, tended to spend a higher percent of their time producing adaptors than did all other groups ($F_{1,35} = 4.05$, $p < .06$, by an a priori contrast). This general tendency must be qualified, however, because group and story condition significantly interacted for adaptors, ($F_{6,70} = 2.42$, $p < .05$). Only in the angry condition did the negative-affect schizophrenics produce significantly more adaptors than each of the other three groups ($p < .01$ for each comparison by Newman–Keuls multiple comparisons). Second, the three patient groups did not differ in the percent of time they engaged in illustrating gestures. Third, normals always spent more time employing illustrators, but again group and story condition interacted significantly, $F_{6,70} = 2.85$, $p < .025$. Normals' use of illustrators was significantly greater than all three patient groups only in the sad story condition ($p < .001$ for each comparison by Newman–Keuls). Fourth, normals were the only subjects who modulated their pattern of gestures as a function of the emotional experience being recounted. The relative pattern of illustrator–

adaptor use for the three psychiatric groups was constant across the three story conditions: depressed patients and positive-affect schizophrenics consistently spent little time engaged in either gesture type, whereas negative-affect schizophrenics consistently spent more time engaged in adaptors.

The results of these gesture studies have direct implications for the affectivity scales. First, because the number of illustrators has been found to correlate significantly with depression as well as blunted affect (Kiritz, 1971, reported in Ekman & Friesen, 1974), and because the frequency of illustrators discriminated neither prone from nonprone subtypes of schizophrenics (Grand *et al.*, 1975) nor negative-affect schizophrenics from either depressed patients or positive-affect schizophrenics (Knight *et al.*, 1984), "paucity of expressive gestures" (Andreasen, 1979) is a questionable differential indicator of affective flattening. Second, the finding that negative-affect schizophrenics produced significantly more adaptors than both depressives and positive-affect schizophrenics (Grand *et al.*, 1975; Knight *et al.*, 1984) indicates that items like "decreased spontaneous movements" (Andreasen, 1979) might have the effect of lowering the affective-flattening scores of the very patients it was intended to select and increasing these scores for patients it was intended to exclude. Third, the finding that the discriminatory power of gesture type was moderated by story condition (Knight *et al.*, 1984) suggests that taking into account the assessment of the intentionality of emotional expression might substantially increase the ability of behavioral indicators to differentiate affective deficits.

Voice Characteristics

It has long been known that affective state is encoded in voice in numerous ways (Scherer, 1979). If affective flatness is indeed a discriminating construct it should be reflected in some voice characteristics. Abrams and Taylor (1978), searching the archives of clinical wisdom, found "unvarying, monotonous voice" for their SEB. Andreasen (1979) made three of the nine items on the AFS voice measures—"lack of vocal inflections," "slow speech," and "increased latency of response."

Early empirical studies using qualitative judgments of vocal characteristics (Cohen, 1961; Markel, Meisels, & Houck, 1964; Sharp, 1963) were unable to find any distinguishing characteristics of schizophrenics' speech. Two studies using physiological measures (Saxman & Burke, 1968; Spoerri, 1966) were slightly more successful in finding some differences. Spoerri (1966), however, concluded that there were no typical schizophrenic speech patterns, and Saxman and Burke's (1968) fundamental frequency level deviation differences between schizophrenics and normals could have been simply an artifact of reading speed.

Alpert and Anderson (1977) were the first to investigate the relation of voice quality to flat affect. They divided 30 schizophrenics into flat and nonflat subgroups and measured their voice amplitude while they were reading high- and low-imagery words that were embedded in a paragraph. As predicted, nonflat schizophrenics read high-imagery words with significantly greater amplitude than low-imagery words, whereas flat-affect schizophrenics read both with equal amplitude. Thus, flat-affect schizophrenics seemed to lack emphasis in their speech prosody. In a subsequent study (reported in Alpert, 1982), when the recorded speech of nonflat patients was electronically compressed to reduce the range of the amplitude selectively, naive raters judged such compressed speech samples as flatter.

Andreasen, Alpert, and Martz (1981) used Alpert's speech measures as concurrent validators of Andreasen's (1979) AFS. A sample of 61 psychiatric in-patients (19 manics, 15 depressives, and 27 schizophrenics) was divided into flat and nonflat subgroups on the basis of AFS scores. Analyses of two pooled samples of spontaneous speech revealed several differences between these subgroups. Flat-affect patients' speech samples were significantly less variable in both amplitude and frequency than those of nonflat-affect patients, and they showed a significantly faster rise time, defined as the time required for a word to reach its peak amplitude. The utterances of flat-affect patients tended to be shorter and to contain fewer syllables, and flat-afffect patients tended to pause longer between utterances. These results provide some cross-method, convergent validation for the AFS. Patients categorized partially by clinical judgments of lack of vocal inflections, slowed speech, and increased latency of response (three of nine AFS items) showed objectively measured speech patterns that coincided with these selection criteria. The data also demonstrate, however, the failure of the AFS to discriminate between depression and flat affect; 67% of RDC major depressive disorders were classified as flat, whereas 63% of schizophrenics were so classified. Moreover, diagnostic groups did not differ on any acoustic measures.

Alpert (1982) later reported that a subsequent analysis of these data revealed that the vocal acoustic qualities that differentiated flat from nonflat depressives were not the same as those that differentiated flat from nonflat schizophrenics. Only flat schizophrenics showed the constricted range of vocal dynamics. The "flatness" of depressives was more characterized by an increase in pause duration, suggesting more slowed speech. Flat schizophrenics showed no evidence of this increase in pause duration.

Levin, Hall, Knight, and Alpert (in press) employed an alternative method for assessing schizophrenics' speech. As part of the study described earlier (Knight *et al.*, 1984), stereophonic audiotapes of the happy, sad, and angry stories were recorded and segments of these, selected to meet several a priori criteria of length, continuity, and location in the story, were content-filtered with a low-pass filter to ensure that only nonverbal vocal cues remained. Five groups of 10 undergraduates each rated the content-filtered tape clips on 7-point scales, assessing the amount of happiness, sadness, anger, expressiveness, and anxiety perceived present. Each independent group rated all the clips on a different emotion. The ratings were analyzed both to determine whether negative- and positive-affect schizophrenics, depressives, and normals differed in their overall intensity and range of affective expression, and whether their affects were accurate for the context and differentiated appropriately among the story types. The measures of contextual accuracy and differentiation discriminated among groups. In terms of overall level of accuracy, the depressives had the least communicative intonation pattern—showing an appropriate modulation only in their sad stories. Negative-affect schizophrenics and normals both showed an intermediate, moderate level of accuracy, and positive-affect schizophrenics were the most accurate. Although negative-affect schizophrenics and normals were similar in their level of accuracy, the differentiation and pattern of their ratings was quite different. Despite the negative-affect schizophrenics' relative pattern of being rated as slightly happier in the happy story than in the sad or angry stories, as sadder in the sad story, and as angrier in the angry story, they showed poorer differentiation than normals, with only one of these comparisons barely reaching significance. Moreover, they were still perceived, as were the depressives, to be predominantly sad regardless of story type. Thus, the negative-affect schizophrenics and depressives were similar to each other in the pervasive sadness of their intonation, but differed in their accuracy pattern. In contrast to these two groups, the accuracy of the normal controls was reduced by their tendency to communicate happiness regardless of story content. Finally, positive-affect schizophrenics were consistently and significantly rated as manifesting the greatest intensity of a particular emotion in the appropriate story.

These same voice clips are also currently being analyzed using Alpert's voice spectrum acoustic measures, described in Andreasen *et al.* (1981). Preliminary results show support for Alpert's (1982) finding of greater pause duration in depressives than in the other groups, but the other measures have not yet been analyzed.

Several conclusions can be drawn from the results of these experiments. First, the voice spectrum acoustic analysis, especially the measure of range of voice dynamics, shows some promise for differentiating flat affectivity from depression (Alpert, 1982). Further empirical specification is, however, required. Second, slowed speech and increased latency of response seem to select for depression rather than affective flattening (Alpert, 1982; Knight *et al.*, 1984). Andreasen's (1982) decision to drop these two voice characteristics from the affective flattening section of her Scale for the Assessment of Negative Symptoms (SANS) seems quite justified. Third, Levin *et al.*'s results indicate that a comparison of the intended affect (story type) with the communicated affect provided the best discrimination between positive-affect schizophrenics and both depressives and negative-affect schizophrenics. Although accuracy pattern differences emerged between the latter two groups, more research is required to replicate these subtle differences and to determine whether their discriminating power can be improved.

Eye Contact

Andreasen (1979) included poor eye contact as a criterion for affective flattening. Abrams and Taylor (1978) made no direct reference to eye contact in their SEB, but it seems reasonable to assume that looking behavior might contribute to such judgments as avoiding social contact and indifference to staff, visitors, and patients.

Much of the evidence that originally supported the notion that schizophrenics engage in very little looking behavior was based upon methodologically unsatisfactory clinical observations of interview behavior or poorly constructed quasi-experiments (Rutter, 1973). A large number of variables must be taken into account when examining looking behavior (e.g., reliability-of-the-gaze judgment, amount of talking, relative status of those engaged in conversation, nature of conversation, setting of the interview, etc. [cf. Exline & Fehr, 1978; and Rutter, 1973, for reviews]). The failure to control for these and other variables led clinicians and early investigators to unwarranted conclusions about the relative looking behavior of various diagnostic groups. Therefore, we will focus only on those studies that have attempted to eliminate confounding variables.

Rutter has conducted a series of well-controlled studies of the looking behavior of schizophrenics. In his earliest study (Rutter & Stephenson, 1972), he found that in an interview situation both schizophrenics and depressives spent significantly smaller proportion of their time gazing at the interviewer than did their matched controls. This was not due to the amount of time spent talking, since this decreased looking behavior was consistent across speaking, listening, and silence. Schizophrenics' and depressives' looking behavior differed on only one variable—schizophrenics looked in shorter glances. The overall amount of eye contact was the same for both groups.

In his next two studies, Rutter (1976) investigated schizophrenics' looking behavior in free dyadic conversations about impersonal topics. In the first study the schizophrenics engaged in two conversations, one with another schizophrenic and another with a psychiatrically normal control. These interactions were compared to depressive- and neurotic/personality-disorder patient–patient (same diagnostic group) and patient–control dyads. A normal control dyad was also tested. Schizophrenics showed the same pattern of looking behavior whether talking to another schizophrenic or to a normal control. In general, their looking behavior was similar to all three control groups. The few differences that did reach significance indicated that schizophrenics looked *more* than depressives and patients with neurotic or personality disorders. In the second study Rutter compared the looking behavior of long-term (more than 2 years of continuous hospitalization) and short-term, recently admitted schizophrenics as each group was conversing with a nurse. No differences were found between these groups.

Subsequently, Rutter (1977b) varied the content of the conversations in which subjects were engaged—personal topic versus neutral topic. He compared both remitted and acute schizophrenics with normal controls on 10 measures of eye contact, while they were engaged in conversations with a nurse. Although he found consistent differences on these measures between topics, he found no differences between groups on any of the measures. Finally, Rutter (1978) reanalyzed data from three previous studies (Rutter, 1976, 1977a, 1977b), examining the timing of looks as a function of the transitions from one speaker to another during the flow of conversation. No differences were found betweeen schizophrenics and controls or between long-term and short-term schizophrenics.

Exline, Paredes, Gottheil, and Winkelmayer (1979) added the dimension of intended emotion to the study of schizophrenics' eye contact. Their data showed a complex interaction between the affective theme of the speech (happy, sad, or angry), the affective intensity of the verbal content, and diagnostic group (normal or schizophrenic). During intense stories, normals gazed more at the interviewer while telling happy stories and gazed down more when telling sad stories. Schizophrenics gazed relatively more at the interviewer than gazing down regardless of affective theme or intensity. Thus, depending on the theme and intensity of the affect in the segments being compared, one could find schizophrenics with more or less eye contact than normals. This interaction suggests that a simple assessment of eye contact, without considering the nature and intensity of the affect being expressed, is insufficient. Over all conditions the authors found no evidence for a decrease in the total amount of direct gazing for schizophrenics and, in fact, they found schizophrenics' direct gazing to be slightly, but not significantly greater than normals. The important discriminator of schizophrenics from normals in this study was not the absolute amount of direct gazing behavior, but the inconsistency between the pattern of gazing and the intended affect.

The studies on looking behavior in schizophrenics provide no direct evidence about the relation of eye contact to affective flattening that is assumed in the AFS. The finding that schizophrenics do not seem to differ from normals in their overall amount of looking behavior does not exclude the possibility that a subsample of schizophrenics, those with flat affect, might exhibit aberrant gazing behaviors. The failure to find differences in eye contact between long-term and short-term schizophrenics (Rutter, 1976, 1978) is somewhat more problematic for the hypothesized relation of gaze and flatness, because one might expect a higher proportion of affectively deficient schizophrenics in the more chronic subgroup. The admittedly tentative link between "long-term" and "affectively flat" makes the similarities in looking behavior of long-term and short-term subgroups at best a weak refutation. The fact, however, that clinical experience was so wrong about the relation of gazing behavior to schizophrenia in general makes questionable Andreasen's (1979) dependence on such experience to justify the relation between poor eye contact and flatness. Clearly, sounder empirical evidence is required. Exline *et al.*'s (1979) research suggests that comparing the patterns of eye contact across different emotional contexts might be a far better discriminator than a simple overall judgment of poor eye contact. Thus, it would be wise to include manipulation of the intended emotion and the intensity of such emotions in any attempt to validate the eye contact–flatness hypothesis.

Anhedonia, Apathy, Indifference

Early descriptions of schizophrenia (Bleuler, 1911/1950; Kraepelin, 1913/1919) included anhedonia, or a marked deficit in the ability to experience pleasure, as a part of the deterioration of the schizophrenic's emotional life. It was later elevated by Rado (1956, 1962) and Meehl (1962) to a place of central importance in the disorder. Its perceived importance as a component of schizophrenics' affective deficit is reflected in Abrams and Taylor's (1978) decision to include four separate items measuring different aspects of "indifference" in the SEB—one item judged from the patient's behavior ("indifference to surroundings") and three items assessing the patient's self-report of indifference ("lack of affection for family," "unconcern for own present situation," and "unconcern for own future"). Andreasen (1979) excluded the assessment of anhedonia from the AFS, but subsequently included "subjective complaints of emotional emptiness" in her affective-flattening criteria of the SANS.

Although anhedonia has been found to be characteristic of a significant subsample of schizophrenics (Grinker & Holzman, 1973) and has tended to differentiate schizophrenics from mixed samples of nonschizophrenics (Grinker & Holzman, 1973; Schwartz *et al.*, 1978), it also has been found not to be unique to schizophrenia (Harrow *et al.*, 1977). Indeed, some have listed it (or its equivalent) as a key symptom in some depressive syndromes (e.g., Beck, 1967; Klein, 1974). It has been shown in a heterogeneous psychiatric sample to have a small but significant correlation with depression

(Harrow *et al.*, 1977), and in a discriminant-function analysis between schizophrenics and affectives (Kendell & Gourlay, 1970), it ("loss of all pleasure in life") was found tied with one other variable for the lowest discriminant weight in the 38 items entered.

A recent study suggests a way in which the discriminating power of anhedonia might be improved. Brown, Sweeney, and Schwartz (1979) compared the ratings of six RDC schizophrenics and five RDC major-depressive disorders on two ratings of pleasurable activity—the Pleasurable Activity Self-Rating Scale and the Pleasurable Activity Observer-Rating Scale. Their results showed a discrepancy between the reported and observed assessments of pleasure. Schizophrenics *reported* a significantly lower degree of pleasure than depressed patients, but were *observed* to emit a higher degree of pleasurable behavior (observable facial signs of positive affect). Thus, as in the other domains of affect indicators, it seems that the discrepancy between the verbal content (self-report) and the nonverbal behavior (facial expression) promises to produce greater discriminatory power.

Several conclusions about the summative scales can be drawn from these selected studies on anhedonia. First, the discriminant validity of schizophrenics' and depressives' self-reports of the loss of the ability to experience pleasure has not been adequately demonstrated. Indeed, several studies provide data that question the untested assumption of discriminant validity (e.g., Harrow *et al.*, 1977; Kendell & Gourlay, 1970). Second, it seems that *behavioral* indicators of anhedonia, such as the SEB item, "indifference to surroundings," would favor the selection of depressives rather than flat-affect schizophrenics (Brown *et al.*, 1979). Third, measures of the discrepancies between self-reports of anhedonia and behavioral manifestation of pleasure in activities might provide the best discriminators between depression and affective flattening.

Summary: Behavioral Indicators

The empirical studies we have reviewed in four behavioral domains indicate that the two major summative scales of affective flattening have serious discriminant validity problems. Some of the items included on each have been shown to be more likely to select for depression than for flat affect—the SEB behavioral item, "indifference to surroundings" and the AFS items, "decreased spontaneous movements," "slowed speech," and "increased latency of response." For other items the extant empirical literature suggests that they do not differentiate between depression and flat affect—the three SEB "indifference" thought-content items and the AFS item, "paucity of expressive gestures." Depending on how one actually measures SEB items such as "constricted affect" and "unvarying affect," they could also fall into this last category. Depressives were shown not to vary either their gestures (Knight *et al.*, 1984) or their vocal, affectively communicative qualities (Levin *et al.*, in press) across different affective stories. Finally, although only weak, inconclusive evidence questioned the discriminatory power of one AFS item, "poor eye contact," no empirical data were found to support its ability to differentiate depression and flat affect.

In contrast, in all four behavioral domains there were data that suggested that measuring the pattern of behavioral indicators across the intended expression of different emotions might yield affective profiles that discriminate affective flattening from depression. Indeed, if we are allowed a couple of speculative jumps, two interesting patterns emerge from the data already at hand. The jumps involve assuming that the patterns Exline *et al.* (1979) and Brown *et al.* (1979) found for their small samples of generic schizophrenics are characteristic of affectively deficient schizophrenics. Because Exline *et al.* provided no information about their diagnostic criteria, and the RDC criteria used by Brown *et al.* has been found to select patients on the basis of thought-disorder symptoms and not affective deficiencies (Marvinney, Rosenberg, & Knight, 1982), these assumptions must be treated as tentative at best. Yet, the pattern that emerges is consistent across three domains. In the gesture domain, negative-affect schizophrenics emitted the same relative pattern of illustrators and adaptors regardless of the emotion being recounted. This pattern, relatively more adaptors than illustrators, is the same pattern that normals produced only when telling happy stories. In Exline *et al.* (1979), the schizophrenics produced across different emotions and intensities the gaze pattern that normals produced most consistently while telling happy stories—proportionately more direct than downcast gazes. Finally, in Brown *et al.* (1979) the schizophrenics tended to produce slightly pleasurable facial expressions, despite modal self-reports of no pleasure or displeasure. A predominantly sad voice with minimal emotional communication (Levin *et al.*, in press) and possibly with a limited dynamic range of amplitude (Alpert, 1982) might be hypothesized to accompany this constricted and somewhat unvarying "happier" pattern of gestures, gaze, and facial expression. In contrast, depressives' speech was found to be slowed (Alpert, 1982; Knight *et al.*, 1984) and their voices sounded unremittingly sad with poor differentiation of other emotions (Levin *et al.*, in press), their modal facial expressions were neutral, and they emitted very few gestures of any kind. Although there are no data on their gazes, we might speculate that depressives will show the sad pattern, more downward than direct gazes, regardless of the emotional content of their speech. It must be emphasized once again that the "negative-affect schizophrenics" pattern is the result of averaging over flat-affect and inappropriate-affect schizophrenics (Grand *et al.*, 1975; Knight *et al.*, 1984; Levin *et al.*, in press) and over more generically defined schizophrenics (Brown *et al.*,

1979; Exline *et al.*, 1979). It might be that this pattern more reflects inappropriate than flat affect, and that separate profiles will emerge for these two groups.

A LONGITUDINAL PERSPECTIVE

The relative importance of course and prognosis in the diagnostic assessment of schizophrenia has been debated ever since opposing views about this issue were first formulated by the great systematizers of schizophrenia (Bleuler, 1911/1950; Kraepelin, 1913/1919). In a review of 38 follow-up studies, Stephens (1978) concluded that the addition of longitudinal data to cross-sectional data in diagnostic assessment improved prediction of outcomes. The addition of longitudinal data should also be important in the assessment of affectivity. If, as our data suggest, affective flattening is a trait that shows significant temporal stability, information about the course of the disorder should help to distinguish it from depression, which tends to be more episodic. Thus, even those symptoms and behaviors that do not distinguish flat affect and depression in a cross-sectional assessment might add important discriminating information when coupled with data on the duration of such symptoms.

Some data in our follow-up studies support the notion that longitudinal information enhances reliability. Part of the variance in the reliabilities in our affectivity judgments (cf. Table 7) can be accounted for by the different amounts of longitudinal data available for each decision. The two best reliabilities were attained when our assessment sources contained the greatest amount of historical data (the two middle-adult judgments), and our worst judgment (the young adult, 7-year follow-up judgment) occurred when we had only the admission and hospital adaptation reports of a single hospitalization. We had an intermediate level of reliability in our young adult Child Guidance study affectivity judgment, when we had both records describing a subject's adjustment in the armed service, which also contained more "behavioral" than "clinical" information, and the complete admission and discharge descriptions of their first hospitalization. Thus, the young adult Child Guidance records permitted at least some assessment both of the duration of symptoms and of recovery, and provided some information about the continuity of affective functioning over time. This relation of amount of longitudinal data and achieved reliability fits with our impressions, when rating the clinical files, that duration assisted in discrimination, especially in doubtful cases.

Throughout this chapter we have talked about depression and affective flattening as if they only occur independently, as if our task was merely to differentiate which was truly present. Their relation may not be so simple. Although the data are fraught with substantial interpretive controversy (e.g., Goplerud & Depue, 1978, 1979; McGlashan & Carpenter, 1979), a number of studies (Lorr & Klett, 1967; McGlashan & Carpenter, 1976a; von Zerssen, 1980) do exist that suggest that depression is commonly found in acute schizophrenics. Indeed, in a recent study of schizophrenics and paranoid psychoses that carefully excluded schizoaffective disorders, Möller and von Zerssen (1982) found that depressive states occur frequently during acute schizophrenic and paranoid psychoses. Their data over the course of hospitalization also indicated that most of these depressions were neither pharmacogenic (drug-induced) nor postpsychotic. For most patients the depressions seemed to coexist with florid symptoms. In addition, McGlashan and Carpenter (1976a, 1979) found that the presence of depression in the schizophrenics they studied was unrelated to prognostic indicators and did not predict 1-year follow-up adaptation. Although, as we indicated earlier, depression (a positive-affective symptom) has typically been found in good-prognosis schizophrenics, recent data from this and other studies (Carpenter *et al.*, 1978; Gift *et al.*, 1980) suggest the possibility that depression may not be limited to good-prognosis cases.

These data are important to our discussion of depression and affective flattening, for they suggest the possibility that the two symptom complexes might occur together in some patients. Thus, several hypotheses must be considered when we attempt to explain the correlations of depression and affective flattening in our samples. As we suggested previously, the problems in diagnostically discriminating the two could lead to confounded judgments. The judged presence of depression in negative-affect schizophrenics might really be misinterpreted affective flattening and anhedonia, and true depression might only exist in positive-afffect good-prognosis schizophrenics.[4] Alternatively, the continued experience of affective deficits, social withdrawal, isolation, and poor adaptation could conceivably lead to increased depression and the covariance could reflect a real relation. Finally, depression could be a phase in the course of the disorders of some schizophrenics (McGlashan & Carpenter, 1976b) and be unrelated to affective flattening. To untie this Gordian knot of the relation of flat affect and depression requires not only improved cross-sectional specificity, but also longitudinal disentanglement.

Our two follow-up studies provide data that allow some preliminary speculation on the developmental interplay of affect deficit and depression. In our Child Guidance sample we divided the Affect Deficit/Social Incom-

4. It should, of course, be mentioned that the diagnostic composition of good prognosis schizophrenics is controversial, and it is not yet clear what role depression plays in these patients (Goplerud & Depue, 1979; McGlashan & Carpenter, 1979). As Goplerud and Depue (1979) indicate, more data are required to determine whether some portion of these patients are really manifesting bipolar depressive disorders.

petence factor scale presented earlier (cf. Tables 1 and 2) into more theoretically pure Affect Deficit/Withdrawal and Social Incompetence subscales. The former included three of the four symptoms on the empirically derived (Knight *et al.*, 1979) Affect Deficit Symptom Scale—flat affect, apathy, and seclusiveness—plus the Affect-Deficit Clinical Judgment. The latter included poor peer relationships from the original Affect Deficit Symptom Scale, plus Service Performance, Marital Status, and Service Social Adjustment (cf. Tables 1 and 2, inverted here to assess *in*competence). We also made a Depression/Anxiety scale by simply summing all the items on the Depression and Neuroses scales. These three complexes—affect deficit, social incompetence, and depression/anxiety—had different development antecedents. As we indicated in an earlier report (Knight & Roff, 1983), the variables in the young adult Affect Deficit/Withdrawal Scale tended to be predicted by a childhood schizoid factor, with the clinical-judgment subcomponent having the strongest ties to this childhood factor. The young adult Social Incompetence Scale was most strongly predicted by poor school achievement and low intelligence measures (Roff & Knight, 1985). Depression/Anxiety was unrelated to a psychoneurotic childhood symptom scale, and was only predicted by the *lack* of symptoms on a scale measuring soft neurological signs (Roff & Knight, 1985).

The adult, life-span course of these three complexes, which seem to have developed from different childhood sources, suggests a particular cross-temporal pattern for their interrelations. Figure 3 presents three cross-lagged panel analyses (Kenny, 1979) of these scales over the 22 years of follow-up from young to middle adulthood. Several results are noteworthy. First, all three scales showed significant cross-temporal stability. Second, both the Affect Deficit/Withdrawal and Depression/Anxiety scales related to Social Incompetence in ways that were consistent across the 22 years assessed. On the one hand, Affect Deficit/Withdrawal was always significantly related to Social Incompetence and the young-adult scale of each construct predicted the middle-adult scale of the other. On the other hand, Depression/Anxiety did not correlate with Social Incompetence at any time. Third, in contrast to the relations with Social Incompetence, the relation between Affect Deficit/Withdrawal and Depression/Anxiety increased over time. These scales were not correlated in young adulthood, but were significantly correlated in middle adulthood. The positive cross-lagged differential ($r_{A_1D_2} - r_{A_2D_1}$ in Figure 3) suggests that the increase in correlation was more likely due to Affect Deficit/Withdrawal increasing subsequent Depression/Anxiety than the reverse. This differential must be interpreted cautiously, however, because it was a weak difference, $Z(45) = 1.09, p < .15$ (one-tailed) (Peters & Van Voorhis, 1940) and the lack of "stationarity" (i.e., the increase in the synchronous correlations over time) does not allow us to rule out spurious third variable alternative hypotheses (Kenny, 1979).

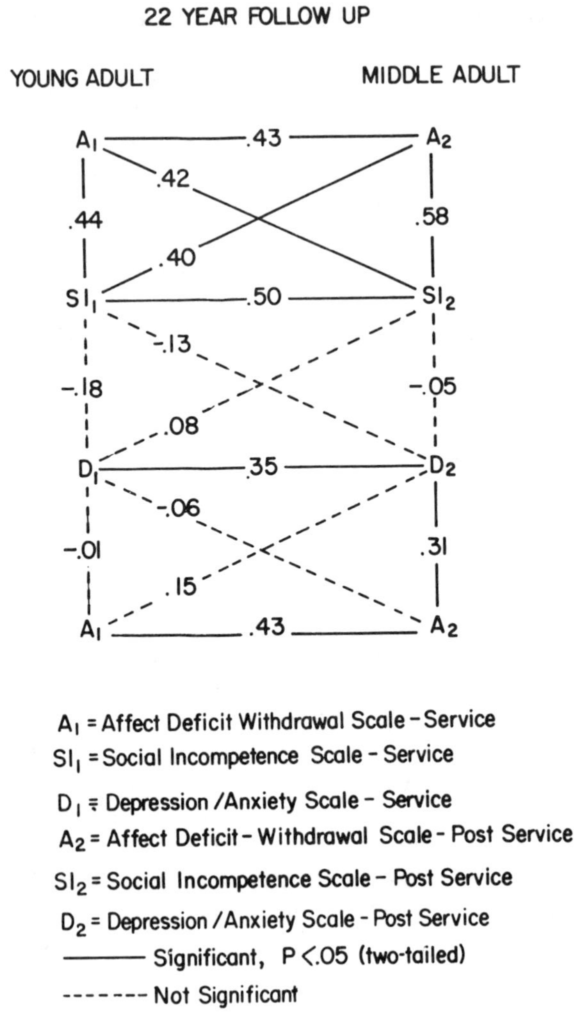

Figure 3. Cross-lagged panel correlations for measures of affect deficit, social incompetence, and depression in young and middle adulthood for the subjects in the Child Guidance Study.

To determine whether this same pattern of results was replicated in our 7-year follow-up study, we chose a set of scales that purportedly measured the same three theoretical constructs, and we repeated analogous triple cross-lagged panel analyses on the follow-up data of this second sample. These analyses are depicted in Figure 4. In young adulthood the three constructs are represented by our Affectivity Deficit Clinical Judgment (Knight *et al.*, 1979), the Phillips (1953) Social Competence Scale, and the Anxious Depression Scale of the Psychotic Inpatient Profile (PIP) (Lorr

& Vestre, 1968). We chose the Anxious Depression Scale on the PIP instead of the Depressive Mood Scale because of its greater descriptive similarity to the Depression/Anxiety Scale in the Child Guidance study. At outcome the three constructs are assessed by the Withdrawal/Affect Deficit Factor Scale (cf. Factor 5 in Table 4), the Social Relationships/Depth Scale (cf. Table 3), and the Depression/Anxiety Factor Scale (cf. Factor 3 in Table 4). The 49 subjects in these analyses are the same subjects that produced the results presented in Tables 5 and 6.

Figure 4. Cross-lagged panel correlations for measures of affect deficit, social incompetence, and depression at initial assessment and outcome for the subjects in the 7-year follow-up study.

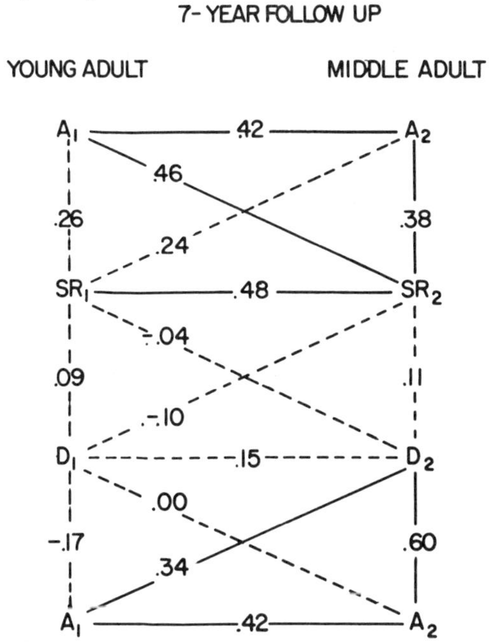

A_1 = Affect Deficit Clinical Judgement

SR_1 = Social Relationships -- Phillips

D_1 = Anxious Depression -- PIP Scale

A_2 = Withdrawal / Affect Deficit -- Factor 5

SR_2 = Social Relationships -- Depth

D_2 = Depression / Anxiety -- Factor 3

——— Significant, $P < .05$ (two-tailed)

------- Not Significant

Despite the differences in the two follow-up samples and the differences in the operationalization of the constructs assessed, the pattern of the relations among these constructs in the 7-year follow-up study is remarkably similar to that found in the Child Guidance study. Affect Deficit tends to correlate consistently with Social Incompetence across time. The correlation in young adulthood between these constructs, $r_{A_1SR_1} = .26$, is significant ($p < .05$), if we apply a one-tailed test, and the predictive correlation, $r_{SR_1A_2} = .24$, just misses the one-tailed cutoff. All the other correlations between these two constructs are highly significant. In contrast, Anxious Depression was, as its corresponding measures were in the previous analysis, completely unrelated to Social Incompetence. Affect Deficit and Anxious Depression also had the same relation as they did in the Child Guidance study. They were unrelated in young adulthood and were significantly related at outcome. Moreover, the cross-lagged differential ($r_{A_1D_2} - r_{A_2D_1}$ in Figure 4) was in the same positive direction, suggesting that affect deficit leads to subsequent depression. In this instance the cross-lagged differential reached one-tailed significance, $Z(49) = 1.75, p < .05$.

As an estimate of the similarity of the pattern of correlations in these two sets of cross-lagged analyses, we calculated a Spearman ρ between the ranks of the 15 corresponding correlations in the two studies. The resulting correlation, $p(13) = .72$, was highly significant, $t = 3.75, p < .01$. We substituted in the 7-year follow-up analyses several alternative measures of the three constructs (e.g., the Depressive Mood PIP scale for the Anxious Depression Scale in young adulthood, a Social Adjustment Scale for the Social Relationships/Depth Scale at outcome, etc.) and recalculated the ρs between the various combinations of alternative measures and the Child Guidance correlations. The pattern remained the same despite such substitutions. The range of ρs was .66 to .76, all significant, $p < .01$.

Thus, across two follow-up samples and a number of operationalizations of these constructs, the same relation between affect deficit, depression, and social incompetence emerged. The finding that the relation between depression and affect deficit increases over time provides a possible explanation for the discrepancies about the prognostic value of depression in schizophrenia. The data suggest that the relation of depression to outcome might vary as a function of the kind of patient sampled and the point in the course of the disorder that depression is assessed. In samples in which good-prognosis cases are more prevalent, the amount of depression might be inflated by the presence of misdiagnosed manic-depressive patients. Depression in such samples might predict better outcome because it is associated with the better prognosis of MDI. When research criteria are more stringent and more MDI cases are excluded, the affect-deficit patients with poorer prognosis might contribute more variance to measures of depression and neutralize depression's good prognosis. Because the relation of depression and affect deficit increases over time, this neutralization effect might be greater in more chronic samples.

The longitudinal data also help us to select among the various alternative hypotheses we suggested earlier about the relation of affect deficit and depression. Neither the hypothesis that their correlation might be an artifact of poor diagnostic discrimination nor the hypothesis that they are unrelated found support. If the artifact explanation were correct, we would expect poorer reliability (i.e., problems discriminating affect deficit and depression) to be associated with a greater correlation between the two complexes. The longitudinal pattern of reliabilities ran directly counter to this explanation—our poorest reliabilities occurred in young adulthood when the two constructs were not related, and we attained our best reliabilities in middle adulthood when depression and affect deficit were found to covary. The fact that in both samples the two constructs became related in middle adulthood disconfirms the hypothesis of their independence. Only the hypothesis that affect deficit leads to a subsequent increase in depression received tentative corroboration. Such a finding indicates, of course, that the task of reliably distinguishing the two constructs in schizophrenics is complicated by the possibility that they may occur together, and that this co-occurrence might increase over the course of the disorder. Thus, progress in our understanding of the role of affect deficit and depression in schizophrenia will require the combined efforts of cross-sectional specificity and longitudinal disentanglement. The data we have reviewed on the prognostic utility of affect deficits indicate that our efforts toward such understanding promise rich rewards.

ACKNOWLEDGMENTS

We wish to thank David Elliott, Judith Sims-Knight, Paula Brown, and Joseph Cunningham for their helpful comments on an earlier version of this chapter.

REFERENCES

Abrams, R., & Taylor, M. A. (1978). A rating scale for emotional blunting. *American Journal of Psychiatry, 135,* 226–229.

Alpert, M. (1982). Encoding of feelings in voice. In P. J. Clayton & J. E. Barrett (Eds.), *Treatment of depression: Old controversies and new approaches* (pp. 217–228). New York: Raven Press.

Alpert, M., & Anderson, L. T. (1977). Imagery mediation of vocal emphasis in flat affect. *Archives of General Psychiatry, 34,* 208–212.

Alpert, M., Hekimian, L. J., & Frosch, W. A. (1966). Evaluation of treatment with recorded interviews. *American Journal of Psychiatry, 122,* 1258–1264.

Andreasen, N. C. (1979). Affective flattening and the criteria for schizophrenia. *American Journal of Psychiatry, 136,* 944–947.

Andreasen, N. C. (1982). Negative symptoms in schizophrenia: Definition and reliability. *Archives of General Psychatry, 39,* 784–788.

Andreasen, N. C., Alpert, M., & Martz, M. J. (1981). Acoustic analysis: An objective measure of affective flattening. *Archives of General Psychiatry, 38,* 281–285.

Astrachan, B. M., Harrow, M., Adler, D., Brauer, L., Schwartz, A., Schwartz, C., & Tucker, G. (1972). A checklist for the diagnosis of schizophrenia. *British Journal of Psychiatry, 121,* 529–539.

Astrup, C., Fossum, A., & Holmboe, R. (1962). *Prognosis in functional psychoses.* Springfield, IL: Charles C. Thomas.

Astrup, C., & Noreik, K. (1966). *Functional psychoses; Diagnostic and prognostic models.* Springfield, IL: Charles C. Thomas.

Beck, A. T. (1967). *Depression: Causes and treatment.* Philadelphia: University of Pennsylvania Press.

Bleuler, E. (1950). *Dementia praecox or the group of schizophrenias* (J. Zinkin, Trans.). New York: International Universities Press. (Original work published 1911)

Boeringa, J. A., & Castellani, S. (1982). Reliability & validity of emotional blunting as a criterion for diagnosis of schizophrenia. *American Journal of Psychiatry, 139,* 1131–1135.

Brown, S. L., Sweeney, D. R., & Schwartz, G. E. (1979). Differences between self reported and observed pleasure in depression and schizophrenia. *Journal of Nervous and Mental Disorders, 167,* 410–415.

Carpenter, W. T., Bartko, J. J., Strauss, J. S., & Hawk, A. B. (1978). Signs and symptoms as predictors of outcome: A report from the International Pilot Study of Schizophrenia. *American Journal of Psychiatry, 135,* 940–945.

Cohen, A. (1961). Estimating the degree of schizophrenic pathology from recorded interview samples. *Journal of Clinical Psychology, 17,* 403–408.

DeWolfe, A. S. (1968). Self-reports and case histories of schizophrenic patients: Reliability and validity of Phillips Scale ratings. *Journal of Clinical Psychology, 24,* 415–418.

Ekman, P., & Friesen, W. V. (1972). *Emotion in the human face.* Oxford: Pergamon Press.

Ekman, P., & Friesen, W. V. (1974). Nonverbal behavior and psychopathology. In R. J. Friedman & M. M. Katz (Eds.), *The psychology of depression: Contemporary theory and research* (pp. 203–223). Washington, DC: Winston.

Endicott, J., Nee, J., Fleiss, J. F., Cohen, J., Williams, J. B. W., & Simon, R. (1982). Diagnostic criteria for schizophrenia: Reliabilities and agreement between systems. *Archives of General Psychiatry, 39,* 884–889.

Exline, R. V., & Fehr, B. J. (1978). Applications of semiosis to the study of visual interaction. In A. W. Siegman & S. Feldstein (Eds.), *Nonverbal behavior and communication* (pp. 117–157). Hillsdale, NJ: Lawrence Erlbaum Associates.

Exline, R. V., Paredes, A., Gottheil, E. G., & Winkelmayer, R. (1979). Gaze patterns of normals and schizophrenics retelling happy, sad and angry experiences. In C. E. Izard (Ed.), *Emotions in personality and psychopathology* (pp. 533–561). New York: Plenum Press.

Farina, A., Garmezy, N., & Barry, H., III (1963). Relationship of marital status to incidence and prognosis of schizophrenia. *Journal of Abnormal and Social Psychology, 67,* 624–630.

Farina, A., Garmezy, N., Zalusky, M., & Becker, J. (1962). Premorbid behavior and prognosis in female schizophrenic patients. *Journal of Consulting Psychology, 26,* 56–60.

Feighner, J., Robins, E., Guze, S., Woodruff, R., Winokur, G., & Munoz, R. (1972). Diagnostic criteria for use in psychiatric research. *Archives of General Psychiatry, 26,* 57–63.

Freedman, N., Rosen, B., Engelhardt, D. M., & Margolis, R. (1967). Prediction of psychiatric hospitalization. 1. The measurement of hospital proneness. *Journal of Abnormal Psychology, 72,* 468–477.

Gift, T. E., Strauss, J. S., Kokes, R. F., Harder, D. W., & Ritzler, B. A. (1980). Schizophrenia:

Affect and outcome. *American Journal of Psychiatry, 137,* 580–585.

Goplerud, E., & Depue, R. A. (1978). The diagnostic ambiguity of postpsychotic depression. *Schizophrenia Bulletin, 4,* 477–480.

Goplerud, E., & Depue, R. A. (1979). Affective symptoms, schizophrenia, and the conceptual ambiguity of postpsychotic depression. *Schizophrenia Bulletin, 5,* 554–559.

Grand, S., Freedman, N., Steingart, I., & Buchwald, C. (1975). Communicative behavior in schizophrenia: The relation of adaptive styles to kinetic and linguistic aspects of interview behavior. *Journal of Nervous and Mental Disease, 161,* 293–306.

Grinker, R. R., & Holzman, P. S. (1973). Schizophrenic pathology in young adults. *Archives of General Psychiatry, 28,* 168–175.

Harris, A., & Metcalfe, M. (1956). Inappropriate affect. *Journal of Neurology, Neurosurgery and Psychiatry, 19,* 308–313.

Harrow, M., Bromet, E., & Quinlan, D. (1974). Predictors of posthospital adjustment in schizophrenia: Thought disorder and schizophrenic diagnosis. *Journal of Nervous and Mental Disease, 158,* 23–36.

Harrow, M., Grinker, R. R., Holzman, P. S., & Kayton, L. (1977). Anhedonia and schizophrenia. *American Journal of Psychiatry, 134,* 794–797.

Hautaluoma, J. (1971). Symptoms, antecendents, and outcomes of psychosis: A cluster-analytic study. *Journal of Consulting and Clinical Psychology, 37,* 332–344.

Hawk, A. B., Carpenter, W. T., and Strauss, J. S. (1975). Diagnostic criteria and 5-year outcome in schizophrenia: Report from the International Pilot Study of Schizophrenia. *Archives of General Psychiatry, 32,* 343–356.

Huber, G., Gross, G., Schuttler, R., & Linz, M. (1980). Longitudinal studies of schizophrenic patients. *Schizophrenia Bulletin, 6,* 592–605.

Jansson, B. (1968). The prognostic significance of various types of hallucinations in young people. *Acta Psychiatrica Scandinavica, 44,* 401–409.

Kant, O. (1937). Study of a group of recovered schizophrenic patients. *Psychiatric Quarterly, 15,* 262–283.

Kendell, R. E., & Gourlay, J. (1970). The clinical distinction between the affective psychoses and schizophrenia. *British Journal of Psychiatry, 117,* 261–266.

Kenny, D. A. (1979). *Correlation and causality.* New York: Wiley.

Kim, J., & Kohout, F. J. (1975). Special topics in general linear models. In N. H. Nie, C. H. Hull, J. G. Jenkins, K. Steinbrenner, & D. H. Bent (Eds.), *Statistical package for the social sciences* (pp. 368–397). New York: McGraw-Hill.

Klein, D. F. (1974). Endogenomorphic depression. *Archives of General Psychiatry, 31,* 447–454.

Knight, R. A. (1968). *The effect of punishment on the performance of schizophrenics: A review of the literature.* Unpublished manuscript, University of Minnesota, Minneapolis.

Knight, R. A., Levin, S., & Miklowitz, D. (1984). [Gesture patterns in the expression of affect in schizophrenic and affective disorder patients]. Unpublished raw data.

Knight, R. A., & Roff, J. D. (1983). Childhood and young adult predictors of schizophrenic outcome. In D. Ricks & B. Dohrenwend (Eds.), *Origins of psychopathology: Research and public policy* (pp. 129–153). London & New York: Cambridge University Press.

Knight, R. A., Roff, J., Barrnett, J., & Moss, J. (1979). Concurrent and predictive validity of thought disorder and affectivity: A 22-year follow-up of acute schizophrenics. *Journal of Abnormal Psychology, 88,* 1–12.

Kraepelin, E. (1919). *Dementia praecox and paraphrenia* (R. M. Barclay, Trans.). Edinburgh: E. & S. Livingston. (Original work published 1913)

Langfeldt, G. (1937). The prognosis of schizophrenia and the factors influencing the course of the disease. *Acta Psychiatrica et Neurologica Scandinavica Supplement, 13,* 1–228.

Langfeldt, G. (1969). Schizophrenia: Diagnosis and prognosis. *Behavioral Science, 14,* 173–182.

Levenstein, S., Klein, D., & Pollack, M. (1966). Follow-up study of formerly hospitalized voluntary psychiatric patients: The first two years. *American Journal of Psychiatry, 122,* 1102–1109.

Levin, S., Hall, J. A., Knight, R. A., & Alpert, M. (in press). Verbal and nonverbal expression of affect in speech of schizophrenic and affective disorder patients. *Journal of Abnormal Psychology.*

Lewine, R. R. J., Fogg, L., & Meltzer, H. Y. (1983). Assessment of negative and positive symptoms in schizophrenia. *Schizophrenia Bulletin, 9,* 368–376.

Lorr, M., & Klett, C. J. (1967). *Manual for the inpatient psychiatric scale* (rev. ed.). Palo Alto, CA: Consulting Psychologists Press.

Lorr, M., & Vestre, N. D. (1968). *Psychotic inpatient profile manual.* Los Angeles: Western Psychological Services.

Markel, N. N., Meisels, M., & Houck, J. E. (1964). Judging personality from voice quality. *Journal of Abnormal and Social Psychology, 69,* 458–463.

Marvinney, D. A., Rosenberg, E., & Knight, R. A. (1982, April). *The identification of schizophrenics: Differential selection by five research diagnostic systems.* Paper presented at the meeting of the Eastern Psychological Association, Baltimore.

McGlashan, T. H., & Carpenter, W. T. (1976a). An investigation of the postpsychotic depressive syndrome. *American Journal of Psychiatry, 133,* 14–19.

McGlashan, T. H., & Carpenter, W. T. (1976b). Postpsychotic depression in schizophrenia. *Archives of General Psychiatry, 33,* 231–239.

McGlashan, T. H., & Carpenter, W. T. (1979). Affective symptoms and the diagnosis of schizophrenia. *Schizophrenia Bulletin, 5,* 547–553.

Meehl, P. E. (1962). Schizotaxia, schizotypy, schizophrenia. *American Psychologist, 17,* 827–838.

Möller, H. J., & von Zerssen, D. (1982). Depressive states occurring during the neuroleptic treatment of schizophrenia. *Schizophrenia Bulletin, 8,* 109–117.

Odegaard, O. (1964). Pattern of discharge from Norwegian psychiatric hospitals before and after the introduction of psychotropic drugs. *American Journal of Psychiatry, 120,* 772–778.

Overall, J. E., & Gorham, D. R. (1962). The Brief Psychiatric Rating Scale. *Psychological Reports, 10,* 799–812.

Peters, C. C., & Van Voorhis, W. R. (1940). *Statistical procedures and the mathematical bases.* New York: McGraw-Hill.

Phillips, L. (1953). Case history data and prognosis in schizophrenia. *Journal of Nervous and Mental Disease, 117,* 515–525.

Pope, H. G., & Lipinski, J. F. (1978). Diagnosis in schizophrenia and manic-depressive illness. *Archives of General Psychiatry, 35,* 811–828.

Rado, S. (1956). *Psychoanalysis of behavior: Collected papers* (Vol. 1). New York: Grune & Stratton.

Rado, S. (1962). *Psychoanalysis of behavior: Collected papers* (Vol. 2). New York: Grune & Stratton.

Roff, J. D. (1981). Reminder: Reliability of global judgments. *Perceptual and Motor Skills, 52,* 315–318.

Roff, J. D., & Knight, R. A. (1985). *Affect deficit and depression in schizophrenia: A longitudinal perspective.* Manuscript submitted for publication.

Roff, J. D., Knight, R., & Wertheim, E. (1976). A factor analytic study of childhood symptoms antecedent to schizophrenia. *Journal of Abnormal Psychology, 85,* 543–549.

Rutter, D. R. (1973). Visual interaction in psychiatric patients: A review. *British Journal of Psychiatry, 123,* 193–202.

Rutter, D. R. (1976). Visual interaction in recently admitted and chronic long-stay schizophrenic patients. *British Journal of Social and Clinical Psychology, 15,* 295–302.

Rutter, D. R. (1977a). Speech patterning in recently admitted and chronic long-stay schizophrenic patients. *British Journal of Clinical Psychology, 16,* 45–55.

Rutter, D. R. (1977b). Visual interaction and speech patterning in remitted and acute schizophrenic patients. *British Journal of Social and Clinical Psychology, 16,* 357–361.

Rutter, D. R. (1978). Visual interaction in schizophrenic patients: The timing of looks. *British Journal of Social and Clinical Psychology, 17,* 281–282.

Rutter, D. R., & Stephenson, G. M. (1972). Visual interaction in a group of schizophrenic and depressive patients. *British Journal of Social and Clinical Psychology, 11,* 57–65.

Saxman, J. H., & Burke, K. W. (1968). Speaking fundamental frequency and rate characteristics of adult female schizophrenics. *Journal of Speech and Hearing Research, 11,* 194–203.

Scherer, K. R. (1979). Nonlinguistic vocal indicators of emotion and psychopathology. In C. E. Izard (Ed.), *Emotions in personality and psychopathology* (pp. 495–528). New York: Plenum Press.

Schneider, K. (1959). *Clinical psychopathology* (M. W. Hamilton, Ed. and Trans.). New York: Grune & Stratton.

Schwartz, D. M., Grinker, R. R., Harrow, M., & Holzman, P. S. (1978). Six clinical features of schizophrenia. *Journal of Nervous and Mental Disease, 166,* 831–838.

Sharp, F. A. (1963). Judgements of psychosis from vocal cues. *Journal of Speech and Hearing Disorders, 28,* 371–374.

Spitzer, R. L., Endicott, J., & Robins, E. (1978). *Research diagnostic criteria.* (Available from Biometrics Research, New York State Psychiatric Institute, 722 West 168th Street, New York, New York 10032).

Spoerri, T. H. (1966). Speaking voice of the schizophrenic patient. *Archives of General Psychiatry, 14,* 581–585.

Stephens, J. H. (1978). Long-term prognosis and follow-up in schizophrenia. *Schizophrenia Bulletin, 4,* 25–47.

Stephens, J. H., Astrup, C., & Mangrum, J. C. (1966). Prognostic factors in recovered and deteriorated schizophrenics. *American Journal of Psychiatry, 122,* 1116–1121.

Strauss, J. S., Bartko, J. J., & Carpenter, W. T., Jr. (1981). New directions in diagnosis: The longitudinal process of schizophrenia. *American Journal of Psychiatry, 138,* 954–958.

Strauss, J. S., & Carpenter, W. T., Jr. (1972). The prediction of outcome in schizophrenia. I. Characteristics of outcome. *Archives of General Psychiatry, 27,*739–746.

Strauss, J. S. & Carpenter, W. T., Jr. (1974). Prediction of outcome in schizophrenia. II. Relationships between predictor and outcome variables. *Archives of General Psychiatry, 31,* 37–42.

Ullmann, L. P., & Giovannoni, J. M. (1964). Development of a self-report measure of the process-reactive continuum. *Journal of Nervous and Mental Disease, 138,* 38–42.

von Zerssen, D. (1980). Psychopathometrische Verfahen und ihre Anwendung in der Psychiatrie. In V. H. Peters (Ed.), *Die Psychologie des 20 Jahrhunderts* (pp. 149–169). Zurich: Kindler.

Warner, W. L., Meeker, M., & Eells, K. (1949). *Social class in America, a manual of procedure for the measurement of social status.* Chicago: Science Research Associates.

Zigler, E., & Phillips, L. (1961). Social competence and outcome in psychiatric disorder. *Journal of Abnormal and Social Psychology, 63,* 264–271.

Zubin, J., Sutton, S., Salzinger, K., Salzinger, S., Burdock, E. I., & Peretz, D. (1961). A biometric approach to prognosis in schizophrenia. In P. H. Hoch & J. Zubin (Eds.), *Comparative epidemiology of the mental disorders* (pp. 143–203). New York: Grune & Stratton.

COMMENTARY

Dr. Kurt Salzinger:* The two papers that we've just listened to both dealt with affect, and I wish to remind you of a series of studies that Dr. Portnoy, then Pisoni, and I conducted over 20 years ago (Salzinger & Pisoni, 1958, 1960, 1961; Salzinger & Portnoy, 1964). We examined affect by counting the number of self-referred affect statements and found, first, that one can, in fact, do this reliably, second, that in the course of an interview, if one reinforces self-referred affect statements one can increase their frequency, and if one subsequently stops reinforcement, such statements decrease to a baseline operant level, and third, that in a 6-month follow-up study it was the conditionability of affect and not the operant level of affective expression that predicted which schizophrenics would be released from the hospital.

Dr. Knight: Your data, indicating that poor-prognosis schizophrenics showed less conditionability of their affect, are very interesting in light of the data I have just reviewed. The research I reviewed showed that an important discriminating characteristic of negative-affect schizophrenics' affective expression was that their gestures, voice characteristics, and gaze patterns remained relatively constant despite interviewer demands for different emotional expressions. In your data, poor-prognosis schizophrenics' self-referred affective statements did not change as a function of the interviewer's reinforcement of such statements. Both of these findings support the point that Lewine and Sommers (cf. Chapter 14 in this volume) have just made about the measurement of negative symptoms. Negative symptoms must be assessed across both different situations and different domains of the interviewer's behaviors (or maybe even across different interviewers) because all these data suggest that we will achieve greater discriminability if we assess affective expression in the context of specific demanded and intended affects.

Dr. Salzinger: Yes, but the point I am making is that we do not know that what we are talking about here is affect. I think it is conditionability. We know that this thing will vary as a function of the interviewer. That is another reason that you get low reliability. We do know that conditionability of affect relates to outcome. Therefore, we know that it is not just affect alone, because if one looks simply at the operant level, it will not relate to outcome. These older studies might shed some light on what it is you are studying.

Dr. Knight: I think that some of the data I have reviewed support your notion that simply assessing the operant level of a particular behavior is

* New York, New York.

less likely either to discriminate flat affect from depression or to predict outcome than an approach that takes the situation into account. Thus, we have to assess more than the operant level. As far as what underlying construct is being assessed, affectivity or conditionability, I would hypothesize that, for several reasons, it is more likely to be the former. First, the constellation of behaviors that has thus far been found deficient in negative-affect schizophrenics includes multiple behavioral domains—gestures, voice, gaze, and facial expressions—that all relate to affective encoding. Second, if it were conditionability that accounted for the predictive validity of the various measures of affectivity, why is its predictive power limited to such measures? Should not conditionability also infuse other symptom domains such as thought disorder with artifactual predictive validity? If conditionability is responsible for our results, it should be able to explain why so many studies have found, on the one hand, that affective variables have been such good predictors and, on the other hand, that cognitive variables have been such poor predictors. Third, in our research, those who have been assessed as affectively deficient after their first psychotic break have been shown to have manifested behavioral patterns in childhood and adolescence that are theoretically consistent with an affective deficit.

I must hasten to add, however, that in a review I did a number of years ago of the positive-reinforcement and punishment literature (Knight, 1968), I found evidence to support the notion that schizophrenics in general were less responsive to positive reinforcement that controls, and were more affected both by the contingency and the information content of reinforcers. Although I found little evidence that this was related to prognosis, your data point in that direction. Thus, the issue of conditionability that you mention is an important one, and how interviewer behavior might influence schizophrenics' affective responses should be assessed.

Dr. Salzinger: It is important to stress that when you have an interview, which is the source of most of the data on affectivity, you never have an operant level. The only time you have an operant level is when the interviewer decides not to reinforce. That is not the natural condition in a clinical interview. In the clinical interview, you have a mix-up of reinforcement for one response class or another. When an interviewer is unaware of the nature or frequency of his or her reinforcements, the effect of these reinforcements cannot be traced. Thus, I think that in the study of affectivity this important methodological issue must be addressed. I would urge those of you doing research on this problem to look at this important variable of reinforcement.

Dr. Knight: I would like to add one more point. The assessments of affectivity that I presented from our follow-up studies were generated not only from the reports of clinical interviews, but also from ward notes, interviews of family members, descriptions of the patient's performance in the armed service, etc. In addition, the clinical interviewers in our studies were all different and presumably had different reinforcement patterns. Thus, our affectivity judgments had predictive validity that was independent of the reinforcement schedule of any particular interviewer. Still, both interviewer behavior and the kind of emotion the interviewer attempts to elicit are extremely important variables that we should attempt to control in future studies.

REFERENCES

Salzinger, K., & Pisoni, S. (1958). Reinforcement of affect responses of schizophrenics during the clinical interview. *Journal of Abnormal and Social Psychology*, *57*, 84–90.

Salzinger, K., & Pisoni, S. (1960). Reinforcement of verbal affect responses of normal subjects during the interview. *Journal of Abnormal and Social Psychology*, *60*, 127–130.

Salzinger, K., & Pisoni, S. (1961). Some parameters of the conditioning of verbal affect responses in schizophrenic subjects. *Journal of Abnormal and Social Psychology*, *63*, 511–516.

Salzinger, K., & Portnoy, S. (1964). Verbal conditioning in interviews: Application to chronic schizophrenics and relationship to prognosis for acute schizophrenics. *Journal of Psychiatric Research*, *2*, 1–9.

16

Positive and Negative Family History for Schizophrenia: Differentiating Variables

SOLOMON C. GOLDBERG
Medical College of Virginia

In the search for objective markers of deficit of schizophrenia, it might be expected that patients with a positive family history would show the greater deficit. This has been demonstrated in the case of the Continuous Performance Test (CPT), first by Orzack and Kornetsky (1971) and, more recently, by Walker and Shaye (1982). Both studies find greater deficit in the positive-family-history schizophrenics.

HYPOTHESIS

The result that would be difficult to explain would be to find that a particular deficit marker was *more* prevalent in the negative family history cases. One would have to consider that the negative family history cases have a qualitatively different and environmental etiology from those with a positive family history. This is in keeping with an assumption that the etiologies of the schizophrenics are heterogeneous, and that some may be genetic in various ways and other nongenetic. Any particular schizophrenic patient may have one etiology, or both genetic *and* nongenetic etiologies, leading to his clinical manifestations.

Our view of negative family history schizophrenia has best been stated in Kendler and Hays's paper (1982a) on this same dichotomy. They conclude: "Although genetic factors are probably of greater etiological importance in familial schizophrenia, environmentally induced brain dysfunction may be more important in sporadic schizophrenia" (p. 1557). It will be our purpose to determine how far this view can be projected before it runs afoul of other facts it cannot accommodate.

Our hypothesis views negative family history schizophrenia as arising primarily from an environmental etiology.

In the remainder of this chapter, we shall present an array of discriminators between positive and negative family history schizophrenia and attempt to argue that one of the unifying threads for negative family history schizophrenia is organic impairment arising possibly through birth complications and early-life infections. For some of these discriminators there is more empirical evidence than for others. Some of the discriminators are more objective, such as CT scans, and others are clearly soft, such as a history of pregnancy and birth complications.

Imperfect Measurement of Family History

In employing a dichotomy, such as negative versus positive family history schizophrenia, there are a number of problems that render the distinction less than perfect. Because of the difficulty in obtaining diagnoses on all family members, there is a chance of misclassifying a true positive family history case as negative. The extent to which fewer than all family members are interviewed or diagnostic information is obtained through informants of unknown quality, the number of misclassifications should increase. The failure to characterize "near cases" of schizophrenia or subclinical vulnerability in a family would also lead to misclassification. Finally, because of a prevalence of 1%, the chances of finding an afflicted family member is small. Thus, some patients with a truly negative family history may still be genetically implicated. A variety of misdiagnoses could lead to false positives. Any misclassification would attenuate the relationship with other variables hypothesized to be relevant to the dichotomy.

SUPPORTING EVIDENCE

The results of Kendler and Hays (1982a) show the characteristics of positive family history schizophrenics to be (*a*) greater thought disorder and (*b*) a nearly significant trend to be more female. Negative family history cases on the other hand (*a*) are more likely to be male, (*b*) have a greater number of EEG abnormalities, and (*c*) have a history of premorbid inferiority feelings. These characteristics of sporadic cases suggest the possibility of underlying organic impairment for the following reasons. Pasamanick and Knobloch (1961), as well as worldwide vital statistics, show greater prevalence of organic impairment in male than in female births in the general population. If one posits organic impairment for negative family history cases, the hypothesis would require a higher proportion of males than females, as is the case. However, gender itself is a weak discriminator and requires larger sample size to show its effect. Premorbid inferiority feelings is not the same variable as poor premorbid status but both are signs of early disturbed behavior that has been related by other investigators to organicity. EEG abnormalities are more self-evidently neurological. Although EEG abnormalities can be found in many normals, the difference between positive and negative family history patients is in the theoretically expected direction.

Continuous Performance Test (CPT)

There are other workers who have employed the positive–negative family history dichotomy fruitfully. Orzack and Korentsky (1971) showed greater deficit in the CPT of schizophrenics with a family history of mental illness. This result was more recently replicated by Walker and Shaye (1982). Adding further credibility to this result are the preliminary findings of Rutschmann, Kornblatt, and Erlenmeyer-Kimling (1977) on children at high genetic risk for schizophrenia. These children, compared to matched controls, have begun to show a CPT deficit even though none is yet clinically schizophrenic. These studies strongly implicate the CPT as a deficit in schizophrenia with positive family history.

Premorbid Competence

Quitkin, Rifkin, Tsuang, Kane, and Klein (1980) find a nearly significant ($p = .09$) trend for a greater degree of premorbid asociality (poor premorbid adjustment) in negative family history schizophrenics. The lack of complete significance of the trend is attributed to the probability of misclassifying some positive history cases as negative because of imperfect ascertainment. Why should premorbid asociality be an attribute of negative family history? Premorbid asocials are described as odd kids who were always strange, never had friends, and were frequently scapegoated. Whatever went awry probably occurred very early in life. A result that is not consistent with Quitkin's is the Kety and Rosenthal finding that their genetic evidence applied more to chronic than to acute schizophrenics (Kety, Rosenthal, & Wender, 1968).

Concordance in MZ Twins

In a much earlier set of papers, Rosenthal (1959), in reviewing the major studies concerned with MZ twin concordance rates in schizophrenia, finds

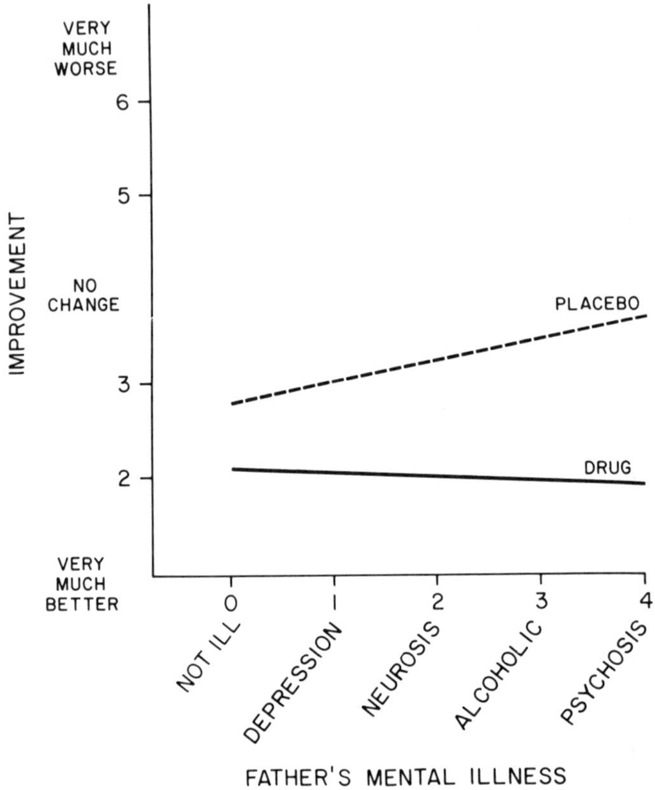

Figure 1. Drug–placebo differences for patients with a mentally ill father.

a significantly greater family history for schizophrenia in concordant MZ twins than in discordant MZ twins. On a theoretical basis alone, because MZ twins are genetically identical, schizophrenia in only one of them is likely to be environmentally determined.

Response to Neuroleptics

There is a clinical lore that negative family history cases of schizophrenia may be less responsive to neuroleptics than positive history cases. Some support for this is provided by Cole, Goldberg, and Davis (1966) in finding greater drug–placebo differences for patients with a mentally ill father (Figure 1). A nonsignificant trend in the same direction was obtained for the patient's mother. The smallest drug–placebo differences were obtained when the parents had no detectable illness and the largest when the parents had a psychotic illness.

PREDICTIONS FROM THE HYPOTHESIS

The foregoing is the extent of the variables in the literature that relate to the presence or absence of a family history for schizophrenia. However, there are other variables of interest about which the theory makes specific predictions.

Sex versus Response to Neuroleptics

For instance, because being female and being responsive to neuroleptics are characteristics of positive family history cases, it should follow that females should be more responsive to drug treatment. The results of Goldberg, Schooler, Davidson, and Kayce (1966) on symptom reduction for inpatients and Goldberg, Schooler, Hogarty, and Roper (1977) on time until relapse for outpatients show this very clearly. Although drug exceeds placebo for both sexes, the *size of the drug–placebo difference* is significantly larger for females. Males are not nonresponders but rather poor responders.

Premorbid Competence versus Response to Neuroleptics

Because poor premorbid status is associated with having a negative family history, it should follow that poor premorbids should show less drug response. This has been demonstrated by Klein and Rosen (1973) using the Premorbid Asociality Scale and by Cole *et al.* (1966) (Figure 2), in which "never married" is regarded as being poor premorbid compared to ever having been married. The drug–placebo difference is larger for patients who were ever married. In that study a scale of premorbid competence was not employed. Marital status was used in its place, because other studies have shown that being married is associated with good premorbid competence. One study by Goldstein (1970) reports findings opposite to these.

Age at Onset versus Response to Neuroleptics

Another expectation from the theory is that negative family history cases became ill earlier and hence earlier onset patients should respond less well to neuroleptics. In support of this prediction, Cole *et al.* (1966) (Figure 3) find greater drug–placebo differences in patients with a later age onset.

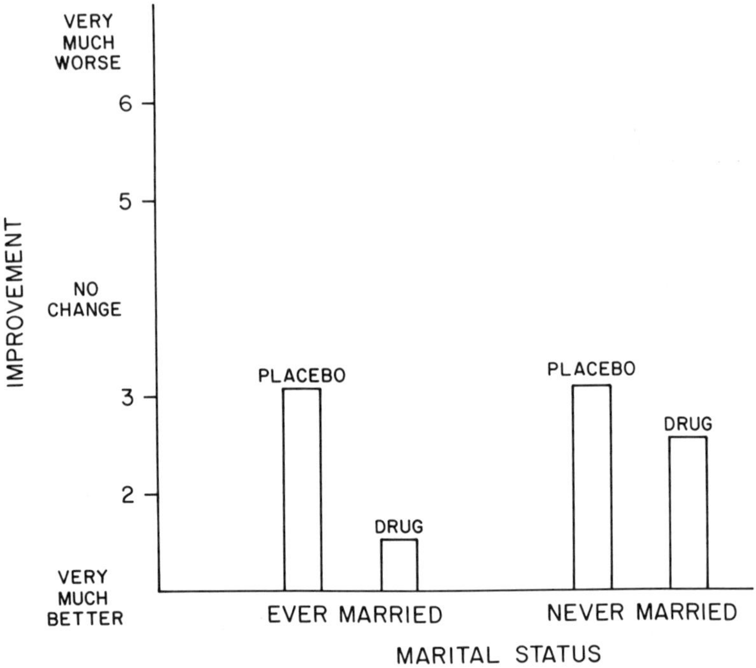

Figure 2. Drug–placebo differences as a function of marital status.

CT Scan versus Response to Neuroleptics

Weinberger *et al.* (1980) and Schulz, Sinecrop, Kishore, and Friedel (1983) have shown that patients with larger "ventricular brain ratios" (VBR) tend to respond less to neuroleptics. The larger VBR patient is almost definitional of the negative family history case whom the theory expects to be suffering an organic deficit.

Some of the CT scan data can be confusing in interpretation because, on the one hand, VBR has been shown to be heritable, and Reveley, Clifford, and Reveley (1982) have shown that in discordant MZ twins, the schizophrenic twin will have the larger VBR. The fact that VBR is heritable has tempted some to conclude that this is the inherited defect in schizophrenia. However, if one accepts that the instance of discordance in MZ twins indicates a negative family history case with organicity, then the fact that the proband has the larger VBR is eminently plausible.

CT Scan and Neuropsychology

The relationship between VBR and impairment on neuropsychology testing shown by Golden *et al.* (1980) and Donnelly, Weinberger, Waldman, and

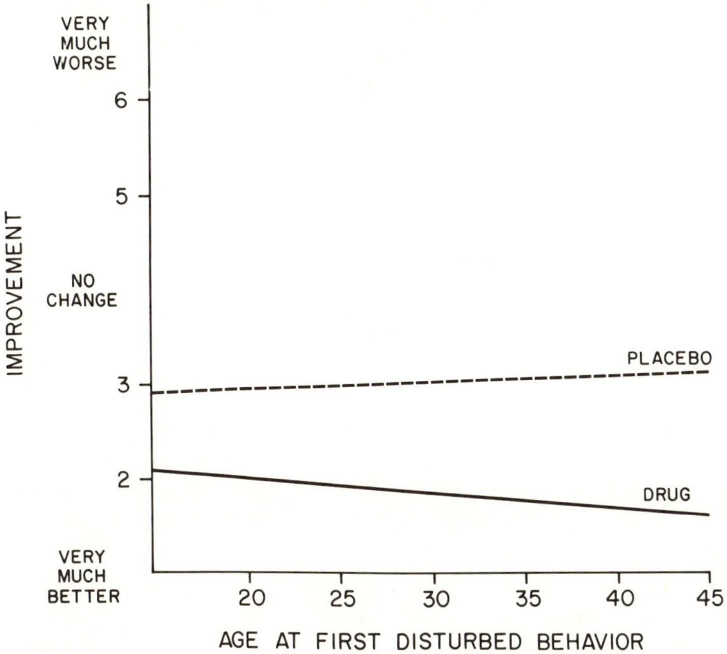

Figure 3. Drug–placebo differences as a function of age of disturbed behavior onset.

Wyatt (1980) has similar implications as with VBR. That is, organic impairment as measured by neuropsychology assessments, such as the Luria–Nebraska, is indicative of the sporadic case. In a much earlier paper, Belmont, Birch, Klein, and Pollack (1964) show organic signs on the Rorschach to be associated with premorbid asociality. Their data also show, as our hypothesis expects, the poor premorbids to be primarily male.

Premorbid Competence and Soft Neurological Signs

Quitkin, Rifkin, and Klein (1976) find an association between premorbid asociality and soft neurological signs, again supporting the link between negative family history schizophrenia and organic impairment.

Negative Symptoms, CT Scan, and Neuroleptic Response

Johnstone, Crow, Frith, Husband, and Kreel (1976) and Crow (1980) have shown a relationship between "positive versus negative" symptoms and VBR. Consistent with our hypothesis, they maintain that negative symptoms tend to be chronic and are not responsive to neuroleptics. We agree that negative family history schizophrenics with enlarged ventricles probably

Table 1. Drug Effects on Negative Symptoms

	Placebo pre–post change standard scores	Drug pre–post change standard scores
Attitudinal apathy (N = 214)	0.353	1.234
Motor retardation (N = 245)	0.114	.849
Social participation versus withdrawal (N = 302)	0.788	1.776

Note. All drug–placebo differences, $p < .01$.

have a different set of symptoms from positive family history schizophrenics, but we disagree that they are necessarily the so-called negative symptoms. An earlier study by Goldberg, Klerman, and Cole (1965) shows that some negative symptoms such as motor retardation, attitudinal apathy, and social withdrawal did show large and significant drug effects (Table 1).

In that study, the symptoms that did not show a significant drug effect were (*a*) guilt, (*b*) looks sad, (*c*) resistive, (*d*) feelings of unreality, (*e*) nonauditory hallucinations, (*f*) delusions of grandeur, (*g*) disorientation, and (*h*) memory deficit. Although some of these do indeed look like negative symptoms, the hallucinations and delusions are not. Indeed, some of the symptoms, such as feelings of unreality, nonauditory (visual and olfactory) hallucinations, disorientation of time, place, and person, and memory deficit for recent events, have an "organic" quality to them. We would propose that many of the defect symptoms associated with enlarged ventricles are understandably those one would expect with organicity.

CT Scan, Family History, and Birth Complications

Very recently, Murray, Reveley, Reveley, Shur, and Lewis (in press) have shown increased ventricular size only in negative family history schizophrenics. Further, all schizophrenics with birth complications had a negative family history and five out of six came from pairs of MZ twins that were discordant for schizophrenia. Contrary to our hypothesis, they find later age of onset associated with larger ventricles. Nasrallah, Tippin, McCalley-Witters, and Kuperman (1982), on the other hand, have reported larger ventricles with positive family history schizophrenics mainly in his process nonparanoid (hebephrenic and catatonic) group.

Amphetamine Challenge

The work of Angrist (1982) and van Kammen, Docherty, Marder, Rayner, and Bunney (1982) have shown that patients whose symptoms exacerbate when challenged with amphetamine are more likely to relapse if neuroleptics are discontinued. An as-yet-untested prediction from the theory is that the nonexacerbating patients should be the negative family history cases. Kornetsky (1976) has shown them to be "chronic" rather than "acute" cases. If we were dealing with objective tests, such as reaction time and WAIS block design rather than clinical symptoms, amphetamine challenge should result in exacerbating reaction time but not block design.

A summarizing table of the proposed discriminators between sporadic and familial schizophrenia is presented for orientation in Table 2. The overall hypothesis underlying the table is that a major unifying principle for negative family history schizophrenia is environmentally induced brain dysfunction. Each of the variables in the table provides the opportunity to disprove the hypothesis empirically. Another expectation from the table is that the entire list of variables should be significantly intercorrelated in the hypothesized direction. Thus, if one did not have good data on family history, a test of the proposed hypothesis would be in terms of their intercorrelations. For all the elements in the table there is at this stage only variable evidence and much more research is needed to test these assertions.

Although we hypothesize that organicity underlies much of negative family history schizophrenia, there are some indications that some of these patients may be bipolar who, because of their delusions, hallucinations, and thought disorder, have been misdiagnosed as schizophrenic. These patients are a separate and important issue. Pope and Lipinski (1978) make

Table 2. Hypothesized Discriminators between Positive and Negative Family History Schizophrenia

Negative family history	Positive family history
Male	Female
Earlier onset	Later onset
Poorer premorbid status	Better premorbid status
More history of birth complications	Less history of birth complications
Discordance in MZ twins	Concordance in MZ twins
Less thought disorder	More thought disorder
More memory deficit, disorientation, visual and olfactory hallucinations	Less memory deficit, disorientation, visual and olfactory hallucinations
More EEG abnormalities	Fewer EEG abnormalities
More neurological soft signs	Fewer neurological soft signs
More signs of "brain damage" on neuropsychology tests	Fewer signs of "brain damage" on neuropsychology tests
Larger VBR on CT scan	Smaller VBR on CT scan
Less CPT deficit	More CPT deficit
Less responsive to neuroleptics	More responsive to neuroleptics
Less exacerbation when challenged with amphetamine	More exacerbation when challenged with amphetamine

a reasonable case to this effect in that some diagnosed schizophrenics who respond only moderately to neuroleptics often respond well to lithium. These are not the organically impaired cases, even though they have a negative family history for schizophrenia.

ETIOLOGY AND TREATMENT

Our hypothesis is that the organic impairment of negative family history cases often arises from birth complications, as is suggested by Murray *et al.* (in press) and the earlier work of Pollin and Stabenau (1968), but may also arise from other early-life infections. However, is it reasonable to expect that a nonspecific event, such as the anoxia of birth complications, would give rise to mental symptoms as specific as schizophrenia? Why not other mental disorders? Anoxia and infections may have very variable effects for reasons we do not understand yet. Why one case would result in schizophrenic symptoms and others in childhood hyperactivity may be a matter of the locus of the lesion. Slater, Beard, and Glithero (1963) have shown schizophrenic symptoms in a group of unequivocal epileptics, implying an organic base for the schizophrenic symptoms. Slater considered whether the epilepsy and schizophrenia were possibly concurrent but independent. If they were independent, the prevalence of schizophrenia would be no greater than in the general population. The fact that the prevalence was considerably greater implies that the two were associated. Yet it is not understood why all epileptics do not show schizophrenic symptoms.

Is negative family history schizophrenia a qualitatively different type of schizophrenia or is it a quantitative dimension? Crow argues against there being positive and negative symptom types, partly because most patients are not purely positive or negative but a mixture of the two. We would propose that positive and negative family history schizophrenia represent two different etiologies, one of which is a genetic diathesis and the other environmental stress. Each is a quantitative continuum. A patient with schizophrenia may have either one or both components in varying amounts. There are now a few studies showing that schizophrenic mothers are more likely to have birth complications. Their offspring, if clinically schizophrenic, could have features of both positive and negative family history schizophrenia.

Treatment?

Given that negative family history cases are not responsive to neuroleptics, how should they be treated?

First, it is important that such cases be identified early so that they are not exposed to the risks of neuroleptics without any of the benefits.

ECT seems an unlikely treatment for organic impairment. The experience of many treatment centers with neuroleptic failures is to try next a course of ECT because they cannot think of what else to do. This has resulted in a considerable amount of uncontrolled clinical experience indicating that ECT is not noticeably effective in such patients. On the other hand, there has been the opposite experience with depression, where ECT has been found effective for drug nonresponders.

Aside from the search for effective treatments in the form of new drugs and behavioral interventions, the major research needs now are to test more specifically the variety of predictions made here. One possible way of doing so, discussed earlier, is to determine the relationship between family history and each of the variables presumed to be related to it. Although logically straightforward, this approach suffers the disadvantage of dealing with single variables that are weak discriminators. For instance, Kendler and Hays find both EEG abnormalities and premorbid inferiority feelings in negative family history cases, but the two discriminators are not related to each other. Murray *et al.* find enlarged ventricles and birth complications mainly in negative family history cases, but schizophrenics with large ventricles did not have significantly more birth complications. A different approach is to treat the list of discriminators as a multivariate composite by means of discriminant function, because it is possible for any patient to be some combination of genetic diathesis and environmental stress rather than exclusively and purely one or the other. A factor analysis as another multivariate approach would be expected to yield a bipolar factor with negative family history, larger ventricles, birth complications, etc., loading on one pole and positive family history, CPT, and worsening on amphetamine on the other pole.

Finally, on a more speculative and exploratory basis, the possibility arises that organic impairment may result in other psychiatric disorders, such as character disorders (Quitkin *et al.*, 1976) and childhood hyperactivity. Similar phenomenologies may arise from different etiologies and vice versa. Genetically transmitted disorders may have "phenocopies" with nongenetic etiologies. There is the likelihood that the organic etiology is not specific to schizophrenia alone. The question may then be raised of how to explain that variability.

REFERENCES

Angrist, B. (1982). *Amphetamine challenge as a predictor of relapse in schizophrenics discontinued from neuroleptics*. Poster presentation at the 1982 meetings of the American College of Neuropsychopharmacology, San Juan, Puerto Rico.

Belmont, I., Birch, H., Klein, D. F., & Pollack, N. (1964). Perceptual evidence of CNS dysfunction in schizophrenia. *Archives of General Psychiatry, 10*, 395.

Cole, J. O., Goldberg, S. C., & Dais, J. M. (1966). Drugs in the treatment of psychosis: Controlled studies. In P. Solomon (Ed.), *Psychiatric drugs* (pp. 153–180). New York: Grune & Stratton.

Crow, T. J. (1980). Molecular pathology of schizophrenia. More than one disease process. *British Medical Journal, 1*, 66–68.

Donnelly, E. F., Weinberger, D. R., Waldman, I. N., & Wyatt, R. J. (1980). Cognitive impairment associated with morphological brain abnormalities on computed tomography in chronic schizophrenic patients. *Journal of Nervous and Mental Disease, 168*, 305–308.

Goldberg, S. C., Klerman, G. L., & Cole, J. O. (1965). Changes in schizophrenic psychopathology and ward behavior as a function of phenothiazine treatment. *British Journal of Psychiatry, 111*, 120–133.

Goldberg, S. C., Schooler, N. R., Davidson, E. M., & Kayce, M. N. (1966). Sex and race differences in response to drug treatment among schizophrenics. *Psychopharmacologia, 9*, 31–47.

Goldberg, S. C., Schooler, N. R., Hogarty, G. E., & Roper, M. (1977). Prediction of relapse in schizophrenic outpatients treated by drug and sociotherapy. *Archives of General Psychiatry, 34*, 171–184.

Golden, C. J., Moses, J. A., Zelazowski, R., Graber, B., Zatz, L. M., Horvath, T. B., & Berger, P. A. (1980). Cerebral ventricular size and neuropsychological impairment in young schizophrenics. *Archives of General Psychiatry, 37*, 619–623.

Goldstein, M. J. (1970). Premorbid adjustment, paranoid states and patterns of response to phenothiazines in acute schizophrenia. *Schizophrenia Bulletin, 3*, 24–37.

Johnstone, E. C., Crow, T. J., Frith, C. D., Husband, J., & Kreel, L. (1976). Cerebral ventricular size and cognitive impairment in chronic schizophrenia. *Lancet, 2*, 924–926.

Kendler, K. S., & Hays, P. (1982a). Familial and sporadic schizophrenia: A symptomatic, prognostic and EEG comparison. *American Journal of Psychiatry, 139*, 1557–1562.

Kendler, K. S., & Hays, P. (1982b). Schizophrenia with premorbid inferiority feelings: A distinct subgroup. Archives of General Psychiatry, *39*, 643–647.

Kety, S. S., Rosenthal, D., & Wender, P. H. (1968). The types and prevalence of mental illness in the biological and adoptive families of adopted schizophrenics. In D. Rosenthal & S. S. Kety (Eds.), *The transmission of schizophrenia* (pp. 345–362). Oxford: Pergamon Press.

Klein, D. F., & Rosen, B. (1973). Premorbid asocial adjustment and response to phenothiazine treatment among schizophrenic inpatients. *Archives of General Psychiatry, 29*, 480.

Kornetsky, C. (1976). Hyporesponsivity of chronic schizophrenic patients to dextroamphetamine. *Archives of General Psychiatry, 33*, 1425–1428.

Murray, R. M., Reveley, A. M., Revley, M. A., Shur, E., & Lewis, S. (in press). Genetic and Environmental Influences in Schizohprenia. In T. Sakai & T. Tsuboi (Eds.), *Genetic aspects of human behavior*. Tokyo: Igaku-Shoin.

Nasrallah, H. A., Tippin, V., McCalley-Whitters, M., & Kuperman, S. (1982). Neurologic differences between paranoid and nonparanoid schizophrenia, Part III. Neurologic soft signs. *Journal of Clinical Psychiatry, 43*, 310–312.

Orzack, M. H., & Kornetsky, C. (1971). Environmental and familial predictors of attention behavior in chronic schizophrenics. *Journal of Psychiatric Research, 9*, 21–29.

Pasamanick, B., & Knobloch, H. (1961). Epedemiological studies on the complications of pregnancy and birth process. In G. Caplan (Ed.), *Prevention of mental disorders in children*. New York: Basic Books.

Pollin, W., & Stabenau, J. R. (1968). Biological, psychological and historical differences in a series of monozygotic twins discordant for schizophrenia. In D. Rosenthal & S. S.

Kety (Eds.), *The transmission of schizophrenia* (pp. 317–322). Oxford: Pergamon Press.

Pope, H. G., & Lipinski, J. F. (1978). Diagnosis in schizophrenia and manic depressive illness. *Archives of General Psychiatry, 35*, 811–828.

Quitkin, F. N., Rifkin, A., & Klein, D. F. (1976). Neurological soft signs in schizophrenia and character disorders. *Archives of General Psychiatry, 33*, 845–853.

Quitkin, F. N., Rifkin, A., Tsuang, M. T., Kane, J. M., & Klein, D. F. (1980). Can schizophrenia with premorbid asociality be genetically distinguishable from other forms of schizophrenia? *Psychiatry Research, 2*, 99–105.

Reveley, A. M., Clifford, C. A., & Reveley, M. A. (1982). Cerebral ventricular size in twins discordant for schizophrenia. *Lancet*, 1i, 540–541.

Rosenthal, D. (1959). Some factors associated with concordance and discordance with respect to schizophrenia in monzygotic twins. *Journal of Nervous and Mental Disease, 129*, 1–10.

Rutschmann, J., Kornblatt, B., & Erlenmeyer-Kimling, L. (1977). Sustained attention in children at risk for schizophrenia. *Archives of General Psychiatry, 34*, 571–575.

Schulz, S. C., Sinecrop, P., Kishore, P., & Friedel, R. O. (1983). Treatment response and ventricular brain enlargement in young schizophrenic patients. *Psychopharmacology Bulletin, 19*, 510–512.

Slater E., Beard, A. M., & Glithero, E. (1963). The schizophrenia-like psychoses of epilepsy. *British Journal of Psychiatry, 109*, 95–150.

van Kammen, D. P., Docherty, J. P., Marder, S. R., Rayner, J. N., & Bunney, W. E. (1982). Longterm pimozide pretreatment differentially affects behavioral response to dextroamphetamine in schizophrenia. *Archives of General Psychiatry, 39*, 275–281.

Walker, E., & Shaye, J. (1982). Familial schizophrenia: A predictor of neuromotor and attentional abnormalities in schizophrenia. *Archives of General Psychiatry, 39*, 1153–1156.

Weinberger, D. R., Bigelow, L. B., Kleinman, J. E., Klein, F. T., Rosenblatt, J. E., & Wyatt, R. J. (1980). Cerebral ventricular enlargement in chronic schizophrenia: An association with poor response to treatment. *Archives of General Psychiatry, 37*, 11–13.

General Discussion

Dr. Brendan Maher:* Before we begin the general discussion, let us take one or two questions addressed specifically to Dr. Goldberg.

Dr. Burt Angrist†: I think one might expect people with intact brains to have more of a normal amphetamine response than people with organicity, which I think is the basis of your hypothesis.

Dr. Solomon C. Goldberg‡: I'm not hearing you. I think you'd be better off without the microphone.

Dr. Angrist: You might expect people with intact brains to have a brisker amphetamine response than people with damaged systems, but I think there are some data that might cut the other way. People with encephalitis lethargica were notoriously intolerant to L-dopa psychoses. Dr. Carpenter, I think, yesterday said that his deficit patients had a higher rate of relapse when they were taken off neuroleptics than the nondeficit ones. Finally, I hear the addicts who are shooting that dopaminergic neurotoxin NMPTP on the West Coast are showing, when doctors go to treat their Parkinsonism with agonists, essentially the whole constellation of a lifetime of L-dopa's complications, all being compressed within the first year, including psychosis. So one might also guess that there might be some relationship between damage and instability, and that could make things go the other way. I don't know how it will go. It certainly should be done.

Dr. Goldberg: It hasn't been done to my knowledge, unless somebody knows of someone doing amphetamine challenge by positive and negative family history.

Dr. Donald F. Klein§: I can talk to that point. You sort of identified the childhood asocials, with the possibility of their being in the negative-family-history group, and that has certainly been our experience. These people stick out in their families like sore thumbs. In the study that Quitkin *et al.* did, not a single one of the childhood asocials had a positive family

* Cambridge, Massachusetts.
† New York, New York.
‡ Richmond, Virginia.
§ New York, New York.

history. The reason it was only at the trend level was because family history was fairly low in the other schizophrenics also.

We gave imipramine to 100 schizophrenics, and 6 of them had a psychotic exacerbation. Of the 6 who had a psychotic exacerbation, 5 were childhood asocials. That was highly significant, even though it was a small sample. Further, in reviewing the literature, there is an old paper buried somewhere by Pilkington on treating mental deficiency with imipramine. He reported very clearly that it was the mentally deficient who showed schizoid personalities over and above their mental deficiency who had a psychotic exacerbation with imipramine. So I go right along with Burt [Angrist]. It is possible that you are correct, but I'm not clear about the idea that there would be less exacerbation when challenged with amphetamine. Certainly imipramine goes the other way. While we are scratching around for straws that can support your hypothesis, I think you left out Dan Weinberger's finding, that when they measured their subjects with regard to premorbid asociality, which he did with using a variation of Rachel Gittelman's scale, there was a clear relationship between the history of premorbid asociality and the VBR ratio.

Finally, one more point. You said that Mike Goldstein, who is here and can speak for himself, had a finding that went against the relative superior benefit of drug in the nonasocial patient. I think that Mike's finding was that in the asocial patients, drug had more effect with regard to psychological tests, but not with regard to clinical behavior. There the findings were rather indifferent one way or the other. Maybe Mike might want to speak to that.

Dr. Michael J. Goldstein:* Yes. Actually, that's not the case. There are about three studies now that have indicated that the premorbid variable does relate to drug response, but I think it is a very complicated issue, because dose response issues are very much involved. For example, in our Ventura County study, there was clearly a dose response, with the poor premorbids doing poor on the low dose and relapsing. Also, in the van Kammen and Marder studies, when patients were withdrawn from their ongoing medication, it was the poor premorbids who relapsed very quickly and required much higher dose level in order to achieve clinical stability than the good premorbids.

So basically the trend of the evidence suggests that the premorbid variable does interact with the drug response, but it is probably some interaction with dose levels, with the poor premorbids requiring higher dose levels to get a more marginal clinical response than you will get with the lower dose level with a good premorbid patient. So I don't think it is such

* Los Angeles, California.

a simple issue of just saying there's a response or not as a function of the premorbid history.

By the way, Sol [Goldberg] I don't know if that never-married part of your study was just males. Was that just males?

Dr. Goldberg: No.

Dr. Goldstein: Because that is nested in the sex-difference factor. 70%–80% of schizophrenic women marry and only 30% of males, so I think you are replicating the same finding that you got for your sex differences with the ever-married variable. I really don't think you can use it.

The other thing about premorbid adjustment is that, in sex differences, it depends whether you use an absolute or a relative scale. For example, males and females differ on most premorbid scales on the average, with very few females showing real asocial patterns. They occur, but they are pretty rare, and it is predominantly a male pattern of the schizoid loner. If you put them on relative distributions, however, of relatively poor premorbid for each sex distribution, you do get the same findings and the same interaction with the phenothiazine drug treatment.

Dr. Barnabe:* I would like to ask Dr. Goldberg whether there have been any studies done on brain electrical activity mapping tests, BEAM tests, which are computerized EEGs. This seems to be a much more sensitive measure than the normal EEG we do, because it is computerized EEG that cuts across the brain like a CT scan, which would pick up some of the episodic discontrol of schizophrenic patients that usually occurs. It might have something to do with the epileptic theory.

Dr. Goldberg: No, we haven't, and the reports of Kendler and Hayes that I mentioned were, I believe, of an eyeball analysis of the EEG rather than any kind of computerized analysis. It was a clinical evaluation of the EEG, but it still seemed to show up.

Dr. Barnabe: The other point I would like to comment on is the prototypical positive and negative etiology. You did say that negative is probably due to genetic reasons and positive due to environmental stress.

Dr. Goldberg: The other way.

Dr. Barnabe: Oh, I'm sorry, the other way. But if you would like to integrate your theories to catch the mixed type, which is really the greatest number, and you look at prototypical negative and prototypical positive in a population, what usually happens is that you have a continuum on which there are a very small number of positives and a very small number of negatives, and you have a mixture in between. Would it be theoretically possible that the genetic analysis has something to do with an immune system that has been proven in environmental stress? You know that a lot

* Bronx, New York.

of environmental stress does diminish the immune system of individuals—and I was wondering if that could be an integrated theoretical model to test some hypotheses and maybe some findings. I'm not sure.

Dr. Goldberg: I'm afraid I hadn't thought of the immune system, for a very good reason, which is that I know nothing about it. If you look at positive and negative family history for schizophrenia, most schizophrenics don't have a visible family history for schizophrenia. They seem to be mostly negative, but that does not mean that in any individual case there isn't a genetic component that can be carried by family members who themselves are not schizophrenic.

Dr. Henry Nasrallah:* I would like to comment on your CT comparison between our studies and the Reveleys. We found family history in first-degree relatives to be associated with very large ventricular enlargement, that is, above 2 standard deviations from the control mean, and we only had males in our sample. In contrast, the Reveleys had both males and females and, as you said, they did not look into first-degree relatives only, but into family history of all psychopathology at all levels.

Dr. Goldberg: Did you use spectrum disorders in the family history?

Dr. Nasrallah: We looked at that and did not come up with anything significant. Only schizophrenia in first-degree relatives came out with a significance. I would like to add to your mini-review of the subject the study of Weinberger and his colleagues of 10 schizophrenic patients and their nonschizophrenic siblings, and 10 matched controls. The schizophrenic sample had the largest ventricles. Their nonschizophrenic siblings (not twins) had an intermediate VBR, all of them larger than normals. So there does seem to be a familial transmission of VBR size.

Dr. Goldberg: Oh, yes.

Dr. Nasrallah: As to whether it is a marker for schizophrenia, that is a very vague issue at this point.

Dr. Goldberg: I think it is possible for a variable to be highly heritable as, say, intelligence, and still, if you inflict a head trauma you can alter one's intelligence. This blow is a stress of the physical environment. So it doesn't mean that high heritability excludes the effects of environment.

Dr. Nasrallah: I'd like to make another comment with respect to the male/female dichotomy that you used. I think that is a very useful one, and it is going to become more useful as we learn about gender differences in schizophrenia. I would like to refer to a recent study that I did, and it's in press in *Acta Psychiatrica Scandinavica*, in which we looked at the season of birth, dividing the patients into males and females, and into paranoid and nonparanoid subtypes. This has never been done. Most of the studies

* Iowa City, Iowa.

lump everybody together, despite the fact that these two variables are important. What we found was that the nonparanoid females had the highest frequency of winter births, that is, cold-month births.

Dr. Goldberg: The nonparanoid?

Dr. Nasrallah: The nonparanoid females, which would have a higher family loading for schizophrenia as well. You have to remember that being born in cold months does not necessarily associate with brain injury causing the schizophrenia; there is another model that posits that being born with schizophrenia genes may protect you from dying, if you are born into cold months with injury, infection, or other brain insults. That is the "protective model" rather than the "insult model," and that is something to consider when you have the high-genetic-loading females born in winter months.

Dr. Maher: Thank you.

Dr. Joseph Zubin:* I want to make two brief points. First, according to the European studies, the nonfamilial schizophrenias seemed to be more severe. I don't see that on your table at all. The second point, if you take into consideration the penetrance of schizophrenia, is that you'd expect a certain number of families not to have any phenotypes, even though they may have the genotypes. I wonder—you may have done this—have you made a distribution by size of family and obtained the probabilities of expected phenotypes based upon some penetrance value, say, a .25 penetrance, whatever you find to be the most scientific expectation? It may be that when you do that by size of family and by the expectancy of penetrance, you will find that your entire distribution is what you'd expect from your own predictions including the proportion of zero phenotypes (the nonfamilial). Then the genetic model may be tenable. Geneticists would love that. On the other hand, if you find there is an excess of probands without any phenotypes in their families, then of course, environmentalists would love it. So I think it would be a good thing to try and see how it works out.

Dr. Goldberg: Yes. I don't have those.

Dr. Maher: We can take some questions or discussion addressed to the other speakers, and I will begin myself by asking of Dr. Lewine if you want to come up to the table. I have been intrigued by a kind of "throw-away" line that you had in your talk where you said, "Is hoarding to be understood as a lack of altruism?" Of course, the message of that, I think, is that when the patient is *not* doing what he ought to be doing, he is inevitably doing something else; in this respect, there are no negative symptoms, there are only positive symptoms. The patient is always doing something. I wonder to what extent you feel there is a failure on our part to recognize the linguistic implications of words like **dis***order*, **in***coherence*. They imply a kind of absence or lack of something (rather than a presence of something else).

* Pittsburgh, Pennsylvania.

This seems slightly inappropriate when referring to organisms or people who are always actually doing one thing or another.

Dr. Lewine: I won't pretend to be a linguist or to be too complex, but essentially, I do believe that we have come to realize in words like *incoherence* absences of things that may well be, as Hughlings Jackson suggested, release from cortical inhibition of a more positive source of processes, so that in some sense the distinction positive and negative is a trivial one. What we may have are a series of cortical insults, or release from inhibition of various levels of cortical control, all sorts of processes that are positive in the sense that they are there.

I'm not sure yet how strongly I believe in a positive–negative distinction. To be quite honest with you, there is a difference between my coauthor and myself on that point. I think right now I continue to believe it is a useful heuristic if not a completely valid linguistic one.

Dr. Maher: Any other questions?

Ms. Alison A. Sommers:* I'm Dr. Lewine's coauthor. Dr. Lewine and I are in substantial agreement with both Dr. Zubin's and Dr. Knight's concerns regarding negative symptoms. In fact, I'd like to expand on Dr. Zubin's comments: Negative symptoms as currently measured do resemble what are putatively other constructs such as *institutionalization*; what has been variously called *postpsychotic depression*, *revealed depression*, and *akinetic depression*; and psychomotor aspects of extrapyramidal symptoms, as well as schizotypal personality and "poor premorbid personality." I will leave aside the question as to whether any of those are distinguishable from each other.

At present we don't really know what negative symptoms are, either epistemologically or empirically. What is called for, we believe, is a series of construct validation studies to explicate the network of relationships between schizophrenic negative symptoms and other variables presumed on theoretical grounds to be related (positively or negatively) to negative symptoms. NIMH has recently funded such a study, or at least part of such a study on which Dr. Lewine and I have recently embarked. I also would like to suggest that other negative-symptoms researchers might find it useful to reread Cronbach and Meehl's old but still very useful 1955 *Psychological Bulletin* article describing the structure of construct validation. Some of their suggestions regarding internal validity, for example, speak to Dr. Knight's comments.

His comments today also represent what I think may be the first thrust toward what Meehl called boot-strapping and the development of a new generation of negative symptoms scales, or perhaps a new way of defining negative symptoms altogether. We hope that you will be continuing along those directions and you certainly have our agreement.

* Chicago, Illinois.

SECTION FIVE

TREATMENT AND OUTCOME

17

The Course of Schizophrenia: An Evolving Concept

COURTENAY M. HARDING AND JOHN S. STRAUSS
Yale University School of Medicine

INTRODUCTION

For the last eight decades, the course of schizophrenia (especially for persons with repeated episodes) has been described as (1) predictable by diagnosis, (2) progressing to uniformly poor functioning, (3) increasingly following a straight line over time, and (4) afflicting a passive person considered to be at the mercy of the disorder (e.g., Kraepelin, 1902; American Psychiatric Association, 1980).

In this chapter we have gathered some evidence which suggests that the course of schizophrenia is a more complex, dynamic, and *heterogeneous* process than has been heretofore appreciated or predicted by diagnostic specificity. The longitudinal picture of course, generated by long-term follow-up studies, reveals *nonlinear* patterns and trends with significant *improvement* in functioning across time for over half of the subjects. Further, the individual has been documented as an *active, developing person* in interaction with his or her environment. These important modifiers reshape the course of illness and the person's life in which schizophrenia is but a part.

THE EVOLUTION OF CONCEPTS ABOUT THE COURSE OF SCHIZOPHRENIA

From Homogeneity to Heterogeneity in the Course of Schizophrenia

From Kraepelin (1902) to the DSM-III (American Psychiatric Association, 1980), the course of schizophrenia has been assumed to be a homogeneously poor one. Described as a slow, downward progression to a marginal or deteriorated state after repeated episodes, the disorder acquired the adage: "Once a schizophrenic, always a schizophrenic," now considered to be an axiom.

Indeed, until the 1980s, evidence from follow-up studies was contradictory and confusing (e.g., Bellak, 1948; Shapiro & Shader, 1979; Stephens, 1970). However, in the last decade, several studies of various lengths have been achieved with more systematic approaches to sample selection, diagnostic criteria, and assessment of outcome.

In studies such as those by Bland and Orn (1978), Hawk, Carpenter, and Strauss (1975), and the World Health Organization (1979), short-term outcome, as a marker within the trajectory of long-term course, was found to be widely heterogeneous within and across samples.

Long-term follow-up studies also revealed there could be significant improvement or recovery for at least half of each cohort across time (Bleuler, 1972; Ciompi, 1980; Ciompi & Müller, 1976; Harding, 1984; Huber, Gross, & Schüttler, 1979; Tsuang, Woolson, & Fleming, 1979). In analyses from the Vermont Study recently completed, 21 to 58 years after first admission for those 82 cases retrospectively diagnosed as meeting the criteria for DSM-III schizophrenia, the findings of improvement continue to hold, including the same proportions of recovery (Harding, 1984).

The long-term follow-up studies focused not only on improvement as group means across all areas of functioning, but also on differential degrees of improvement across various domains of functioning within each subject. As specifically detailed by Harding, Brooks, Ashikaga, Strauss, and Landerl (in press), some individual subjects were working and relating well, but haunted by persistent hallucinations or delusions. Other scenarios revealed people who worked, but had no friends and no symptoms, whereas other subjects had a constellation composed of no work, no symptoms, but warm, intimate relationships.

This differential kind of functioning was vividly described by the team of Strauss and Carpenter (1974, 1977) as "open-linked" systems. Their concept was generated from several analyses related to outcome in schizophrenia carried out in the Washington Field Center of the World Health Organization's International Pilot Study of Schizophrenia. As part of that prospective follow-up study, the investigators analyzed the Washington Center data to determine the relationships among outcome characteristics, the prognostic value of various diagnostic systems, and the prognostic value of characteristics other than diagnosis. In analyzing predictors of outcome other than diagnosis, open-linked systems were found in which each domain of functioning (work, social relationships, severity of symptoms, and duration of time spent out of hospital in the year before entering the study) predicted to some degree the level of functioning a person would display in the corresponding domain 2 and 5 years after the episode (Strauss & Carpenter, 1977). In addition, work experience prior to episode increased the likelihood of being able to work post-episode (see Figure 1). The existence of open-linked systems was documented in the findings of the Rochester First Ad-

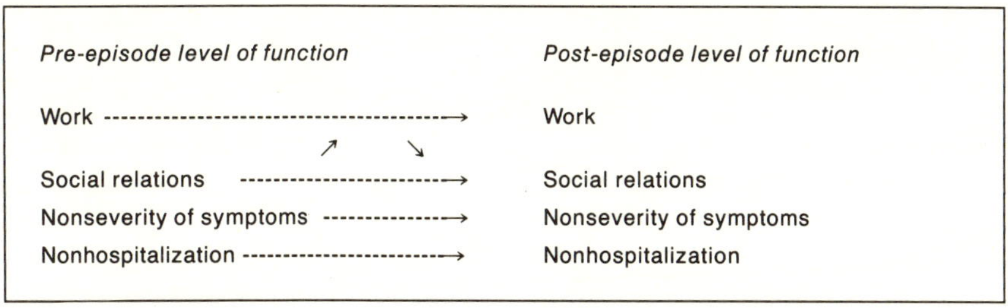

Figure 1. Open-linked systems in the course of schizophrenia (Strauss & Carpenter, 1974, 1977).

mission Study for the outcomes of other psychiatric disorders as well (Strauss, Kokes, Ritzler, & Van Ord, 1978).

Thus, the concept of homogeneity in the course of schizophrenia has evolved to one in which the disorder has been shown to have (1) a markedly heterogeneous course as it progresses across time, (2) heterogeneous levels of capabilities across various domains of functioning (work, relationships, and symptoms) emerging within specific individuals, and (3) predictor–outcome relationships suggesting the existence and persistence of open-linked systems that constitute the course of schizophrenia as well as that of other psychiatric disorders.

From Predictability by Diagnostic Classification to Nonspecificity

Two ways to reduce the heterogeneity in schizophrenia (also among those mentioned by Carpenter in Chapter 13 of this volume) have been to narrow the diagnostic criteria in order to obtain the core disorder, or to reclassify entirely those illnesses that looked like schizophrenia but remitted. In the first strategy, a variety of diagnostic classifications has been devised to select for "true" or "core" schizophrenia (e.g., American Psychiatric Association, 1980; Feighner *et al.*, 1972; Langfeldt, 1937; Schneider, 1959; Spitzer, Endicott, & Robins, 1975). In the second strategy, remitting schizophrenia has been variously renamed such as the *schizophreniform psychoses* by Langfeldt (1939), the *reactive psychoses* by Jaspers (1923/1963), or as *cycloid psychoses* by Leonhard (1961).

None of these strategies appeared to have been fully effective. When testing the same cohort diagnosed by various systems, outcomes persist in being heterogeneous (e.g., Bland & Orn, 1978; Harding, 1984; Hawk, Carpenter, & Strauss, 1975; Vaillant, 1978). Evidence grows in support of Vaillant's contention that "prognosis and diagnosis are two different dimensions of psychosis" (1975, 1978).

From Linearity to Nonlinearity in Course as Assessment Strategies Changed

Course is a longitudinal concept indicating a flow across time. Yet most follow-up studies have based their design on cross-sectional assessments, one at an arbitrary baseline (such as index hospitalization) and one at an equally arbitrary subsequent time period (such as at 1 year, or at 5 years, or at 10 years). These cross-sectional assessments have provided a valuable but limited picture, a static snapshot that is labeled *outcome*. The field has come to accept "outcome" as a real and significant entity. However, "outcome" might also be viewed as an investigator's artifact. In a 10-year follow-up, the 5-year point is simply a marker of time in the 10-year course. In the 20-year follow-up, both 5 and 10 years are markers of course. Thus, "outcome" can be considered a marker along a continuum of a moving trajectory. To illustrate this point further, the following figures present graphically what happens when the assessment time-frame is changed. Utilizing a legacy from Meyerian Life Charts (Meyer, 1919), Leighton and Leighton's adaptation (1949), and Vaillant's longitudinal charts (1980), a 62-year sweep of a subject's life course has been illustrated across five domains of functioning (see Figure 2).

In this exploratory illustrative technique, the white areas signify good functioning or good situation, crosshatch depicts intermediate, and black portrays poor levels. The vertical lines delineate major life events. A strong picture of patterns and trends across a life-course trajectory emerges. Figure 3 portrays a 1-year slice out of the same schematic presentation as would be seen in a 2-year follow-up study. Figure 4 reveals the narrow span of data obtained by two cross-sectional points in time in a typical long-term follow-up design. Many inferences have been made regarding how patients got from point I (Index) to point N (Now). Given the full data from Figure 2 as a contrast to Figures 3 and 4, one could only conclude that "two cross-sectionals do not a longitudinal make."

The subject whose life was depicted in the above figures was selected at random from the 269 people, once profoundly ill, long-stay, state-hospital patients, who were followed by Brooks and colleagues for 30 years (Brooks & Deane, 1965; Chittick, Brooks, Irons, & Deane, 1961; Harding & Brooks, 1980) in the Vermont Longitudinal Project. Analyses of data from this study are being carried out to identify and understand the implications of year-by-year patterns of function as they emerge for subclusters of subjects (Harding, Strauss, Ashikaga, & Brooks, 1984).

In the Bonn studies, headed by Huber and his associates (Huber, Gross, Schüttler, & Linz, 1980), 502 schizophrenics were followed up at an average of 21.4 years. The German team identified 73 kinds of course, which were clustered to represent 12 types. Bleuler (1972) followed along his Burgholzli sample for 23 years, and Ciompi and Müller (1976) in the Lausanne In-

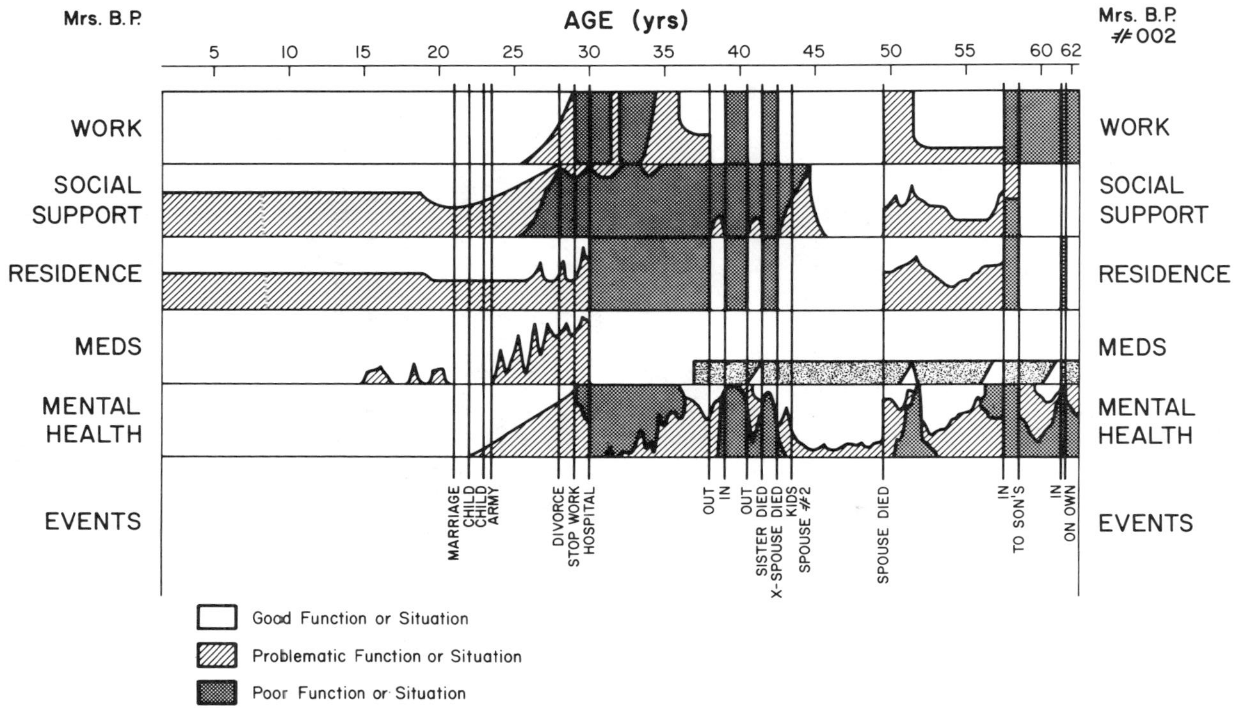

Figure 2. Six sets of patterns and trends across a life trajectory: 62 years of a subject's life.

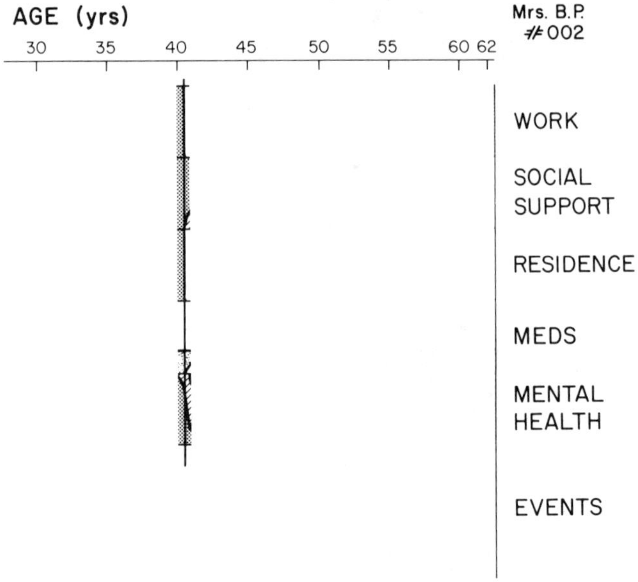

Figure 3. A 1-year slice from the subject's 62 years.

vestigation followed up patients for an average of 36 years. These two well-known very long term follow-up investigations each isolated in a schematic fashion eight types of course, with two types of onset (acute or chronic), two types of course (undulating or simple), and two types of "end state" (recovery or mild, and moderate or severe) (Ciompi, 1980). Their schematics represent a clear attempt to trace patterns of course in schizophrenia, and are the beginning of an important search for targeting different trajectories.

However, these patterns of course must be considered as relative overviews of the processes involved in the evolution of disorder, when compared to the measurements completed every two months by Strauss and his associates in the Yale Longitudinal Study. This study has been an intensive follow-along investigation in which subjects were interviewed periodically over a 2-year period following discharge from a psychiatric hospitalization. Basic clinical and demographic data were collected from the subjects while they were still on the in-patient unit. Subsequently the subjects were followed along, with a semistructured interview given every 2 months for the first year, and then a follow-up interview 2 years after discharge (Strauss, Hafez, Lieberman, & Harding, 1985).

The Yale Longitudinal Study began to chart the interactions between these persons and their environments that might influence the course of disorder and recovery. These interactions were viewed as taking place across several life contexts: family, friends, work, and treatment, as well as within

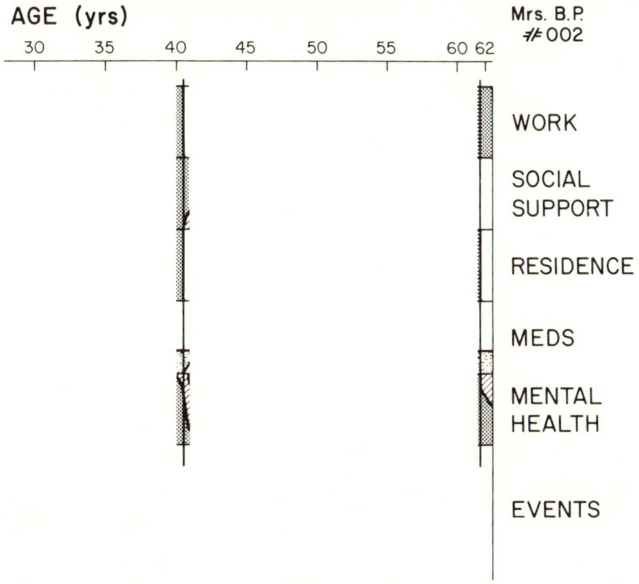

Figure 4. A typical longitudinal study: Two cross-sectional slices out of the subject's 62 years of life.

the person, affecting his or her symptoms, self-esteem, need for structure, degree of involvement, ability to have social relations, and the meaning of events (see Table 1).

One of the first findings from these intensive and repeated observations was that the course did not follow a straight line. This finding contradicts the type of reports generated from single-point follow-up outcome studies, which tend to give the impression that relatively few vacillations occur during the follow-up period. When assessment of subjects is conducted at more frequent time intervals, however, the major changes that do occur become apparent (see Figure 5).

Careful review of these changes suggests that recognizable phases in the course of disorder can be identified (Strauss *et al.*, 1985). These phases

Table 1. The Yale Longitudinal Study

Active, developing person
Person–environment interaction
Across contexts (family, friends, work, and treatment)
Across components (self-esteem, structure, involvement, social relations, meaning, and symptoms)
Across time (nonlinear course, identifiable phases of recovery, phases of environmental response)

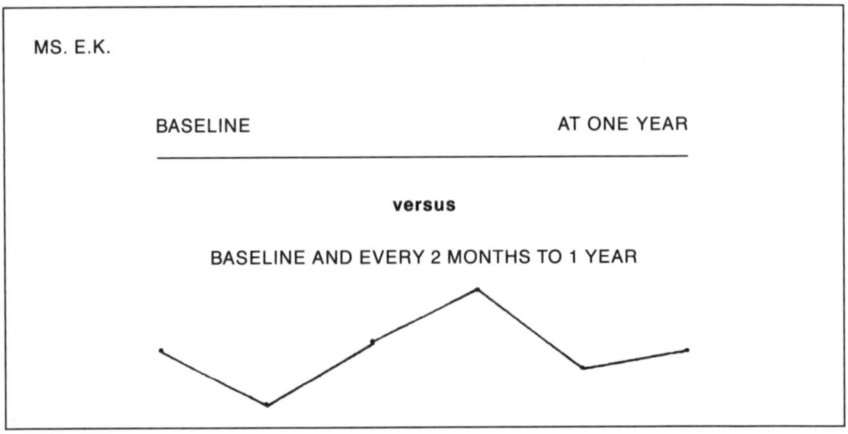

Figure 5. The differences in data dependent upon frequency of observation.

have considerable implications for understanding the course of disorder, as well as for treatment and research. All of these investigations are (1) reshaping the concept of a linear course of schizophrenia into one with the multiple possibilities, and (2) sharpening our appreciation for the hidden complexities involved.

From a Passive Victim to Active Shaper of Own Course

In the Yale Longitudinal Study, several hypotheses have been suggested by the data collected so far. It appears that the subjects in this study are very active in shaping the course of their disorder, not only in their compliance (collaboration) or noncompliance with treatment, but also by possibly controlling their own psychotic symptoms (Breier & Strauss, 1983). Further, the subjects demonstrate that they are also continuing to develop as human beings. Acquisition of new skills in relating to people and in working, as well as shifts in attitudes and perspectives, have been commonly noted.

The interaction of many individual and environmental characteristics influencing the course of schizophrenia is also suggested by some of the more intensive long-term follow-up studies. The Vermont Longitudinal Research Project, mentioned previously, is nearing completion and has provided an extensive prospective follow-along of subjects combined with a retrospective follow-back (Harding & Brooks, 1984). This strategy supplies information that gives a picture across 21–58 years lived after first admission (e.g., that of Mrs. B.P., shown in Figure 2). The cohort was a middle-aged, poorly educated, lower-socioeconomic group, mostly single, and mostly schizophrenic (Chittick *et al.*, 1961). The clinicians who worked with these

Table 2. Clinical Descriptions of *The Vermont Story* Cohort at Time of Selection in the Mid-1950s

Very slow
Poor concentration
Impaired memory
Confused
Touchy and suspicious
Temperamental and unpredictable
Overdependent
Chronic physical disabilities
Peculiarities of appearance, speech, and behavior
Constricted sense of time, space, and other people
Goalless or unrealistic goals
Prolonged reaction time
Impaired ability to perform precise or skilled activity

Note. Derived from Chittick, Brooks, Irons, and Deane (1961, pp. 30–31).

subjects described in vivid terms their characteristics in the 1950s when they were selected (Table 2). The description lists many negative symptoms and portrays a group of subjects who were hospitalized over a long period (average 6 continuous years, with a range to 20+ years) and were profoundly ill and disabled as well. Utilizing a comprehensive design described elsewhere (Harding & Brooks, 1980, 1984), information was generated 20 to 25 years later in a reliable, replicable manner on 97% of the cohort. Those living subjects diagnosed as DSM-I schizophrenics (N = 149) and those meeting DSM-III criteria for schizophrenia (N = 82) were assessed using a number of structured scales and schedules. These findings are described at length elsewhere (Harding, 1984), and an overview is shown in Table 3. The current picture of the functioning of these subjects is a startling contrast to their previous levels, described during their index hospitalization (as shown in Table 2).

After several hours of repeated personal interviews with these subjects and with people who had known them well, in addition to two sets of prospectively gathered records, individual life histories have been generated.

Table 3. Current Status of Subjects Meeting DSM-I and DSM-III Criteria for Schizophrenia

Most subjects:
Resided in community
Were actively involved with friends and family
Were productive and law-abiding citizens
Were symptom-free

From these histories, plus anecdotal evidence from the subjects themselves, it appears that their individual courses have been shaped by an interactive combination of personality characteristics, psychopathology, environmental supports, treatment, and luck; by growth, development, hard work, and persistence.

CONCLUSION

Our understanding of the course of schizophrenia has been an evolving concept. The complexities and dynamic qualities of schizophrenia have become increasingly apparent. *Outcome* has come to mean a definitive status when, in fact, it reflects only a fleeting moment of time, a marker of course, and needs to be looked at from the standpoint of patterns and trends rather than cross-sectional points. Course needs to be assessed across contexts, and across individual components of a developing person. Course appears to be shaped by the person–environment interaction and by the goodness of fit between those two. Course has not been found to be linear, becomes more heterogeneous as assessment time passes, and is not yet predictable by strictness of diagnostic criteria. From this data-based conceptual evolution, a new appreciation of the person with schizophrenia emerges as one who can be very active, continues to develop, and may function better over time.

ACKNOWLEDGMENTS

This research was supported by NIMH Grants No. MH29575 and MH00340.

REFERENCES

American Psychiatric Association. (1980). *Diagnostic and statistical manual of mental disorders* (3rd ed.). Washington, DC: APA.

Bellak, L. (1948). *Dementia praecox*. New York: Grune & Stratton.

Bland, R. C., & Orn, H. (1978). 14-year outcome in early schizophrenia. *Acta Psychiatrica Scandinavica, 58*, 327–338.

Bleuler, M. (1972). *Die schizophrenen Geistesstörungen im Lichte langjähriger Kranken - und Familiengeschichten*. Stuttgart: Thieme (S. M. Clemens, Trans., *The schizophrenic disorders, long-term patient and family studies* (pp. 1–502) New Haven, CT: Yale University Press)

Breier, A., & Strauss, J. S. (1983). Self-control of psychotic disorders. *Archives of General Psychiatry, 40*, 1141-1145.

Brooks, G. W., & Deane, W. N. (1965). Chronic mental patients in the community. *Diseases of the Nervous System, 25*, 85–90.

Chittick, R. A., Brooks, G. W., Irons, F. S., & Deane, W. N. (1961). *The Vermont Story.* Burlington, VT: Queen City Printers.

Ciompi, L. (1980). Catamnestic long-term study on the course of life and aging in schizophrenics. *Schizophrenia Bulletin, 6*(4), 606–618.

Ciompi, L., & Müller, C. (1976). *Lebensweg und Alter der Schizophrenen. Eine katamnestische Lanzeitstudie bis ins Senum.* Berlin: Springer-Verlag. (E. Forsberg, Trans., *The life course and aging in schizophrenia: A catamnestic longitudinal study into advanced age.* Underhill, VT: Longitudinal Research Project, 1984)

Feighner, J., Robins, E., Guze, S., Woodruff, R., Winokur, G., & Muñoz, R. (1972). Diagnostic criteria for use in psychiatric research. *Archives of General Psychiatry, 26*, 57–63.

Harding, C. M. (1984). *Long-term outcome functioning of subjects rediagnosed as meeting the DSM III criteria for schizophrenia.* Doctoral dissertation, University of Vermont, Burlington.

Harding, C. M., & Brooks, G. W. (1980). Longitudinal assessment of a cohort of chronic schizophrenics discharged twenty years ago. *Psychiatric Journal of the University of Ottawa. 5*(4), 274–278.

Harding, C. M., & Brooks, G. W. (1984). Life assessment of a cohort of chronic schizophrenics discharged twenty years ago. In S. Mednick, M. Harway, & K. Finello (Eds.), *The handbook of longitudinal research* (Vol. 2, pp. 375–393). New York: Praeger Press.

Harding, C. M., Brooks, G. W., Ashikaga, T., Strauss, J. S., & Landerl, P. D. (in press). Aging and social functioning in once chronic schizophrenic patients 21-58 years after first admission. The Vermont Story. In G. Hudgins & N. Miller (Eds.), *Schizophrenia, paranoia, and schizophreniform disorders in later life.* New York: Guilford Press.

Harding, C. M., Strauss, J. S., Ashikaga, T., & Brooks, G. W. (1984, May). *Social competence and life course after psychoses.* Presented at the annual meeting of the American Psychiatric Association in a symposium entitled "Social Factors and the Course of Mental Disorder," Los Angeles.

Hawk, A. B., Carpenter, W. T., & Strauss, J. S. (1975). Diagnostic criteria and five-year outcome in schizophrenia. *Archives of General Psychiatry, 32*, 343–347.

Huber, G., Gross, G., & Schüttler, R. (1979). *Schizophrenie. Verlaufs und sozialpsychiatrische Langzeituntersuchungen an den 1945 bis 1959 in Bonn hospitalisierten schizophrenen Kranken* (Monographien aus dem Gesamtgebiete der Psychiatrie, Vol. 21). Berlin: Springer-Verlag.

Huber, G., Gross, G., Schüttler, R., & Linz, M. (1980). Longitudinal studies of schizophrenic patients. *Schizophrenia Bulletin, 6*(4), 592–605.

Jaspers, K. (1963). *General psychopathology* (J. Hoenig & M. Hamilton, Trans.). Manchester, England: Manchester University Press. (Original work published 1923)

Kraepelin, E. (1902). Dementia praecox. In E. Kraepelin, *Clinical psychiatry: A textbook for students and physicians* (6th ed., A. E. Diefendorf, Trans.). New York: Macmillan.

Langfeldt, G. (1937). The prognosis in schizophrenia and the factors influencing the course of the disease. *Acta Psychiatrica et Neurologica Scandinavica, Supplement 13.*

Langfeldt, G. (1939). *Schizophreniform states.* Copenhagen: Munksgaard.

Leighton, A. H., & Leighton, D. D. (1949). *Gregorio, the hand trembler: A psychobiological personality study of a Navaho Indian.* Peabody Museum Papers, Cambridge, MA: Harvard University Press.

Leonhard, K. (1961). Cycloid psychoses: Endogenous psychoses which are neither schizophrenic nor manic depressive. *Journal of Mental Science, 107*, 633–648.

Meyer, A. (1919). The life chart. In *Contributions to medical and biological research.* New York: Hoeber and Co.

Schneider, K. (1959). *Clinical psychopathology* (M. W. Hamilton & E. W. Anderson, Trans.). New York: Grune & Stratton.

Shapiro, R., & Shader, R. (1979). Chapter II. Selective review of results of previous follow-up studies of schizophrenia and other psychoses. *Schizophrenia: An international pilot study*. Chichester, England: Wiley.

Spitzer, R. L., Endicott, J., & Robins, E. (1975). *Research diagnostic criteria (RDC)*. New York: Biometrics Research, New York State Psychiatric Institute.

Stephens, J. H. (1970). Long-term course and prognosis in schizophrenia. *Seminars in Psychiatry, 2*(4), 464–485.

Strauss, J. S. (in press). Psychiatric diagnosis: A reconceptualization. In G. Klerman & T. Millon (Eds.), *Contemporary directions in psychopathology: Toward a DSM-IV*. New York: Guilford.

Strauss, J. S., & Carpenter, W. T., Jr. (1974). The prediction of outcome in schizophrenia. II. Relationships between predictor and outcome variables. *Archives of General Psychiatry, 31*, 37–42.

Strauss, J. S., & Carpenter, W. T., Jr. (1977). Prediction of outcome in schizophrenia. III. Five year outcome and its predictors. A report from The International Pilot Study of Schizophrenia. *Archives of General Psychiatry, 34*, 159–163.

Strauss, J. S., Hafez, H., Lieberman, P., & Harding, C. (1985). The course of psychiatric disorder. III. Longitudinal principles. *American Journal of Psychiatry*, 142(3), 289–296.

Strauss, J. S., Kokes, R.F., Ritzler, B.A., Harder, D.W., & VanOrd, A. Patterns of disorder in first admission psychiatric patients. *Journal of Nervous and Mental Disease*, 1978, *166*, 611–625.

Tsuang, M. T., Woolson, R. F., & Fleming, J. A. (1979). Long-term outcome of major psychoses. I. Schizophrenia and affective disorders compared with psychiatrically symptom-free surgical conditions. *Archives of General Psychiatry, 36*, 1295–1301.

Vaillant, G. E. (1975). *A ten-year follow-up of remitting schizophrenia*. Presented at the 129th annual meeting of the American Psychiatric Association, Anaheim, CA.

Vaillant, G. E. (1978). A 10-year follow-up of remitting schizophrenics. *Schizophrenia Bulletin, 4*(1), 78–85.

Vaillant, G. E. (1980). Adolf Meyer was right: Dynamic psychiatry needs the life chart. *Journal of the National Association for Private Psychiatric Hospitals, 11*(4), 4–14.

World Health Organization. (1979). *Schizophrenia: An international follow-up study*. Chichester, England: Wiley.

COMMENTARY

Dr. Marty Harrow:* We have four different samples we have followed up prospectively as part of the Chicago Follow-Up Study, and we are getting somewhat different results than Courtenay [Harding]. We are finding much poorer outcomes among the schizophrenics we are studying. I like to characterize Courtenay's project as the smiling faces. Our schizophrenics might represent the frowning faces. In other words, in four different samples our schizophrenics are doing poorly. One of the samples was started by Roy Grinker 10 years ago, and 10 years later the subjects are still doing poorly. Also, two other points: As far as the strictness of criteria, we have found

* Chicago, Illinois.

considerable difference between DSM-II schizophrenics and DSM-III schizophrenics. The psychosis of DSM-III schizophrenics seems to persist to a much greater extent than is the case with DSM-II schizophrenics. Five, 6, 7, 8 years later, a moderate percentage of them are still delusional, even though they are outside the hospital, and most are not functioning well at all. It is not that all of them are doing poorly, but many are. I'm just saying that other prospective studies are finding only a small percentage of schizophrenics truly recovered. Maybe in another 20 years our schizophrenics will improve and function well, and maybe not. But for people who have not worked in our society for 10 years, as is the case with many of our schizophrenics from the Chicago Follow-Up Study it is still unlikely that after another 10 years they are going to go back to work.

The other point I can make is that the sex ratio in Dr. Harding's study shows a slightly larger percentage of females than males. We have found that when you use DSM-III criteria, you are eliminating people with affective syndromes, and you no longer classify them as schizophrenics. Basically, the great majority of those people no longer classified as schizophrenics are females who are functioning moderately well at follow-up. Once you eliminate those, you find a larger percentage of males and a larger percentage of people who are responding more poorly to treatment and just doing poorly.

Dr. Harding: Dr. Harrow brings up many interesting points. To tackle his last one first, in our DSM-III rediagnostic work, we ended up with half females, half males, 41 of each. I think that what we were trying to bring out about the course of disorder, was that 12 years isn't long enough to see major recovery in groups, whole groups of people. You just have not stayed around long enough, and I think that is an essential ingredient. That's why I pointed out that we can't compare findings from 5-year and 12-year and 20-year follow-up studies and lump them all together and say this is "outcome." I think it is very different at different periods of time in the career of a person. That is one point.

This group was an extremely chronic group, had been profoundly ill, have met the stricter criteria, and their findings are still coming across as being 27% at the top in functioning levels, 40% in the middle range, and 30% plus at the bottom. These results are very similar to the findings of the Europeans, who had different criteria for schizophrenia. It is just amazing to me, that all of our signals about recovery are coming out very similarly; enough so to perhaps override the differences in methodology.

Dr. Irwin Feinberg:* I was very pleased to hear this presentation. When I first went to work in the NIMH program at St. Elizabeths Hospital, I was amazed to see a number of patients get well who had had severe,

* San Francisco, California.

typically schizophrenic symptomatology, both of the negative and the positive kind, who had been continuously ill for 20 or 30 years. When they got well, they were not, by the way, people who showed terrible ravages of having been in some isolated situation for years. Instead, they were remarkably normal. I don't know what the percentages of such recoveries are, and I don't think that the exact percentages are terribly important. I think what is important is that there is no evidence at this time that *any* symptom of schizophrenia is irreversible. That fact is one of the most encouraging aspects of research into this terrible illness. Your data are nicely consistent with my much more limited personal experience. Whatever the exact percentages of late recovery turn out to be, the occurrence of such recovery is the basic and most important fact. I think that some of the talk about deficit states, with the implication of neurologic irreversibility, is unfortunate, for no symptom of schizophrenia has been proved to be irreversible.

Dr. Harding: Thank you, Dr. Feinberg. I would like to say that when we look at who is symptomatic today, one of the pieces of information I got on the telephone last night was that we have only eight people out of this group who are considered definitely schizophrenic now. That is 10%! We have another 17 (or 21%) who are probable. These figures leave about 68% who have *no* symptoms of schizophrenia (positive or negative) in this group at this point in time.

Dr. Bruce Dohrenwend:* This is a remarkable set of results. I do, however, have a couple of questions. First, you ended up with 149 DSM-I live schizophrenics. Could you tell us more about how many you started with in the cohort and whether there is any reason to believe that those lost to follow-up are different? Second, the members of your cohort were discharged into a very expensive and focused service program. I wonder if you would comment on the extent to which you think we are observing the natural course of the disorder; that is, would the outcome have been the same without that intensive early start? Of course, this is a difficult question to answer without a control group.

Dr. Harding: We had 269 people who were in The Vermont Story cohort in the late 1950s. Twenty to 25 years later, 71 (26%) were deceased, 13 (5%) refused participation, 7 (3%) were not located, and 178 (66%) were alive and interviewed. The families of the deceased were also interviewed to document functioning up to the time of death. Thus, 97% of this cohort was located and accounted for.

As to the diagnostic work, there were 213 (79%) out of the original 269 subjects who met the more loosely formulated DSM-I criteria for schizophrenia. When removing those who had died (57) or were lost to follow-up (7), we arrived at the 149 live DSM-I group inquired about by

* New York, New York.

Dr. Dohrenwend. Our early analyses have used this cohort until the rediagnostic work could be completed by Alan Brier and John Strauss. Their work, just finished last week, revealed that 118 (55%) subjects met the DSM-III criteria for schizophrenia. When the deceased and lost-to-follow-up subjects were removed, we came to the 82 alive DSM-III subjects mentioned by us in the presentation. It is of great interest to us that in our preliminary data runs, the proportions of recovery are just about the same no matter how we slice the pie—for the DSM-I's, for the DSM-III's, for the deceased, and for the refusals.

As far as the rehabilitation effort, because we took everybody out of the bottom of that state hospital, and therefore were unable to find a matched control, we cannot say for sure whether rehabilitation made a difference. We are trying to pull a matched sample out of Augusta State Hospital from 1955 and run the same protocol with them. They did not get the rehabilitation effort, and we would like to see if there is any significant difference in course. By the way, the program was comprehensive but not necessarily expensive. For example, it cost $21 a week in 1955 to keep someone out in a halfway house. These subjects had jobs during the recession period in 1958, which I find very interesting.

18

Expressed Emotion and Schizophrenic Relapse: Implications from the Pittsburgh Study

GERARD E. HOGARTY
University of Pittsburgh School of Medicine

Four published studies (Brown, Birley, & Wing, 1972; Brown, Monck, Carstairs, & Wing, 1962; Vaughn & Leff, 1976; Vaughn, Snyder, Freeman, Jones, & Falloon, 1984) conducted by British investigators in England and in California have indicated that an attitude called *expressed emotion* (EE), shown by a key relative toward a schizophrenic member of the family shortly after hospital admission, is subsequently associated with relapse in the nine months following hospital discharge.[1] In Pittsburgh, we have attempted an independent validation of the concept in a larger and more broadly defined sample, results of which represent a qualified replication of the British work. In fact, a close examination of past studies suggests that the basis for generalization might not extend much beyond observations drawn from the Pittsburgh data. Studies in Denmark, India, and elsewhere in the United States are currently in progress. The substance of the published studies indicates that critical comments (or the analog hostility) and, to a lesser extent, emotional overinvolvement, are the essential EE components that are predictive. Among the three previous studies that employed a common methodology, 48% to 58% of patients returning to high-EE households relapsed by nine months, compared to 16% or 17% of patients returning to low-EE households. In the first investigation conducted by Brown *et al.* (1962), a somewhat different methodology was employed, wherein 76% of high-EE patients "deteriorated," compared to 28% of low-EE patients. In the previous studies, the amount of face-to-face contact with the key relative was observed to interactively influence relapse in high-EE households (increasing relapse in high-EE households and having no effect in low-EE homes). Drug compliance, for the most part, was shown to have an independent main effect on relapse in past trials. The conclusion drawn from these earlier investigations, however, was that EE was "the best single predictor" of schizophrenic relapse, at least in the first 9 months following hospital discharge (Vaughn & Leff, 1976).

THE PITTSBURGH STUDY

Because the formal results and methodologic detail of this trial will be published elsewhere, it is only possible to comment on findings in very general terms. Among 159 patients followed for 1 year post-discharge, the *only* main effects among selected variables and relapse were (1) drug compliance and (2) the number of prior hospitalizations. Relapse rates on and off drug, in fact, are nearly identical to those observed in placebo-controlled studies (Hogarty, 1984). No variable among the 13 tested explained the relapse of these noncompliant patients, beyond the fact that they failed to take medication. However, because the thrust of our interest in EE was an attempt to understand the relapse of drug-maintained patients, an extensive analysis was carried out for the 114 patients maintained on antipsychotic medication, most often fluphenazine decanoate. In this subsample, there was again but a single unqualified main effect on relapse: the number of prior hospitalizations. Only Brown *et al.* (1962), report a main effect of prior hospitalization on relapse. However, a number of interactions were found that essentially involved expressed emotion and relapse. We observed that high expressed emotion predicted relapse for male patients but not female patients; RDC schizophrenic patients but not RDC schizoaffective disorders; younger patients (under 25) but not older patients; and, in a more qualified sense, patients exiting hospital still psychotic compared to patients able to achieve a good remission of psychotic symptoms while hospitalized. Effects were tested in a multivariate manner and the results, in our opinion, represent largely unconfounded effects. However, a closer examination of the individual cases that operated against the hypothesis (i.e., low-EE patients on drug who relapsed) revealed that the failure of EE to predict relapse applied essentially to a small group of older, schizoaffective females who were, for the most part, divorced or separated prior to or at the end of study. Interpersonal stressors other than EE were observed in these cases, sufficiently severe, in the judgment of the treating clinicians, to have accounted for the patients' relapse. Other variables of importance, principally the amount of face-to-face contact prior to and following hospital discharge, the patient's race, the rapidity of onset for the index episode, a family history of mental disorder, the presence or absence of mentally ill relatives in the household, and paranoid subtype all failed to show an association with relapse, alone or interactively. It is the absence of a relationship between face-to-face contact and relapse that is the principal difference, we feel, between past studies and the Pittsburgh trial.

As such, we provide supporting evidence for the predictive value of EE, although important qualifications are offered. In view of the claims made for broader relevance of EE in prior studies, a brief review of the existing evidence and support for such claims seems warranted if, for no other reason, than to attempt a reconciliation of differences that to us seem more apparent than real.

Sex

In the original Brown *et al.* (1962) study, all 128 patients were male, thus precluding any test of the EE-and-sex question. However in the Brown *et al.* (1972) replication, among the 101 patients studied, 53 were female. In this trial, relapse among men (50%) was over two times that of women (21%). Thus, with only 12 females judged to have relapsed, it is hard to generalize to the replication of EE for each sex, especially when no data are provided regarding the distribution of EE households by the sex of the patient. These authors claim a significant EE effect for each sex, but use a statistic (gamma) that one could argue is a less appropriate measure of association needed to approach the question. We do know from other trials, principally the Pittsburgh study, that high EE is likely to be associated with being a male patient, and low EE with being a female patient. Further, females are more often married than males, and at least for those patients maintaining intact marriages, the relapse rate among married patients is less than among the never married. In Brown *et al.* (1972), relapse among unmarried patients (42%) was nearly double that of the married patients (26%).

In a 1976 replication conducted by Vaughn and Leff (1976) involving 37 patients, 59% (22 patients) was female and 41% (15 patients) was male. Again, the relapse rate for men is "double that for women." By extrapolation (because explicit data are not provided), it appears that 7 of 15 men (47%) relapsed, but only 4 of 22 women (18%). Eight percent of married patients relapsed, but 42% of the unmarried relapsed. None of the 9 married women relapsed. Further, distributions of EE and sex are not provided, but one could possibly infer that EE, sex, and perhaps marital status also are confounded in this trial: married women tended to be in low-EE homes and unmarried men tended to be in high-EE homes. With an overall relapse rate of only 28% in this study, the EE replication might mostly speak to the 0% relapse rate among married women (who might tend to reside in low-EE households), and an excessive relapse rate (54%) attributed to unmarried men (who might tend to reside in high-EE households). At any rate, it would be difficult, indeed, to generalize the predictive validity of EE to females, with only 4 relapsed female patients in this trial.

In the California study of Vaughn *et al.* (1984), only 24%, or 13 of 54 patients, is female. Further, among 7 high-EE females, only 1 patient relapsed, and among 6 low-EE females only 1 patient relapsed as well. Much like the British trials, the relapse rate for men was three times that for women. As such, the California study provides no evidence that expressed emotion is a relevant factor in predicting the outcome of schizophrenic females. Overall, there is little support for EE and female relapse.

Schizophrenia versus Schizoaffective Disorder

In the RDC system (Spitzer, Endicott, & Robins, 1978), a diagnosis of schizoaffective disorder requires that patients concurrently meet criteria for schizophrenia *and* for a major affective disorder as well. It is nearly impossible to directly approach the question of whether EE replicates for schizophrenic patients with a significant affective component, because three of the four prior studies employed the Present State Examination and its CATEGO classification system (Wing, Cooper, & Sartorius, 1974). Patients included in these studies variably met classes "S" (a more Schneiderian-type schizophrenia), "P" (paranoid state), or "O" (other). The first investigation by Brown *et al.* (1962) used operational criteria for schizophrenia. A comparative study of the RDC and the CATEGO systems seems to indicate that all RDC *schizophrenic* patients would be included in the CATEGO system, but not all CATEGO class "S," "P," and "O" patients would meet RDC criteria for schizophrenia (Kendell, Brockington, & Leff, 1979). What little evidence exists that is addressed to the question can be found in the Brown *et al.* (1972) study. Patients judged to have "typical schizophrenia" (half the sample) relapsed at a greater rate than those of "probable" or "doubtful" schizophrenia, although the authors contend that the relationship between EE and relapse remains when clinical state is controlled. No distributions by EE, relapse, and clinical state are provided, however.

In the Vaughn and Leff (1976) trial, no distinctions among CATEGO classes are provided, although symptom constructs such as Grandiose Delusions and Residual Schizophrenia were more likely found among *high-EE* patients who *relapsed*. However, this trial did report a considerably higher relapse rate (53%) among 30 neurotically depressed patients, two-thirds of whom were married women. Among these patients, *very little* stress in the form of EE was associated with a relapse, suggesting the role of other factors.

Otherwise, in the California study (Vaughn *et al.*, 1984), nearly all patients met the "S" classification for schizophrenia. However, one-third of the "nonrelapsed" patients did experience a rehospitalization during the 9 months after discharge, usually for reasons related to prominent affective symptomatology. By inference, therefore, a proportion of this sample might likely have met RDC criteria for schizoaffective disorder. The EE designation for these affectively impaired, rehospitalized patients is not known, but one might ask whether low-EE and female patients are prominently represented, as in the Pittsburgh sample. On balance, then, what little evidence does exist regarding EE, relapse, and schizophrenic subtype seems to indicate that the strength of the EE prediction is associated with more distinct definitions of schizophrenia.

Age

Information regarding the relationship between age, EE, and relapse is sparse. In the Brown *et al.* (1962) study, patients who were very young at the time of *first* hospital admission more often deteriorated during the course of study than others, but age at discharge had no relationship to outcome. In their replication study, Brown *et al.* (1972) indicated that current age at hospital admission (under 45) was highly associated with relapse. Of interest, age was also associated with sex, indicating that the sample was composed largely of younger male patients and older female patients. No information was provided regarding the distribution of age, EE, and relapse. In Vaughn and Leff (1976), the mean age for the schizophrenic sample is provided (33.1 years), with a note that only sex and marital status among various demographic variables were shown to be related to relapse as a main effect. However, the mean age of schizophrenic men (28.1) was considerably less than that of the whole sample, indicating, again, a population of younger men and older women.

In the California study (Vaughn *et al.*, 1982) age is not mentioned and, apparently, during the testing of demographic variables, age was not associated with outcome. Thus, all we can say is that in one study, age has a main effect on relapse, and in our own trial there is an interactive effect between age, expressed emotion, and relapse. It is the association between age and sex in the Brown *et al.* (1972) and Vaughn and Leff (1976) studies, and the subsequent associations between sex and expressed emotion that provide tentative support for the Pittsburgh results—that younger males and older females come from quite different EE households and experience quite different outcomes.

Illness Severity at Hospital Discharge

It is something of a curiosity that an important observation first reported by Brown *et al.* (1962) had not been tested in subsequent investigations of expressed emotion. In this early trial, ratings of EE were made *after* hospital discharge, and patients rated a day or two prior to leaving hospital were judged to be either free or nearly free of symptoms, moderately ill, or severely ill. Patients in these latter categories had an increased risk of deterioration *if* they returned to households high in expressed emotion (principally emotional overinvolvement) and experienced high face-to-face contact with the relative as well. Although we have not tested various components of EE as they interact with clinical state, the Pittsburgh results confirm an interactive effect between expressed emotion, clinical state, and relapse, although the effect is independent of face-to-face contact. In many regards, this earliest investigation of expressed emotion is the richest in terms of theoretical explanations for the rationale and mechanism of action underlying the EE concept. Brown *et al.* (1962), for example, speculated that in one-third of cases, EE might be due to the *clinical state* of the patient, in another third, to abiding characteristics of the relative, and, for the remaining third, to an interaction between these two factors. Surprisingly, in the Brown *et al.* (1972) replication, illness at discharge is not an independent variable tested for its interactive effects with expressed emotion, although 39% of patients in this trial either had persistent schizophrenic symptoms or experienced a Type II relapse (a marked exacerbation of persistent symptoms).

In the California study, patients who were ill at discharge appear to have been removed from the principal EE analyses.

In the Vaughn and Leff (1976) trial, 10 of 11 relapsed patients were of Type I (deteriorated from a nonschizophrenic state at discharge to schizophrenic), indicating that very few patients were ill at hospital discharge. Typically, in the United States at least, as in-patient days become fewer as a function of insurance coverage (a trend likely to escalate as DRGs find broader application in psychiatry), one would predict that the clinical state of the schizophrenic patient at discharge will become an increasingly important predictor of outcome, in terms of its interaction with the emotional climate of the household to which the patient returns.

Thus, what little evidence exists regarding EE and illness severity at discharge does support the observation from the Pittsburgh sample.

DISCUSSION AND INTEGRATION

An interpretation of the Pittsburgh results might lead one to conclude that the variables associated with EE that argue *against* the hypothesis (schizoaffective disorder, older age, and good remission of symptoms at discharge) represent, in practice, second-order variables better explained by the hierarchical characteristic of the remaining nonconfirming variable: patient sex.

Increasingly, "affectivity" among schizophrenic patients seems to be more closely associated with being female (Burbach, Lewine, & Meltzer, 1984); this is not an entirely shocking observation given the preponderance of females among the affective disorders. What seems central to the evolving notions of schizophrenic pathogenesis is the association between expressed emotion, principally criticism, and the relapse of primarily young, "pure" schizophrenic, *male* patients. For the majority of patients, high EE is essentially due to criticism only insofar as a minority of families receive this classification on the basis of emotional overinvolvement (EOI). Still, one could argue that even for those households classified as high on the basis of EOI, this component of EE is itself a variant of criticism, a metacommunication to the effect that the patient is somehow "imperfect," not capable of autonomous or independent behavior, or is otherwise in need of protection. Because four of five existing studies provide no evidence for the relationship between EE and the relapse of female patients (and the fifth does by inference and/or by the application of a questionable statistical procedure), we must look to (1) possible differences in the pathophysiology of schizophrenic disorders by sex, together with (2) the differential nature of the offending stimuli, by sex, capable of exploiting the schizophrenic deficit. This observation requires a response, because it is rare, indeed in the study of schizophrenia ever to find a variable that independently replicates across studies and across continents, namely, criticism and the relapse of schizophrenic men.

Space precludes a comprehensive evaluation of the existing literature, but it is generally agreed that the cognitive and perceptual organization of males and females, including nonverbal perception and judgment, is different (Maccoby & Jacklin, 1974; Rosenthal, Hall, Matteo, Rogers, & Archer, 1979), and that such differences not only persist but tend to increase over time. Some have argued that these later differences might be attributed to the differential socialization of children by sex, but clear intrinsic differences appear to exist (Sagi & Hoffman, 1976), perhaps as a basis for the survival of the species, given the essential role of mothering in identifying and responding to the nonverbal needs of infants (Rosenthal *et al.*, 1979). Further, central elements of schizophrenic pathophysiology have consistently implicated the patient's inability to process information correctly, a phenomenon that extends from aspects of disordered attention and perception to the functional capacity for correctly identifying, storing, retrieving, integrating, and responding to internally and externally generated stimuli (Anderson, Hogarty, & Reiss, 1980). Considerable evidence exists that male schizophrenic patients have earlier onsets and (in many of the EE studies) have a considerably less favorable outcome than female patients. Perhaps we can infer that the deficits might be more profound or more *functionally significant* among the male schizophrenic patient. Further, abstraction, synthesis, and integration tend to be left-hemisphere functions, more likely the dominant organizing hemisphere for males.

Given these notions as incompletely formulated premises, one must ask how criticism elicits its toxic effect. Criticism, as an organizing principal in human psychopathology, seems to have been only indirectly appreciated as an assault on self-esteem or as the stimulus for self-critical behavior, giving rise, perhaps, to fear and anxiety—the variables that operate at the heart of most theories of personality. To us, it appears that criticism from others elicits the widest range of maladaptive behavior among the diverse mental disorders affecting children, adolescents, and adults, and among otherwise "normal" professors, politicians, and presidents. At a psychophysiological level, criticism from others is an *abstract* concept, which requires that one go beyond the structure of language to the symbolic meaning of *criticism* in order to appreciate the psychological effect. Although the influence of criticism is understudied among nonpatients, it is at once apparent that the first and immediate response is a limbic one—fear, anger, anxiety—a response that has its documentation in a psychophysiologic literature (Tarrier, Vaughn, Lader, & Leff, 1979). Criticism might well represent the source of "activation dysregulation" essential to all severe mental disorders, as recently reviewed by Braden (1984). However, human criticism demands an adaptive response, a *cognitive* exercise that requires an individual to identify, appraise, search past memory stores, and formulate a plan of action that would preserve self-esteem and psychological integrity. Primary processes, or primitive responses, would resolve largely as "limbic discharges," or psychosocial withdrawal. Second-order, more adaptive processes require an extraordinarily difficult exercise in abstracting, integrating, planning, and responding. Herein, perhaps, lies an answer to male schizophrenic (and perhaps to more pure female schizophrenic) vulnerability to criticism: the essential limbic-frontal-temporal cortical structures *most* needed to appropriately respond to criticism might well represent the cognitive functions *most* impaired in "pure" schizophrenia. Not only are recent autopsy studies supportive (Crow, 1984) but, when faced with difficult abstracting tasks involving the frontal lobe, the brains of some schizophrenic patients seem to actually "turn off" (Weinberger, 1984).

And what of female schizoaffective patients? Increasingly, and borne out by examination of factors contributing to the relapse of female schizoaffective patients in our own studies, precipitants of relapse for female patients seem more closely associated with an actual or impending loss or disruption of close interpersonal relationships (Paykel, 1974), which might, perhaps, disproportionately influence sex-mediated neuroendocrinologic and neurotransmitter functions.

In our opinion, the consistent observations from the studies of expressed emotion and the schizophrenic relapse of male patients provide empirical support for such speculations and contain clear directions for differential treatment. In Pittsburgh, a new program is being developed, specifically designed as a "therapy of the sexes," in an attempt to capitalize and build upon the important contributions of expressed emotion to the pathophysiology of schizophrenic disorders.

ACKNOWLEDGMENTS

The Pittsburgh Study (EPICS) was supported by Grant MH-535247 from the Psychotherapy Research Branch of NIMH. Supervision of the study, data collection, analyses, and patient care were most generously provided by Carol Anderson, PhD, Joseph McEvoy, MD, and Mark Munetz, MD, co-investigators; Mary Ashley Carter, PhD, Gertrude Bayer, MA, Athena McLean, MS, Kathryn Stockdale, MA, EE raters and research associates; Patricia Bartone, MSN, Rosemary Cather, MSN, Susan Cooley, RNCSMN Ed., and Ann Louise DiBarry, MSN, nurse clinicians; Jack Cahalane, MSW, Carol Javna, PhD, and Douglas Reiss, PhD, family or behavioral therapists; Deborah Greenwald, PhD and Sander Kornblith, PhD, supervising psychologists; Michael Madonia, BA, Richard Ulrich, MS and Kathy Erndl, BA, data processing and analysis; Bridget Virostek, project administrative secretary and preparer of this manuscript, and Jennifer Hogarty, BS, AB, who assisted in the literature review. Finally, we are most indebted to Christine Vaughn, PhD for her untiring efforts in training our EE raters, reviewing tapes, and providing support and direction during this investigation.

REFERENCES

Anderson, C. M., Hogarty, G. E. & Reiss, D. J. (1980). Family treatment of adult schizophrenic patients: A psycho-educational approach. *Schizophrenia Bulletin*, *6*, 490–505.

Braden, W. (1984). Vulnerability and schizo-affective psychoses: A two-factor model. *Schizophrenia Bulletin*, *10*, 71–86.

Brown, G. W., Birley, J. L. T., & Wing, J. K. (1972). The influence of family life on the course of schizophrenic disorders: A replication. *British Journal of Psychiatry*, *121*, 241–258.

Brown, G. W., Monck, E. M., Carstairs, G. M. & Wing, J. K. (1962). Influence of family life on the course of schizophrenic illness. *British Journal of Preventive and Social Medicine*, *16*, 55–68.

Burbach, D. J., Lewine, R., & Meltzer, H. Y. (1984). Diagnostic concordance for schizophrenia as a function of sex. *Journal of Consulting and Clinical Psychology*, *52*, 478–479.

Crow, T. J. (1984, May). *Disturbances in the temporal lobe*. Paper presented at the 137th annual meeting of the American Psychiatric Association, Los Angeles.

Hogarty, G. E. (1984). Depot neuroleptics: The relevance of psychosocial factors. *Journal of Clinical Psychiatry*, *45*, 36–42.

Kendell, R. E., Brockington, I. F., & Leff, J. P. (1979). Prognostic implications of six alternative definitions of schizophrenia. *Archives of General Psychiatry*, *36*, 25–31.

Maccoby, E. E., & Jacklin, C. N. (1974). *The psychology of sex differences*. Stanford, CA: Stanford University Press.

Paykel, E. S. (1974). Life stress and psychiatric disorder. In B. S. Dohrenwend & B. P. Dohrenwend (Eds.), *Stressful life events* (pp. 135–149). New York: Wiley.

Rosenthal, R., Hall, J. A., Matteo, M. R. D., Rogers, P. L., & Archer, D. (1979). *Sensitivity to nonverbal communication: The PONS test*. Baltimore: Johns Hopkins University Press.

Sagi, A., & Hoffman, M. L. (1976). Empathic distress in the newborn. *Developmental Psychology, 12*, 175–176.

Spitzer, R., Endicott, J., & Robins, E. (1978). Research diagnostic criteria: Rationale and reliability. *Archives of General Psychiatry, 35*, 773–782.

Tarrier, N., Vaughn, C. E., Lader, M. D., & Leff, J. P. (1979). Bodily reactions to people and events in schizophrenics. *Archives of General Psychiatry, 36*, 311–315.

Vaughn, C. E., & Leff, J. P. (1976). The influence of family and social factors on the course of psychiatric illness. *British Journal of Psychiatry, 129*, 125–137.

Vaughn, C. E., Snyder, K. S., Jones, S., Freeman, W. B., & Falloon, I. R. H. (1984). Family factors in schizophrenic relapse: a replication. *Archives of General Psychiatry, 41*, 1169–1177.

Weinberger, D. R. (1984, May). *Neuropathological localization in schizophrenia*. Paper presented at the 137th annual meeting of the American Psychiatric Association, Los Angeles.

Wing, J. K., Cooper, J. E., & Sartorius, N. (1974). *The description and classification of psychiatric symptoms: An introduction manual for the PSE and Catego system*. London & New York: Cambridge University Press.

COMMENTARY

Dr. Keith H. Nuechterlein:* Although I didn't directly participate in the UCLA replication of the British work on expressed emotion, I am a member of the clinical research center that carried out the study, and I think that your results are striking in several ways. I think it is important, as you note, to start identifying the characteristics of subjects within the schizophrenic population for whom the expressed emotion concept may have relevance for the course of illness and relapse and those for whom it may not. I think that can be a real contribution.

I am wondering to what extent you feel that the relapse criteria that you are using are very similar to the ones used in the British studies and in the UCLA/Camarillo study, because I know that this has been a point of debate. They used very specific criteria.

Dr. Hogarty: Right. They are similar to those used in the English studies, but in those studies, because patients were kept in hospital or were able to remain in hospital until they made a full recovery, the type of relapse in the UK studies is generally Type I. In our studies, we have both Type I and Type II, because our average length of stay is 21 days for schizophrenia. So we tend to get more Type II relapse.

The criteria changed somewhat to my understanding in the UCLA/ Camarillo study. They are now using rating-scale criteria, if I am correct;

* Los Angeles, California.

an operational definition of change in related components of psychopathology. I'm not sure.

Dr. Nuechterlein: They used rating scales, yes, particularly the Psychiatric Assessment Scale, as well as the Present State Exam.

Dr. Hogarty: I think in that study, another difference would be that they dropped patients who exited hospital in a symptomatic state and who remained symptomatic. I don't think that they could come to a decision as to how to accommodate those people, so they removed them from the analyses.

Dr. Nuechterlein: Well, actually they analyzed it both with them in and with them out, and the British Expressed Emotion findings replicated either way.

Dr. Hogarty: We consider these people as survivors. There are six of them in our trial. So those would be the similarities and differences. By the time we are finished with our analysis, we will use rating-scale criteria. I think that these are parallel criteria for a relapse, and I think they are all very important. We haven't seen any marked differences in the five criteria we have used to date. The results, our interpretations of the results doesn't change any, using different criteria.

Dr. Nuechterlein: It would be nice to try some type of direct replication of criteria across centers, because I really think that could shed more light on differences in results. I think that some investigators in the UCLA group feel that the criteria used in the UCLA/Camarillo study and in your study are significantly different. A direct comparison might be very helpful.

Dr. Hogarty: Well, their criteria are very different than what anyone else has used. I think that they are very important. No one has used those criteria before to my knowledge. They look very good.

Dr. Nuechterlein: Thank you. I appreciate your comments.

Dr. Jack Durell:* Whereas you pointed out the importance of drug noncompliance as the major correlate of—and I say correlate—of relapse, clinically, one gets the impression with many patients that drug noncompliance is an early symptom of relapse. So it becomes interesting to look at drug noncompliance as a dependent variable and try to determine whether one can isolate predictive variables of drug compliance.

Dr. Hogarty: We tried that.

Dr. Durell: And I wonder whether the EE is useful in that respect.

Dr. Hogarty: That's a good question. I mentioned that we eliminated those patients from the analysis. We did put drug noncompliance in early as a dependent variable and tried to explain it. We couldn't explain the relapse of the noncompliance group at all, beyond noncompliance. I think what is important to remember from our placebo controlled studies is that

* Rockville, Maryland.

there is a group of patients who will relapse without medication, maybe 35%, 40% of patients in the first year. There is also a group who will relapse on medication. So there are two different groups.

The group that relapses off medication may very well be a group that is becoming ill and then noncomplies. I think from our past studies we have some evidence that it might be, in fact, the case. However, none of the variables that we have described today can explain noncompliance or the relapse of those patients. There may be other variables, but not these.

Dr. Ming Tsuang:* The literature on high EE and low EE are quite impressive, particularly with acute schizophrenic condition, and the point I would like to make to the investigators in this area is this: It is misleading to denote this high EE/low EE as "environmental." It is also misleading to equate "environmental" strictly with "psychosocial." Probably some biological factors are involved. For instance, there may be a genetic component to this high EE/low EE phenomenon. High EE/low EE are currently described by a very global measurement. Future research should concentrate on distinguishing the psychosocial, biological, and genetic components of the phenomena. As an example, using neuropsychological measurement, such as eye tracking and some other variables, to quantify and characterize this high EE/low EE will be very important research to pursue to tease apart psychosocial and biological components.

Dr. Hogarty: Yes. We are. We are pursuing that. That's a very important observation. This work is being done collaboratively with Mike Goldstein and Bob Asarnow. There are associations between parental communication deviance and information-processing deficits. For those more analytically minded in this group, the vagueness in communication, the difficulties in communication that have been observed for many years in the parents of schizophrenic patients do tend to have a psychophysiologic substrate, as Dr. Tsuang infers. There is also some very preliminary evidence that information-processing deficits are more likely to appear among siblings in high-EE households than among siblings in low-EE households. This work is being done in large part by Dr. Diane Wagner, who is with our program.

So I think that observation is an accurate one, a very important one, and I hope within a year we will be able to report on further observations.

* Providence, Rhode Island

19

Treatment of Schizophrenia: Maintenance Strategies and Pharmacologic Tactics

NINA R. SCHOOLER
National Institute of Mental Health

INTRODUCTION

The purpose of this chapter is to review some recent research on drug treatment in schizophrenia, with particular emphasis on long-term maintenance treatment. In order to set this research into some historical perspective, the first section of the paper will provide a brief overview of changes in the past several years in the nature of the clinical research on drug treatment for schizophrenia. Following that, studies aimed at dosage reduction of antipsychotic drugs will be discussed. The third and final section will examine the role of antidepressants in long-term maintenance treatment for schizophrenia.

THE HISTORICAL CONTEXT OF MAINTENANCE TREATMENT

In a recent review of maintenance antipsychotic treatment for chronic schizophrenia (Schooler & Severe, 1984) we identified 16 studies that provided detailed information regarding symptomatic change. Of these 16, 12 had been conducted with in-patients and only 4 with patients in the community. Only one of the 10 in-patient studies had been carried out after 1970 and only one of the out-patient studies prior to 1970. If this review had been written 10 years ago it would have drawn almost exclusively on research conducted in in-patient settings. Further, patients in those studies had been hospitalized, on the average, over 10 years (Schooler & Severe, 1984). Thus, the research setting is an accurate reflection of the clinical environment for patients at the time.

Studies in the 1960s and early 1970s also reflected a concern with the high end of a dose–response continuum. The basic research question took the following form: Given a patient population that has shown (on the average) a 50% reduction in ratings of psychopathology on 500 mg of chlorpromazine, can we increase the proportion of patients who show change and/or increase the magnitude of change in those patients who have shown some response? This question pre-supposed the assumption that the dose–response curve is linear above the moderate range, so that an increase in dosage should result in improvement in both the response rate and the magnitude of response. Studies by Prien and Cole (1968) and Prien, Levine, and Cole (1969) exemplified this model. In these studies, two dose levels of chlorpromazine and of trifluoperazine were compared to placebo in a 6-month treatment period among long-stay chronic patients. The differences between moderate and high dosage were not substantial. This contrasts to the exceedingly robust effect for drug–placebo differences (Davis, 1975). The basic conclusion to be drawn from studies of increasing dosage is that the dose–response curve is not linear for antipsychotic drugs in the upper range and that therefore such increases in dosage did not purchase concommitant therapeutic gains.

A parallel trend to high-dose studies in maintenance treatment has been the use of "rapid neuroleptization" as a strategy in acutely exacerbated patients, in an effort to avoid or shorten hospitalization. In this model, frequent injections, often hourly, of a high-potency neuroleptic (most often haloperidol) have been compared to standard treatment in terms of symptomatic improvement both during the first few days and then after several weeks of treatment. These studies, reviewed by Cole (1982), are also consistent in finding that dramatic increases in dosage do not parallel improvement in response.

A third kind of study involved fixed-length drug holidays. Some studies that fall under this rubric were primarily concerned with medication-administration schedules and effective use of nursing time by using once-a-day versus multiple daily administration or 4- or 5- versus 7-day administration (Prien, Gillis, & Caffey, 1973). However, a number of studies (Chien, 1975) and, more recently, Shenoy, Sadler, Goldberg, Hamer, and Ross (1981) have examined fixed-length drug-discontinuation periods, with the goal of determining whether patients can be maintained off medication for a specified period under clinical care and then returned to maintenance treatment. In general, results of these studies suggest that periods of 3 weeks (Shenoy *et al.*, 1981) and 3 months (Chien, 1975) are not associated with increased risk of relapse. These studies parallel results of early inpatient withdrawal studies in suggesting that 3 months or less is inadequate to detect a drug–placebo difference (Davis, 1975). However, a recent study with outpatients (Levine *et al.*, 1980) did see drug–placebo differences in relapse during a 3-month drug-withdrawal period.

The role of compliance in out-patient maintenance treatment was a major focus of research with schizophrenic patients during the 1970s. These

Table 1. Relapse Rates for Guaranteed Medication from Prospective Studies Comparing Depot Fluphenazine to Oral Neuroleptics

Study	Patient population	*N*	Study length (months)	Relapse rate (depot fluphenazine)
Crawford and Forrest (1974)	Stable out-patients	29	10	14%
Del Giudice, Clark, and Gocka (1975)	Newly discharged	88	16	NA
Rifkin, Quitkin, Rabiner, and Klein (1977)	Remitted out-patients	73	12	8%
Falloon, Watt, and Shepherd (1978)	Newly discharged	41	12	40%
Hogarty *et al.* (1979)	Newly discharged	105	24	40%
Schooler *et al.* (1980)	Newly discharged	214	12	24%

studies drew their rationale from the clinical observation that, despite significant drug–placebo differences in efficacy, there were relapses and residual symptoms among patients on medication. Could these reflect patient noncompliance with treatment? Might compliance be the key to the problem of limited efficacy that increased dosage had not been? Studies with prospective designs that compared long-acting depot neuroleptic treatment (guaranteeing medication receipt and compliance) to oral administration of medication (allowing patients to noncomply) are presented in Table 1. With the exception of the study by Del Giudice, Clark, and Gocka (1975), all of the studies found no significant difference in relapse between the group in which medication was guaranteed and the group that could have been covertly noncompliant. These studies generally have been interpreted as indicating that noncompliance does not play a major role in relapse of schizophrenic patients. Recently, Kane and Borenstein (1985) have questioned this conclusion, based on a combination of lack of sufficient statistical power and inadequate study length. However, as can be seen in the final column of Table 1, relapse rates on the depot medication ranged from 14% to 40% in the course of 10-to-24-month studies. Regardless of whether these rates are significantly lower than those obtained when patients can covertly reject medication, they represent an accurate estimate of the relapse rate among patients receiving antipsychotic drugs in whom compliance is guaranteed. These rates are substantial and their variability among studies seems to be related to the degree of patient clinical stability, either in terms of time since the most recent hospitalization or degree of remission required for study entry. Newly discharged patients (Falloon, Watt, & Shepherd, 1978; Hogarty *et al.*, 1979; Schooler *et al.*, 1980) show higher rates, 24%-40% in a 12-to-24-month period, than stable or remitted out-patients (Crawford & Forrest, 1974; Rifkin, Quitkin, Rabiner, & Klein, 1977) with rates of 14% and 8% during a 10-to-12-month period.

In summary, this very brief and therefore overgeneralized sketch of maintenance antipsychotic drug treatment in schizophrenia suggests (1) significantly greater efficacy than placebo; (2) lack of a linear dose–response curve above moderate dosage either in acute treatment (rapid neuroleptization) or long-term maintenance; (3) evidence of limited efficacy for some patients even when compliance with medication is assured: and (4) a shift in the setting of studies from the hospital to the community.

Had this paper been written 10 years ago the focus would have been on the results of dosage-increase studies, drug holidays, and length of time and dosage needed to detect drug–placebo differences. The promise of studies in community settings and the role of compliance in assessing treatment effects would have represented the conclusion calling for future research.

DOSE-REDUCTION STRATEGIES

Attention to medication strategies that will reduce the amount of antipsychotic drug received by patients, particularly during long-term treatment, has been a more recent development. The research grows out of a number of clinical concerns. Perhaps the most important of these is the risk of tardive dyskinesia in neuroleptic-treated patients (Kane, Woerner, Weinhold, Wegner, & Kinon, 1982). A logical hypothesis is that the risk of tardive dyskinesia associated with neuroleptic drug treatment can be reduced by reducing drug exposure. A second concern derives from the observation that, especially among long-term treated patients, negative symptoms of passivity, anhedonia, and social withdrawal seem prominent. Such symptoms are believed by some to be drug related—either actually caused by drug treatment or persisting despite treatment.

Two dose reduction strategies have been developed and will be described: (1) continuous low dosage, and (2) intermittent or targeted treatment, which is characterized by the use of medication only during periods of symptom exacerbation rather than continuously.

Both of these strategies are designed for maintenance rather than treatment of acute episodes. Further, both depend on the clinical identification of symptomatic worsening and the increase to standard dosage levels (in the low-dosage strategy) and introduction of medication (in the targeted or intermittent approach). Following episodic treatment to resolve an acute episode, medication dosage is again either reduced to a low dosage or discontinued. Thus, both strategies share a common need to define remission and provide accurate identification of relapse when it occurs.

The nature of these strategies suggests that patient characteristics such as the course of the illness and the speed with which neuroleptic medication is effective will be important in determining which of the dosage-reduction strategies will be more successful. This interindividual variability in course and the interaction of treatment with that course will probably prove to be critical variables as investigators seek to learn which patients are most likely to benefit from dose-reduction strategies and which of these strategies is more appropriate for which types of patients.

Low-Dose Treatment

A review of studies comparing chlorpromazine to placebo in schizophrenia (Cole & Davis, 1968) concluded that a major factor determining whether the study found a significant drug effect compared to placebo was whether dosage was above a threshold of 400 mg chlorpromazine per day. However, none of the studies reviewed by Cole and Davis systematically attempted to evaluate the lower end of the dose–response continuum by comparing a low dose to a higher one. A more recent review of the effect of dosage in maintenance treatment (Baldessarini & Davis, 1980) found no relationship between dose and relapse rate over a wide range (100 to 2000 mg/day chlorpromazine equivalent). None of this latter group of studies involved random assignment to dosage level either.

Table 2 presents four studies that have examined this treatment strategy in community-treated patients. All share in common the use of long-acting injectible fluphenazine decanoate or enanthate in order to ensure delivery of drug treatment and to eliminate the possibility of covert noncompliance, which could blur the experimental dosage distinction.

Table 2. Studies of Low-Dosage Treatment

	Depot fluphenazine (mg/2 weeks)				Relapse rates (%)	
Investigator	Standard dose	Low dose	*N*	Study duration	Standard	Low
Goldstein, Rodnick, Evans, May, and Steinberg (1978)	25	6.25	104	6 weeks	5	16
Kane *et al.* (1983)	12.5–50	1.25–5	125	1 year	7	56
Marder *et al.* (1984)	25–50	5–10	50	1 year	20	22
Hogarty (1984)	20($\bar{X}$)	4($\bar{X}$)	42	1 year	25	23

Goldstein, Rodnick, Evans, May, and Steinberg (1978) conducted the earliest reported study of low-dose treatment. The study compared a low dose of injectible fluphenazine enanthate (6.25 mg every 2 weeks) to a standard dose of the same drug (25 mg every 2 weeks) in newly discharged patients. Patients were also randomly assigned to either six weekly sessions of pragmatic, crisis-oriented family therapy or no family contact. The low-dose treatment was a substitute for a placebo control, which was not feasible in the setting of this research—a community mental health center with hospital stays of less than 2 weeks. After the 6-week study course, and persisting for 6 months, none of the patients in the group that received standard dose and family therapy had relapsed. In this still symptomatic but community-treated patient population, dosage reduction, particularly in the absence of family support, was associated with significant increase in relapse.

A study directly investigating the low-dose treatment strategy was conducted by Kane *et al.* (1983). Patients were included if they were in remission or partial remission for at least 4 weeks on the standard dose. The actual mean time since hospital discharge was over 14 months. The assumption underlying use of low-dose treatment in this study and in the others to be described is that the presence of a small amount of medication functions to attenuate or blunt the process of symptom exacerbation so that increased medication can be introduced before full relapse occurs. The question of whether relapse on medication is a different process or experience than relapse on placebo (or off medication) is an interesting aside that cannot be addressed in detail here. Responsible opinion can be found stating that symptom exacerbation on medication is worse because it represents the breakthrough of symptom expression despite the presence of drug treatment. The counterview holds that symptoms are less severe because the presence of neuroleptic drug attenuates symptom expression.

Use of low-dose treatment also assumes that medication may prevent the development of symptom exacerbation; it serves a true prophylactic role. As shown in Table 2, cumulative relapse at the end of 1 year in the study by Kane and associates was 56% in the low-dose group compared to 7% in those maintained on standard dose. Within the sample studied, neither length of time in remission nor severity of psychopathology as indexed by rating-scale-data predicted relapse. As noted earlier, remission or stable partial remission characterized the entire population. Because this is a patient characteristic that in standard-dose studies seems to be related to a low rate of relapse, these data suggest that even relatively low-risk patients experience increased symptoms when dosage is reduced.

Hogarty (1984) reported on dose reduction in a small sample of patients who achieved reasonable remission of psychotic symptoms, generally 5 or 6 months following discharge. Patients were randomly assigned to standard dose of fluphenazine decanoate ($\bar{X}$ 20 mg every 2 weeks) or to 20% of that dose ($\bar{X}$ 4 mg every 2 weeks). As shown in Table 2, at the end of a year approximately 25% of patients had relapsed regardless of treatment assignment.

Marder *et al.* (1984) examined the question of dose reduction in a sample of male veterans who were symptomatically stable on fluphenazine decanoate (no more than 25 mg/2 weeks) for at least 2 months. Patients were randomized to either continuation of the 25 mg dose or a reduced fixed dose of 5 mg/2 weeks. This dose could be doubled (5 mg to 10; 25 mg to 50) in the event of defined symptom exacerbation. There were no significant differences in relapse either on the original dose or including the increase.

The conclusion reached in these studies of dosage reduction is that, in relatively stable populations, moderate reduction does not increase the risk of relapse (Hogarty and Marder studies), although it does so in more acutely ill patients (Goldstein). However, even in clinically stable patients, reduction to 10% of standard dosage significantly increases risk of relapse (Kane).

The examination of measures of psychopathology and social adjustment suggests that dosage reduction, even within the rather narrow range that has been studied thus far, does have substantial effects. Goldstein and his colleagues found no significant main effects of dosage level upon specific symptoms during their 6-week study period, although symptoms of withdrawal were higher in the standard-dose group. However, men showed significantly more symptoms of hostility and anxious depression in the standard-dose condition, whereas women showed more symptomatology if they received the low dose. They did find a significant reduction in withdrawal symptoms among patients who received family therapy—regardless of dosage. After 6 months, the reduction in withdrawal symptoms for patients who had received family therapy persisted, but only for patients who also received the standard dose. These complex results suggest that the influences of dosage on symptomatic change may be mediated by environmental variables (e.g., family therapy) and organismic variables (sex).

Detailed symptom analyses from the study by Kane and his colleagues are not yet available, but analyses of social functioning after a year of treatment (Kreisman *et al.*, 1984) indicate that among patients who did not experience a relapse during the year of treatment, those who received the low dose showed better functioning on a number of measures than those who received standard dose. This pattern appeared both in ratings made by the patient and in those made by family members.

Marder and associates examined both ratings of psychopathology (Brief Psychiatric Rating Scale [BPRS]) and self-ratings of subjective distress (Symptom Checklist–90). There were no differences between the low- and standard-dose groups in clinicians' ratings of psychopathology (BPRS) among patients who had not relapsed after 3 months treatment. However, self-rated symptoms of obsessive compulsiveness, interpersonal sensitivity, depression, and phobic anxiety were all lower among patients on the reduced dosage. They also were rated as showing less akathisia and retardation.

In general, in patient populations at lower risk for relapse there are significant positive effects of dose reduction on other aspects of functioning (Marder study; subsample in Kane's study who do not relapse). Among patients such as those in Goldstein's study who are at higher risk for relapse, dose reduction is not associated with reduced symptomatology. The importance of predicting which patients are likely to tolerate dose reduction without relapse becomes especially important if there are substantial symptomatic and social-functioning benefits to those patients who can avoid relapse with low-dose treatment.

Intermittent or Targeted Treatment

This maintenance strategy involves treating patients without neuroleptic medication except for periods when prodromal symptoms appear that foreshadow a relapse. The strategy is based on the assumption that neuroleptic medication does not have direct prophylactic properties to prevent relapse, and that the substantial effects in preventing relapse are seen because continuous administration of medication insures that when a relapse begins medication that will treat the florid symptoms is present. If the patient is closely monitored while medication free, such symptoms can be detected in time to introduce medication and prevent a full relapse and hospitalization. In patients whose illness follows an episodic course, intermittent treatment should be as successful as standard dose in preventing relapse.

Two studies report on the efficacy of targeted or intermittent neuroleptic treatment. Both treatment approaches stress the importance of consistent monitoring of patients for signs of impending relapse. Carpenter and Heinrichs (1983), who use the term targeted medication, provide such monitoring through the use of an individual relationship with a therapist/case manager who provides the patient with a framework for dealing with the illness based upon a model of environmental stress and its role in symptom exacerbation. As described in an early report (Carpenter, Stephens, Rey, Hanlon, & Heinrichs, 1982), recently discharged patients are randomly assigned to medication discontinuation or continuation and then followed for up to 24 months. Preliminary results indicate that patients randomized to the low-dose condition do receive less medication and receive it less than a third of the time. Based on a relatively small number of cases, there are no significant differences between groups in either symptoms of psychopathology, social functioning, days in hospital, or number of hospitalizations. Conclusions from this study will be limited by the fact that treatment is not delivered under blind conditions. Thus, although patients assigned to continuous medication receive the same kind of individual case monitoring as those whose medication is discontinued, there may be "special" attention to those who are off medication.

The second study investigating this strategy was reported by Herz, Szymanski, and Simon (1982). They identified subjects who were in relative remission from psychotic symptoms, had been on stable doses of antipsychotic medications for at least 6 months, and lived in close proximity to a significant other person. This last criterion may be especially important, because implementation of intermittent treatment requires identification of early signs of illness. In an earlier study, Herz and Melville (1980) found substantial agreement both among patients and between patients and their families in the report of which symptoms were prominent in the development of an episode. Most frequently reported were "being tense and nervous" (reported by over 70% of patients), followed by other symptoms of dysphoria, such as trouble sleeping (60%), restlessness (50%), loss of interest (59%), and reduced enjoyment (60%). However, only about half of the patients report that the pattern of symptom development is the same for each episode.

The Herz *et al.* (1982) study was an open pilot study for a randomized double-blind clinical trial that is currently underway. Among 19 patients meeting criteria presented above, 14 were effectively discontinued from medication. During the 6 to 8 months of the study, 5 of the 14 (36%) experienced prodromal signs that were treated successfully with medication.

Conclusive data comparing intermittent or targeted medication to standard drug in maintenance treatment are not yet available, but the ongoing work by Carpenter and his colleagues and Herz and his associates address many of the relevant issues, as shown in Table 3. The populations being studied are complementary: recently discharged versus stable. Studying the recently discharged population provides an opportunity to identify patient characteristics most appropriate for the strategy. The stable population represents the group presumptively most suited to the strategy. Both studies include an initial drug-withdrawal period to eliminate patients who cannot

Table 3. Targeted or Intermittent Treatment Studies

Investigator	Patient population	Psychosocial support	Control features	Study length
Carpenter group (Baltimore)	Recently discharged (8 weeks)	Individual case manager	Random nonblind	24 months
Herz group (Buffalo)	Stable out-patients (6 months)	Support group	Random double blind	12 months

tolerate even a brief 4-week period off medication. Both investigators recognize the importance of psychosocial support but provide it in different ways. Carpenter and Heinrichs (1983) utilize a case manager/therapist and individual family sessions to form an alliance with the patient. The Herz study (Herz *et al.*, 1982) relies on patient groups to provide support and aid in identification of prodromata. Both studies utilize random assignment. In the Carpenter study, both patient and staff know which patients are not actually receiving medication. This does mirror the clinical situation realistically, but, as noted above, may result in differential attention between the targeted and continuous groups. The ongoing Herz study is double blind.

Conclusion

The two strategies for dose reduction are based on different assumptions regarding the role of antipsychotic medication in the long-term treatment of schizophrenic patients. None of the studies compares the two strategies, and, therefore, the accuracy of these assumptions remains untested. A study directly comparing intermittent or targeted, low-dose, and standard-dose medication is being undertaken as a collaborative multicenter study by the National Institute of Mental Health (Schooler & Keith, 1984). This study, in conjunction with the work described previously, should provide answers to many questions about the role of dose-reduction strategies in the treatment of schizophrenia.

ROLE OF ADJUNCTIVE ANTIDEPRESSANTS IN MAINTENANCE TREATMENT

Treatment of a depressive syndrome that arises in the context of maintenance antipsychotic treatment of schizophrenia has long been considered a difficult clinical problem. The concept of a postpsychotic depressive episode affecting as many as 25% of patients has been described (McGlashin & Carpenter, 1976), and the contribution of this condition to subsequent relapse has been recognized (Mandel, Severe, Schooler, Gelenberg, & Mieske, 1982). However, conclusions regarding the role of antidepressant drug treatment for schizophrenic patients have been generally negative (Siris, van Kammen, & Docherty, 1978; Donaldson, Gelenberg, & Baldessarini, 1983.)

Siris *et al.* (1978) concluded that the efficacy of antidepressants in schizophrenia had not been adequately evaluated because most studies had been hampered, either by inclusion of patients regardless of whether or not they were experiencing depressive symptoms or by the use of fixed ratios of antidepressant to antipsychotic (e.g., amitriptyline–perphenazine), probably because the fixed-ratio combination is marketed.

Siris *et al.* (1985) have recently reported results of a study that rectifies the design problems of prior work in this area. Patients had recovered from recent episodes of schizophrenia or schizoaffective disorder, according to the Research Diagnostic Criteria (RDC). They were stabilized on fluphenazine decanoate and benztropine. Benztropine was used to treat akinesia, which can be difficult to distinguish from depressive symptoms on purely phenomenological grounds. Patients were also required to meet rating criteria on the Hamilton Depression Scale for 3 weeks, with the further stipulation that the last rating not be the lowest. This criterion was designed to exclude patients who were improving spontaneously. Patients were randomly assigned to receive either adjunctive imipramine or a placebo for 6 weeks. Significantly greater overall improvement was seen for the imipramine group compared to placebo. Further, there were significant differences in improvement in 6 of 11 symptoms of depression. No differences between the groups were seen in terms of ratings of psychosis or side effects. These results are based on a very small sample of 28 patients. The study is being extended both in terms of number of patients and length of treatment period.

The importance of this clinical trial is twofold. First, it provides evidence of the efficacy of a treatment that may be of substantial clinical utility. Second, it serves as an example of an effective research strategy that identifies very precisely a narrow target population and then studies a specific treatment strategy in that restricted population. The results of this study obviously should not be generalized to the broader population of schizophrenic patients. With that caveat, this small study provides firmer evidence regarding the role of antidepressants in the treatment of schizophrenia than does the preexisting literature of the past 25 years.

SUMMARY

This article has not attempted to review in its entirety the broad area of drug treatment for schizophrenia, in terms of either clinical issues or research paradigms. A major omission has been the development of renewed interest in the interaction and combination of psychosocial treatments, particularly techniques that involve families as well as patients, with drug treatment for schizophrenia. Some issues of relevance to this topic are dealt with in other chapters of this volume.

The chapter has identified two important stylistic trends in treatment clinical trials in schizophrenia: the large-scale clinical trial with broad inclusion criteria exemplified by the dose-reduction studies, and the finely tuned and focused study exemplified by the study of adjunctive imipramine in depressed schizophrenic patients.

Both research strategies will play important roles in our developing understanding of drug treatment for schizophrenia, and it is with enthusiasm that we can look forward to the answers that will be forthcoming.

REFERENCES

Baldessarini, R. J., & Davis, J. M. (1980). What *is* the best maintenance dose of neuroleptics in schizophrenia? *Psychiatry Research*, *3*, 115–122.

Carpenter, W. T., & Heinrichs, D. W. (1983). Early intervention, time-limited, targeted pharmacotherapy of schizophrenia. *Schizophrenia Bulletin*, *9*, 533–542.

Carpenter, W. T., Stephens, J. H., Rey, A. C., Hanlon, T. E., & Heinrichs, D. W. (1982). Early intervention vs continuous pharmacotherapy of schizophrenia. *Psychopharmacology Bulletin*, *18*, 21.

Chien, C. P. (1975). Drugs and rehabilitation in schizophrenia. In M. Greenblatt (Ed.), *Drugs in combination with other therapies* (pp. 13–34). New York: Grune & Stratton.

Cole, J. O. (1982). Antipsychotic drugs: Is more better? *McLean Hospital Journal*, *7*, 61–87.

Cole, J. O., & Davis, J. M. (1968). Clinical efficacy of the phenothiazines as antipsychotic drugs. In D. H. Efron, J. O. Cole, J. Levine, & J. R. Wittenborn (Eds.), *Psychopharmacology: A review of progress 1957-1967*. Washington, DC: U.S. Government Printing Office.

Crawford, R., & Forrest, A. (1974). Controlled trial of depot fluphenazine in out-patient schizophrenics. *British Journal of Psychiatry*, *124*, 385–391.

Davis, J. M. (1975). Overview: Maintenance therapy in psychiatry. I. Schizophrenia. *American Journal of Psychiatry*, *132*, 1237–1245.

Del Giudice, J., Clark, W. G., & Gocka, E. F. (1975). Prevention of recidivism of schizophrenics treated with fluphenazine enanthate. *Psychosomatics*, *16*, 32–36.

Donaldson, S. R., Gelenberg, A. J., & Baldessarini, R. J. (1983). The pharmacologic treatment of schizophrenia: A progress report. *Schizophrenia Bulletin*, *9*, 504–527.

Falloon, I., Watt, D. C., & Shepherd, M. (1978). A comparative controlled trial of pimozide and fluphenazine decanoate in the continuation therapy of schizophrenia. *Psychological Medicine*, *8*, 59–70.

Goldstein, M. J., Rodnick, E. H., Evans, J. R., May, P. R. A., & Steinberg, M. R. (1978). Drug and family therapy in the aftercare treatment of acute schizophrenics. *Archives of General Psychiatry*, *35*, 1169.

Herz, M. I., & Melville, C. (1980). Relapse in schizophrenia. *American Journal of Psychiatry*, *137*, 801.

Herz, M. I., Szymanski, H. V., & Simon, J. C. (1982). Intermittent medication for stable schizophrenic outpatients: An alternative to maintenance medication. *American Journal of Psychiatry*, *139*, 918.

Hogarty, G. E. (1984). Depot neuroleptics: The relevance of psychosocial factors. *Journal of Clinical Psychiatry*, *45*, 34–42.

Hogarty, G. E., Schooler, N. R., Ulrich, R., Mussare, F., Ferro, P., & Herron, E. (1979). Fluphenazine and social therapy in the aftercare of schizophrenic patients: Relapse analyses of a two-year controlled trial. *Archives of General Psychiatry, 36*, 1283–1294.

Kane, J. M., & Borenstein, M. (1985). Non-compliance in the outpatient treatment of schizophrenia. *Psychopharmacology Bulletin.*

Kane, J. M., Rifkin, A., Woerner, M., Reardon, G., Sarantakos, S., Schiebel, D., & Ramos-Lorenzi, J. (1983). Low dose neuroleptic treatment of outpatient schizophrenics. I. Preliminary results for relapse rates. *Archives of General Psychiatry, 40*, 893–896.

Kane, J. M., Woerner, M., Weinhold, P., Wegner, J., & Kinon, B. (1982). A prospective study of tardive dyskinesia development: Preliminary results. *Journal of Clinical Psychopharmacology, 2*, 345–349.

Kreisman, D., Blumenthal, R. L., Kane, J. M., Borenstein, M., Woerner, M., Rifkin, A., & Reardon, G. (1984). *Patient and family response to standard low doses of medication in outpatient schizophrenics.* Poster presented at the American Psychopathological Association Meeting, New York.

Levine, J., Schooler, N. R., Severe, J. B., Escobar, J., Gelenberg, A., Mandel, M., Sovner, R., & Steinbook, R. (1980). In F. Cattabeni (Ed.), *Long-term effects of neuroleptics* (pp. 483–493). New York: Raven Press.

Mandel, M. R., Severe, J. B., Schooler, N. R., Gelenberg, A. J., & Mieske, M. (1982). Development and prediction of postpsychotic depression in neuroleptic treated schizophrenics. *Archives of General Psychiatry, 39*, 197–203.

Marder, S. R., von Putten, T., Mintz, J., Lebell, M., McKenzie, J., & Faltico, G. (1984). Maintenance therapy in schizophrenia: New findings. In J. M. Kane (Ed.), *Drug maintenance strategies in schizophrenia* (pp. 31–49). Washington, DC: American Psychiatric Association.

McGlashin, T. H., & Carpenter, W. T. (1976). Postpsychotic depression in schizophrenia. *Archives of General Psychiatry, 33*, 231–241.

Prien, R. F., & Cole, J. O. (1968). High dose chlorpromazine therapy in chronic schizophrenia: Report of the National Institute of Mental Health-Psychopharmacology Research Branch Collaborative Study Group. *Archives of General Psychiatry, 18*, 482–495.

Prien, R. F., Gillis, R. D., & Caffey, E. M. (1973). Intermittent pharmacotherapy in chronic schizophrenia. *Hospital & Community Psychiatry, 24*, 317–322.

Prien, R. F., Levine, J., & Cole, J. O. (1969). High dose trifluoperazine therapy in chronic schizophrenia. *American Journal of Psychiatry, 126*, 53–61.

Rifkin, A., Quitkin, F. Rabiner, C. J., & Klein, D. F. (1977). Fluphenazine decanoate, fluphenazine hydrochloride given orally, and placebo in remitted schizophrenics. I. Relapse rates after one year. *Archives of General Psychiatry, 34*, 43–47.

Schooler, N. R., & Keith, S. J. (1984). *Treatment strategies in schizophrenia protocol.* Rockville, MD: National Institute of Mental Health.

Schooler, N. R., Levine, J., Severe, J. B., Brauzer, D., DiMascio, A., Klerman, G. L., & Tuason, V. B. (1980). Prevention of relapse in schizophrenia. *Archives of General Psychiatry, 37*, 16–24.

Schooler, N. R., & Severe, J. B. (1984). Efficacy of drug treatment for chronic schizophrenic patients. In M. Mirabi & L. Feldman (Eds.), *The chronically mentally ill research and services* (pp. 125–142). New York: S.P. Medical & Scientific Books.

Shenoy, R. S., Sadler, A. G., Goldberg, S. C., Hamer, R. M., & Ross, B. (1981). Effects of a six-week drug holiday on symptom status, relapse and tardive dyskinesia in chronic schizophrenics. *Journal of Clinical Psychopharmacology, 1*, 141-145.

Siris, S. G., van Kammen, D. P., & Docherty, J. P. (1978). Use of antidepressant drugs in schizophrenia. *Archives of General Psychiatry, 35*, 1368–1377.

Siris, S. G., Rifkin, A., Reardon, G. T., Doddi, S. R., Foster, P., & Casey, E. (1985). A trial of adjunctive imipramine in postpsychotic depression. *Psychopharmacology Bulletin, 21*, 114–119.

COMMENTARY

Dr. Eugene Paykel:* Gerry Hogarty talked earlier about presenting to a mainly British audience. I am a mainly British member of this audience. I wanted to report a clinical perspective that is a bit different to Nina [Schooler's]. I am a little unhappy with the conclusion that it is already safe to try intermittent medication and low-dose maintenance in the community, although in the long run, I am happy to live with the results of whatever the studies show. I think a lot swings on an issue that we haven't really heard discussed at the meeting so far, and this is whether schizophrenic relapse and schizophrenic symptoms in themselves damage.

When I was starting my training in psychiatry in 1962, I was taught that schizophrenia was an illness that often produced successive episodes and that each episode left a little more damage at the end of it. If that's really the case, then obviously one has to view the risk of having a relapse while off medication very differently than if it is simply a question of having a relapse and getting a restitution back to where the patient was. If the latter happens, I think you can run the risk quite comfortably and it is justified to do so.

Clinically, my impression, being responsible for a service in England where we have many schizophrenics in the community (some of whom I have watched since about 1971 when I went back to England) who are treated mainly by a nurse in the community with depot injections, is that very few patients in fact relapse while on adequate doses of neuroleptics and that many relapse as soon as they come off. Also, for what it's worth, my clinical impression of these patients is that if they stay on medication after a first episode and are undamaged, then they tend not to get damage thereafter, although if they stay on medication after a third or fourth episode, they may already be damaged and stay damaged. I don't think the existing studies answer this question. You've really got to get a group of first-episode patients, follow them up, and see what happens, and none of the follow-ups have quite done that while on adequate medication, but it seems to me very important in the long run to find that out.

Dr. Schooler: I think that is absolutely correct. First of all, I was perhaps eliding my phrases when I used the term relapse as the criterion for introducing medication in the intermittent- or targeted-medication studies. I am confident that both Dr. Carpenter and Dr. Herz would state unequivocally that neither of them regard the criterion at which standard doses, adequate doses of medication are introduced to be that of relapse. The question in the low-dose studies is, of course, somewhat different. I was not suggesting that the evidence we have is such that we should consider these demonstrated treatments clinically. Rather, I was suggesting that the evidence we have

* London, England.

suggests that is appropriate to continue to study these treatments. The evidence regarding them is not such that we ought to preclude further research about them. I think there are other issues besides the ones that you've raised. For instance, it has been suggested that intermittent treatment may be more productive of tardive dyskinesia than continuous treatment. I don't think the evidence we have regarding any of those questions is good enough to preclude studying the treatment approaches.

*Dr. Keith H. Nuechterlein**: I want to ask a question about the potential usefulness of the low-dose strategy, as well as the targeted-medication strategy. I think that these do look like very promising strategies. I am wondering if you could give us any clues at this point as to the domains of measures that you think might be productive in predicting the individuals who would be more responsive to or appropriate for these medication strategies. It seems to me that the literature in the past has suggested that we don't have any good, firm predictors at this point.

Dr. Schooler: Well, there are some very simple ones, I suspect. My own guess is that one of the best predictors is going to turn out to be the dosage from which the patient was shifted to the reduced dose. Certainly the older literature on placebo-controlled studies, the studies done by Prien and Levine and Cole, all suggested that one of the best predictors of likelihood of a nonrelapse on placebo was dosage at the time of randomization, and I think it will turn out to be important in dose reduction as well.

A second variable I think will be relevant as a predictor is going to be stability—the length of time since the last severe episode the patient experienced. Then beyond that, I think the data suggest that there are going to be environmental characteristics that may be important in this regard. Some form of the expressed emotion idea will probably turn out to persist. One of the concerns I have with expressed emotion is that it seems painful to me somehow that the wealth of data that are gathered and that are available about these families and about these patients ends up in a single dichotomous variable. It seems to me that if that dichotomous variable has some power, probably there will be more power in a more detailed exploration of the information that goes into it.

I think the last issue has to do not so much with the prediction of the patient's course, but of the balance of benefit and disadvantage to the patients that will accrue from medication tactics. I think Gene Paykel drew our attention to what is one of the most disconcerting risks, which is that monkeying around with the medication may not be an entirely benign process and the sheer act of having done so may have negative consequences overall. Is improved social functioning in those who do not relapse worth the risk to those who do?

* Los Angeles, California.

20

Interventions with Families and the Course of Schizophrenia

MICHAEL J. GOLDSTEIN AND JERI A. DOANE
University of California, Los Angeles

Interest in the role of the family in schizophrenia has followed a somewhat bipolar course. The euphoria of the 1950s and 1960s was followed by the depressive pessimism of the 1970s. Hopefully, we are in a euthymic period at the present time, when some of the issues that were so affect laden in the past can be viewed with dispassion. Two questions with regard to family factors in schizophrenia remain as important issues that deserve our attention. First, is there evidence that stressors within the family, either of a specific or nonspecific form, antedate the onset of schizophrenia and play a contributory role in the development of the disorder? Second, do attributes of the family environment that follow the onset of schizophrenia influence the short-term course of the disorder?

Evidence concerning the first issue is not easy to come by, although we have been involved in a longitudinal study designed to shed some light on this issue, data from our longer term follow-ups are still being collected at the present time and we are not ready to present preliminary findings. One important factor that limits our ability to obtain more definitive answers concerning the family's contribution to the onset of schizophrenia is the great difficulty in teasing apart gene–environment interactions during the pre-onset period. The lack of a clear-cut marker for the predisposition for schizophrenia limits the researcher's ability to evaluate the subtle interplay between genetic and family stress factors in the pathogenesis of this disorder.

These types of complexities may be part of the reason for the notable shift in emphasis during the last few years toward the second issue, which concerns the family's contribution toward the course of the disorder once it occurs. No doubt interest in this issue has been stimulated by major changes in the delivery of mental health services. Patients are now released from hospitals after very brief periods of inpatient stay, and frequently either find their way back to homes of family members or remain in close contact with them. Observers who noted that schizophrenics vary greatly in their ability to adapt to the community after hospital discharge have questioned whether attributes of the family environment modulate the short-term course of the disorder. Incidentally, by *short-term course* we refer to the patient's symptomatic and social-role functioning over a 1- to-2-year period after an episode of the disorder. The work of Brown and his colleagues in Great Britain was specifically designed to answer this question of whether the family environment influences the course of the patient's illness. A brief review of this work may be helpful.

RESEARCH ON EXPRESSED EMOTION

Brown, Birley, and Wing (1972) attempted to identify attributes of the home environments of relapse-prone schizophrenic patients. They introduced the term *expressed emotion* (EE) to describe attributes of these relapse-prone environments observed during home visits. Two characteristics of such homes were an excessive level of criticism directed at the index patient and/or a quality of emotional overinvolvement (EOI). The original studies indicated that patients from high-EE homes showed more behavioral disturbance during the prodromal phase of their last episode. However, Brown *et al.* (1972) claimed that although this patient attribute also predicted relapse, when a variant of a multiple regression analysis was done, it was not as potent a predictor as the expressed emotion level of the patient's key relatives.

In order to carry out a prospective study of the predictive value of EE status, Brown's colleagues, Vaughn and Leff (1976), shortened the Brown interview technique for eliciting attitudes thought to underlie high levels of criticism and emotional overinvolvement, observed behaviorally in the original home-observation studies. This interview, the Camberwell Family Interview, has become the standard instrument for evaluating the EE status of key relatives. The two studies carried out by Vaughn and Leff, using this assessment device, revealed that patients from families classified as high or low EE did in fact vary markedly in rate of relapse. Patients returning to high-EE homes were 3 to 4 times likely to relapse during the next 9 months than were those returning to low-EE households. These studies also suggested that regular ingestion of neuroleptic medication, or a reduction in face-to-face contact between patient and relatives (Leff, 1976), narrowed the differences in relapse rate for patients from high- and low-EE homes.

The exciting and provocative findings of Vaughn and Leff stimulated a spate of replication studies designed to evaluate whether the predictive validity of the EE measure holds up cross-nationally and cross-culturally. Although these efforts are very understandable, they have focused upon a particular methodology for assessing EE, the Camberwell Family Interview, and lost sight of the original model underlying this research. The original hypothesis of the Brown *et al.* studies was that certain behavior expressed by relatives toward a recently released schizophrenic patient increases the stress level within the home and lowers the patient's threshold for relapse. The interactional behaviors, identified as psychotoxic, were rather specific and they implicated styles of negative affective communication within the family.

But the Camberwell Family Interview is not a measure of intrafamilial affective communication. Instead it measures attitudes toward a patient, expressed within the context of an interview with a mental health professional. These attitudes may or may not be expressed in face-to-face interaction with the patient. We know from years of research in social psychology that there is rarely isomorphism between verbally expressed attitudes and overt interactional behavior. Thus, it is possible that attitudes elicited on the Camberwell Family Interview are imperfectly correlated with interactional behavior and that the predictive validity of the Camberwell-derived EE attitudes in any one study depend upon the degree of attitude–behavior correlation observed in that particular sample. Surprisingly, despite the obvious nature of this issue, it has rarely been addressed in the accumulating literature on EE. Failure to replicate the predictive validity of EE attitudes from the Camberwell does not prove that the affective climate of the family is irrelevant to the course of schizophrenia. However, if similar findings are found for EE-type measures derived from direct obervations of family behavior, it would be strong evidence against this hypothesis.

In our research program, we decided that it was necessary to demonstrate that affective attitudes expressed toward a relative in an interview corresponded with interactional behavior patterns. In order to do this, two things were needed: a standardized situation to evaluate interactional behavior, and a coding system that reflected the behavioral analogues of EE attitudes. For the former, we adapted a version of the direct-interaction task used previously in our prospective longitudinal study (Goldstein, Judd, Rodnick, Alkire, & Gould, 1968) to assess family interaction in a laboratory setting. In this modified version, family members were asked to discuss two emotionally loaded family problems derived from a prior interview. One problem was initiated by the patient and the second by a relative. These discussions were recorded in the absence of an experimenter.

For the latter, we used the Affective Style (AS) coding system developed by Jeri Doane (Doane, West, Goldstein, Rodnick, & Jones, 1981), which was designed to measure affective attitudes expressed toward a relative during a direct interaction task. Some of the codes in this system overlap with the EE dimensions of criticism and emotional overinvolvement. This system was used to code the interactional data in our sample of schizophrenic

Table 1. Negative Affective Style Codes

CRITICISM

1. Personal Criticism
   Unnecessary or overly harsh modifiers; and/or negative reference to broad classes of behavior, and/or negative evaluation of the child's character or nature.
2. Benign Criticism
   Mild; circumscribed; matter-of-fact; directed toward specific incidents or sets of behaviors.

GUILT INDUCTION

Conveys child is to blame or at fault for some negative event and parent has been distressed or upset by the event.

INTRUSIVENESS

Parent implies knowledge of child's thoughts, feelings, or motives without basis for such knowledge.

1. Critical Intrusiveness
   Contains a harsh, critical attribution of intent.
2. Neutral Intrusiveness
   Neutral quality; refers to child's emotional states, ideas, preferences, etc.

patients and their parents. The codes in the AS system are presented in Table 1. As Table 1 shows, there are a number of types of criticisms in this scheme—benign and personal criticisms as well as guilt-induction statements, in which personal criticism is implied. The interpersonal analogue of overinvolvement is reflected in the intrusion code, in which one person speaks as an expert concerning the listener's thoughts, inner states, and motives.

Direct-interaction assessments were done with a sample of schizophrenic patients and their parents. Most of the patients subsequently entered a controlled-treatment study designed by Ian Falloon (Falloon *et al.*, 1982), which contrasted an individual and a family-based therapeutic program, a study that we will return to later in this paper. All parents in this study were assessed by the Camberwell Family Interview as to EE status, but all persons who collected or coded the interactional data were blind as to these EE ratings.

Table 2 presents the total number of negative AS statements (sum of criticisms and intrusive remarks) expressed by the parents across the two interactional tasks. We see that the high-EE relatives express a significantly greater number of criticisms and intrusive statements than low-EE parents ($p < .002$). However, since high-EE relatives attain this status by way of diverse attitudinal patterns (high on criticism, high on criticism and emotional overinvolvement, and high on emotional overinvolvement only), we investigated whether these subtypes within the high-EE group expressed dif-

Table 2. Means and Standard Deviations of Low- and High-EE Parents on Affective Style Total Scores

Parental EE status	*N*	Mean	Standard deviation
Low	28	5.39	3.95
High	34	9.59	5.87

ferent styles of AS as well. Figure 1 presents the frequency of criticism and intrusive statements within the low EE and the different subtypes of high EE. We can see that there is a notable group differentiation such that the subtypes of high-EE attitudes correspond with different patterns of interactional behavior (criticism with critical EE attitudes, and intrusiveness with emotional overinvolvement). These data are also highly significant ($p < .05$).

Although there is a reasonable level of comparability between attitudes expressed on the Camberwell and affective style expressed interactionally, the distributions revealed that the correspondence is far from perfect. The majority of high-EE parents, defined as critical on the Camberwell, are indeed expressive of criticism, but others express none at all. Thus, some high-EE parents are congruent across situations and others appear to dampen or inhibit these high-EE attitudes when in direct confrontation with the patient. Currently, we are investigating whether those high-EE individuals

Figure 1. Mean number of critical and intrusive statements in direct interaction among high- and low-EE parental subgroups.

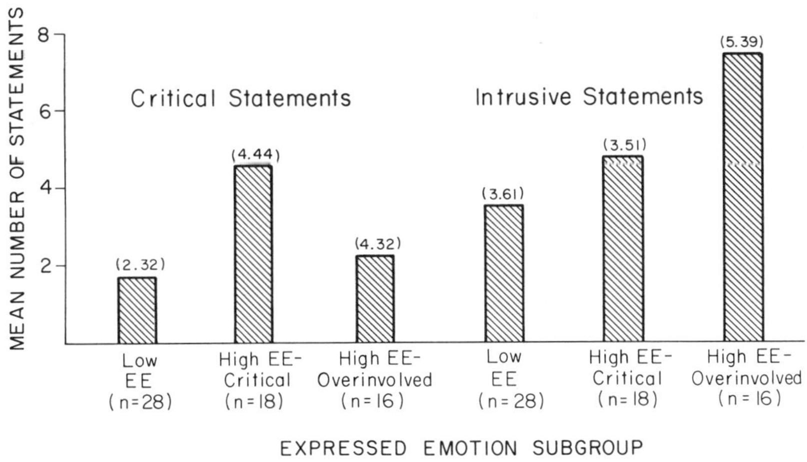

Note: numbers in parentheses are standard deviations.

who do express these negative affective attitudes when interacting with the patient are more likely to have a relapse-prone relative than individuals who express the attitude but not the interactional behavior.

PATIENT ATTRIBUTES ASSOCIATED WITH EE STATUS

We mentioned earlier that Brown *et al.* indicated that certain patient characteristics were associated with both high-EE attitudes and subsequent relapse as well. However, the patient's contribution to the affective climate of the family following hospitalization has received little attention since then. If high-EE attitudes are associated with relapse, is it not possible that this is due to a correlation with a third variable, such as the severity or quality of patient symptomatology at the time of hospital discharge? Leff (1976) reported negative data in this regard when psychiatrist's ratings of the severity of symptoms at discharge were examined.

A similar analysis of symptom ratings, of the sample from the Falloon study (Miklowitz, Goldstein, & Falloon, 1983), revealed parallel findings to those reported by Leff. There were no significant differences between patients from high- or low-EE homes on the Present State Exam (PSE) (Wing, Cooper, & Sartorius, 1974), rated during the most acute phase of the current episode, or on the Brief Psychiatric Rating Scale (BPRS) (Overall & Gorham, 1962), obtained shortly before discharge. Nor were there differences in the number of prior episodes. There were also no differences in ratings of premorbid adjustment on the UCLA Social Attainment Scale (Goldstein, 1978). The latter is particularly important, as premorbid adjustment is an established prognostic indicator and it is important to demonstrate its independence from EE attitudes.

Miklowitz (1983) did find, however, that one high-EE subgroup, the EOI subsample, was associated with ratings of poor premorbid adjustment and high levels of residual symptomatology, as rated on the BPRS at discharge. However, high-EE relatives defined by a highly critical attitude had patient relatives indiscriminable from those from low-EE families in symptom type, severity, or premorbid adjustment.

Symptoms and premorbid adjustment do not exhaust the personal qualities of a schizophrenic individual that can arouse high EE feelings in a relative. Possibly some other more subtle aspects of the schizophrenic's behavior arouse critical or overinvolved feelings in a close relative. Currently, we are investigating whether there are certain key behaviors emitted by the schizophrenic during the direct-interaction task that trigger criticism or intrusiveness by a parent.

In a study currently underway, a coding system termed the Coping Style Scale was applied to the same transcripts that previously had been scored for affective style. This scoring was done by raters blind as to the AS scoring done previously or to parental EE level. The coping style codes covered three broad categories of self-statements expressed by a patient: positive, negative, and autonomous. Positive self-statements refer to statements of worth or pride in some activity or attribute of the patient; negative self-statements are self-critical remarks; and autonomous statements reflect assertions by the patient to follow some self-selected path of action.

Data analyzed so far have revealed that patients from high- and low-EE homes differ markedly in the rate of negative and positive self-statements. As hypothesized, patients from high-EE homes express a significantly higher number of negative self-statements and a lower number of positive self-statements than patients from low-EE homes ($p < .001$). The next step in this study is to carry out sequential analyses to determine whether these self-denigrating remarks trigger parental criticism and intrusiveness or whether they represent reactions to these parental behaviors. Possibly, the sense of ineptitude expressed by these negative self-statements may be particularly infuriating to relatives who see them as one more sign of the frustrating negative symptoms of the disorder.

FAMILY-INTERVENTION PROGRAMS AND THE SHORT-TERM COURSE OF SCHIZOPHRENIA

Although there are a number of unanswered questions concerning the relative contributions of patient and parent to the resultant negative affective climate associated with a poorer short-term course, it is not necessary to have all the answers before approaching this problem from another direction. If there are stress-producing, noxious elements in the family environment that lower the threshold for relapse, then programs designed to modify these aspects of the family environment should produce a more favorable course. In fact, this has been the rationale underlying four major studies, three of which have been completed (Falloon *et al.*, 1982; Goldstein *et al.*, 1968; Leff, Kuipers, Berkowitz, Eberlein-Vries, & Sturgeon, 1982) and one which is close to completion (Anderson, Hogarty, & Reiss, 1981). In each of these studies, patients were kept on maintenance pharmacotherapy throughout the aftercare period. The central research question was whether the addition to regular pharmacotherapy of a family-based therapeutic program could reduce the probability of relapse in the schizophrenic patient relative.

The first of these studies was carried out by myself and colleagues at UCLA. The sample consisted of patients who, for the most part, were undergoing their first lifetime episode of schizophrenia, and the period of the controlled trial was 6 weeks following discharge after a very brief hospitalization. In a 2 × 2 design, patients were randomly assigned to one of two dose levels of injectable phenothiazine (moderate [25 mg] or low [6.25 mg] of fluphenazine enanthate) and to the presence or absence of a crisis-oriented family therapy program. Relapse rates were evaluated at the end of the 6-week controlled trial and at 6-month follow-up.

In the Leff *et al.* and Falloon *et al.* studies, patients were more chronic, and received individually determined maintenance levels of phenothiazine drugs, injectable in the former and oral in the latter; relatives were involved in a longer term, family-oriented program that lasted for a minimum of 9 months. In the Leff study, the family-intervention program was targeted specifically for relatives, and patients were not involved. The format was a multifamily group. In the Falloon study, individual family therapy sessions did involve the patient as well as key relatives and were held in the home. A common feature of the Leff *et al.* and Falloon *et al.* studies was that they selected patients primarily from high-EE homes so that these interventions were targeted toward the most relapse-prone patients and family units. The Goldstein *et al.* study, in contrast, did not select on this variable and took all consecutive patients who applied for treatment in the local community mental health center whose key relatives were living in the area.

Despite the wide variation in samples and the format of treatment, the results of these three studies were remarkably similar. Figure 2 presents the relapse rates for these studies, contrasting patients treated with and

Figure 2. Relapse rates from three studies contrasting a family-intervention program with the absence of such a program (all schizophrenic patients on continuous medication).

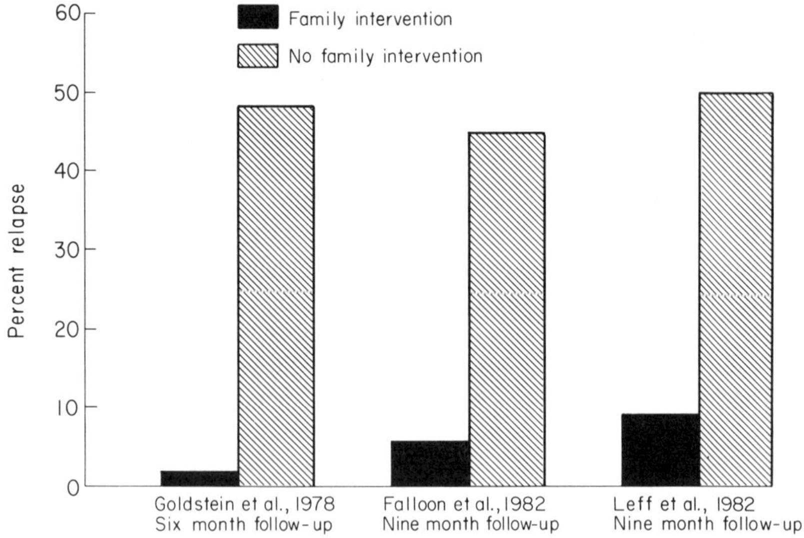

without a family-based intervention. Although no final report has appeared from the Anderson *et al.* study, preliminary reports suggest similar results from that study. Across the three studies, the relapse rate for the family-treated groups are approximately one-fourth of that found in the groups where the relatives did not participate in the focused aftercare intervention program.

The fact that three of the four studies used regular intramuscular neuroleptic medication suggests that the family program added something above and beyond insuring medication compliance. Indeed, it certainly appears that something has happened or changed within the family that has markedly altered the short-term course of the patient's disorder.

ATTEMPTS TO EVALUATE THE IMPACT OF ONE FAMILY-INTERVENTION PROGRAM

The replicated finding that some form of family intervention lowers the risk for relapse in patients already on maintenance pharmacotherapy, does not indicate what processes have been modified by the family program. Most family programs tested in these controlled trials have been comprehensive in nature, providing education for relatives and support for the family system, as well as specific training in altering intrafamilial behavior. A theoretical model that emphasizes the affective climate of the family as a risk factor for relapse would receive greater support if it could be shown that the family programs that reduce relapse, do, in fact, modify this component of family life. In the Leff *et al.* report (1982) there was a suggestion that this was the case, as the majority of participants in the parent-group condition did show a shift in their EE status from high to low, and where this shift did not occur relapse was more likely.

However, as we indicated previously, this merely documents a change in attitudes expressed to an interviewer during a repeat Camberwell Interview, but does not indicate that family behaviors have changed. In Los Angeles, we have attempted this type of evaluation with data from the Falloon *et al.* study cited previously. Before going into the results of our research on changes in affective communication, it is necessary to understand the design of the Falloon *et al.* study. This study involved 39 patients diagnosed as schizophrenic by both the PSE/CATEGO and DSM-III criteria, who were living with one or both parents at the time that they had a major exacerbation of the disorder. Most entered the study after a period of inpatient treatment but a few entered the studies as outpatients. All patients were treated with neuroleptics after leaving the hospital (or placed on medication if they entered as outpatients), and dosages were adjusted until the patient was judged to have stabilized. This ordinarily took 4–6 weeks after maintenance treatment was initiated. At that point, patients were randomly assigned to one or two psychosocial treatment conditions—family management or individual management. All patients selected for the study were considered at high risk for relapse because the homes they returned to were designated as high-EE based on the Camberwell or by virtue of excessive stresses and tensions observed in the family unit.

The family-management condition was carried out primarily in the homes, whereas the individual treatment was done in the clinic. Both treatments followed a common behaviorally oriented model in which communication and problem-solving training were core modules. Neither concentrated on modifying affective communication, although such modification would be expected in the family-management condition as a notable side effect of more effective communication and problem-solving skills. For both forms of treatment, the sessions were held once per week for the first 3 months, then declined to once every 2 weeks for the next 3 months, and finally ended up with monthly maintenance sessions for the final 3 months of the 9-month treatment period. During the total 9-month treatment period, relatives were telephoned every 2 weeks and detailed information was collected regarding any life events or stresses occurring during the previous 2 weeks and how the family coped with them. Reports of these calls were rated blindly on a 10-point scale of coping effectiveness.

Before each family entered its respective psychosocial treatment program, they participated in a pretherapy family-assessment task. This was the direct-interaction task described earlier in this chapter, in which two problems were discussed with an experimenter present. After the first 3 months of treatment, this procedure was repeated. The problems discussed were developed in a similar fashion as for the pretherapy assessment. The problems used were those identified as idiosyncratically relevant to each family at the time each assessment took place.

The interactions were audio-recorded, and verbatim transcripts of these discussions were coded blindly by raters using the Doane Affective Style coding system. Of the 39 families who participated, 3 dropped out and 34 completed both assessments. The total number used in our analyses was reduced to 33 because a father in one family failed to show up for the posttest assessment.

First, we examined whether there was a greater decline in the negative affective style codes of criticism and intrusion for parents in family therapy than for parents of individually treated patients. In order to test this, the total number of these types of parental statements were summed over the two-problem discussion and analysis of covariance was carried out in which the pretherapy scores served as the covariate for the posttherapy scores. These results are presented in Figure 3, where we see that the incidence of negative affective style messages was markedly lower in the family-treated

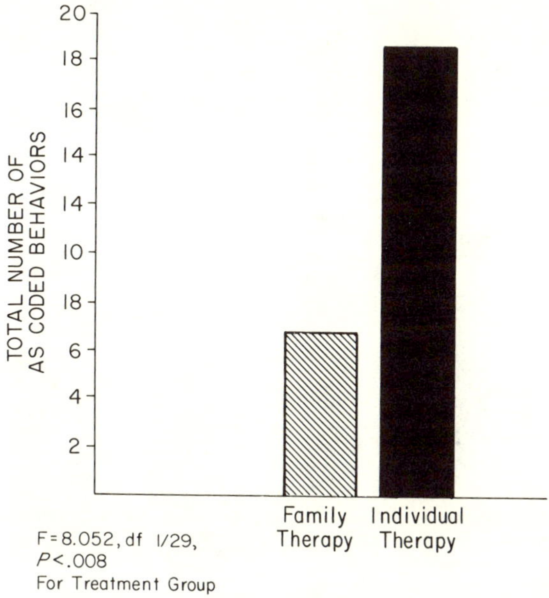

Figure 3. Total number of critical and intrusive affective style (AS) statements at 3 month posttest, by therapy group (adjusted means). (From Miklowitz *et al.*, 1984.)

group ($F_{1,30}$ = 9.41, $p < .005$). A breakdown of the data for criticisms and intrusions revealed highly significant reductions for both types of negative affective communications for relatives in the family, as contrasted with the individual treatment groups ($F_{1,30}$ for criticisms = 5.49, $p < .05$; $F_{1,30}$ for intrusions = 8.1, $p < .01$).

This sample consisted of an equal number of single- and dual-parent families. We then tested whether the contrast between the parents in the family or individual-treatment groups was valid for both types of families. In Figure 4 are pre- and post-AS data for both types of family structures by treatment condition. We see that there is a comparable reduction in the sum of criticisms and intrusions for both types of family structures in the family-treatment condition. Interestingly, although there was little or no change in the level of negative AS statements for single parents in the individual-treatment condition, there are suggestions of a worsening affective climate in the dual-parent families when only the patient is treated. This was quite intriguing, but unexpected, as we had anticipated that the single parents, because of their limited marital support system, might deteriorate more without family treatment.

The pattern of group means suggests the Falloon family-management approach does indeed reduce the average level of negative affective com-

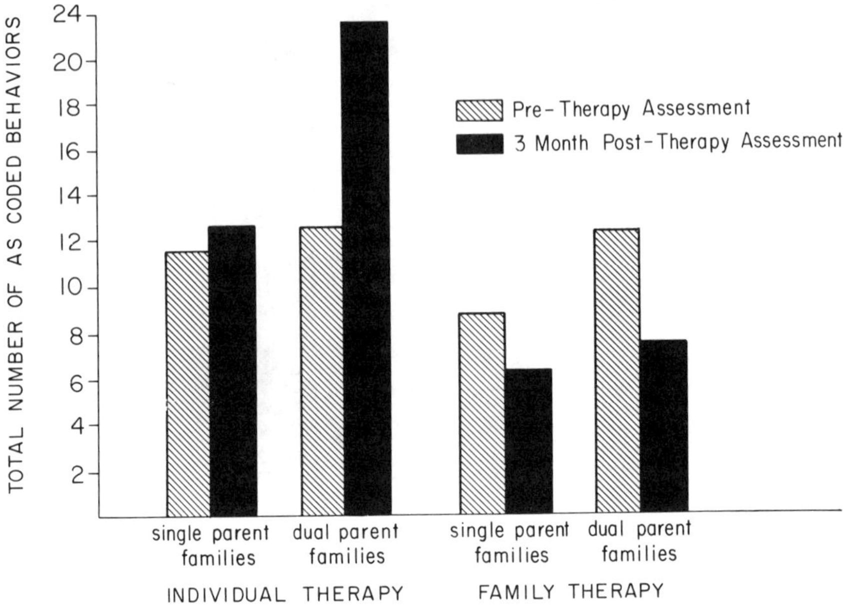

Figure 4. Pre–post changes in affective style (AS) by family composition and therapy group. (From Miklowitz *et al.*, 1984.)

munication in parents of schizophrenics. But, an average does not tell us how many families reduced this behavior in each treatment condition, nor does it establish a precise association between the reduction of negative affective communication in a parent, or parents, and the likelihood of relapse in the patient offspring. In order to deal with these two questions, the 33 families were divided into 3 groups based on the patterns of pre–post AS scores. Because the British work on EE treats criticism and overinvolvement as independent dimensions in defining EE status, we considered the rate of change in criticism separate from the rate of change in intrusiveness. Families were thus classified into three categories; (1) *dual increase*, in which both criticism and intrusiveness increased from pre- to posttest; (2) *dual decrease*, in which both declined during the same period; and (3) a *mixed group*, in which one attribute increased and the other decreased. Figure 5 presents the frequency of each type of family-change pattern by treatment group, and it also presents the number of relapse cases that occurred in each of these pattern-based category groups. First, we see that the dual-increase pattern is found in half of the individual-therapy families but only rarely appears in the family-therapy group. Conversely, the dual-decrease pattern is prominent in the family-treated cases, but less frequent in the individual-therapy condition. The frequency of the mixed pattern does not vary by treatment groups. Thus, there is a clear trend for a reduction in one or both forms of the negative AS behaviors in the family-treatment condition.

All but one of the relapses occurred in the individual-therapy condition, and all but one occurred in the dual-increase or mixed groups. The probability of relapse for individually treated patients in one of these two groups is 67% compared with 25% for the dual-decrease group. These data show that 88% of families in family therapy have a reduction in one or both dimensions of AS, in contrast to 50% of those in the individual-therapy condition. Increases in AS are associated with relapse in that condition as well. What is puzzling is that there are some cases in the family-therapy condition who show the dual-increase pattern ($N = 2$) or the mixed pattern ($N = 6$) who did not relapse. Of course, this reassessment of the families occurred after only 3 months of family therapy and it is possible that, with sustained therapeutic contacts over the subsequent 6 months, changes in the affective climate of these families did occur which prevented relapse.

Data supporting this hypothesis that involve the ratings of coping effectiveness alluded to earlier have recently been reported by Doane, Falloon, Goldstein, and Mintz (1985). Doane *et al.* classified families at the 3-month assessment as relatively benign or negative in AS, on the basis of parental behavior in the interaction task. Her classification was based on whether the parent(s) reduced the number of harshly critical remarks (personal criticisms, guilt-inducing remarks, or critical intrusions) or reduced the number of intrusions below a previously determined cutting score of 6. Within the family-therapy condition, negative-AS status was associated with lower rated coping than the benign-AS families at the 3-month point. However, after 3 more months of family therapy, the differences between

Figure 5. Patterns of change in AS in individual and family therapy.

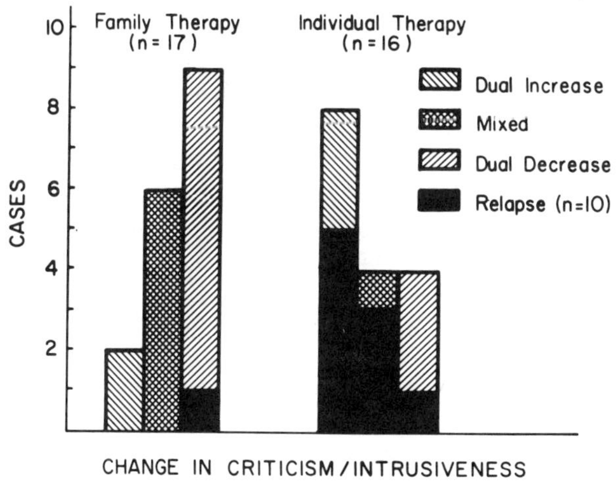

the two AS groups had disappeared and both, in fact, showed significantly higher levels of coping than either AS group in the individual-therapy condition, who had in fact deteriorated in coping. Thus, although there are some families who had not reduced their negative AS by the 3-month point, they do show improvement with sustained family therapy and this improvement in coping is associated with a significantly lower rate of patient relapse than was found in the individual-therapy condition. In the latter condition, there seems to be little change in family coping effectiveness following the 3-month assessment.

DISCUSSION

The various studies summarized in this paper indicate that the affective climate of the family with a schizophrenic young adult offspring relates to the short-term course of the disorder. Further, when family-based interventions are associated with a longer period of community tenure for the patient, parallel reductions in this negative affective climate are noted in direct observations of family behavior. The optimum results were found when both components of the AS system, criticism and intrusiveness, were reduced in frequency during the period from pretest to a 3-month posttest, although benefits were observed when only one component was attenuated.

Whenever one type of family behavior is reduced in frequency, it naturally raises the question of what characterizes the new pattern of family transactions. A key objective of the Falloon *et al.* study was to train family members in a defined set of strategies for dealing with problems inside and outside of the family. A coding system was developed by Doane for recording instances in the direct family interaction tasks where family members utilized these recommended problem-solving strategies (PSS). When pre- and 3-month direct interaction tasks data were contrasted in the number of PSS behaviors expressed, there was a highly significant difference between treatment conditions at 3 months favoring the family-treated group (adjusted mean FT $= 24.59$; adjusted mean IT $= 10.39$, $F = 6.60$, $p > .02$). Also when the pattern of change in AS, presented in Figure 4, was examined for PSS change levels, sharp differences in the 3-month data were found between the dual-decrease group in family therapy and the dual-increase group in individual therapy (mean PSS for dual decrease FT $= +20.0$; mean dual increase IT $= -0.20$). This means that in the former group there were 20 more instances of PSS behavior than was evident at pretest, whereas in the latter there was virtually no change for baseline. The remaining AS-change groups showed slight positive-changes scores that were similar in the two treatment conditions.

These data suggest that a task-centered form of problem solving takes the place of the negative interaction patterns of criticism, blaming, and intrusiveness into the inner state of the patient. When a large reduction in the negative AS behaviors (in the form of reductions in both criticism and intrusiveness) has occurred, a major shift in this more affectively neutral, task-centered behavior is observed; the reverse is noted when hieghtened levels of both forms of AS are evident. These data suggest a marked reciprocity between uncontrolled negative affective expression focused upon the patient, and a more controlled, cognitive form of behavior focused upon common family problems. Because we have only two points in the Falloon study where direct-interaction data were obtained, we cannot speak to the sequential linkage between these two dimensions of family behavior. Does family-based intervention first inhibit negative affective expression thereby permitting the acquisition of problem-solving skills? Or, does the early acquisition of problem-solving skills simply replace negative affective expressions without any specific instructions to limit or inhibit these behaviors? Further studies with repeated observation of the family therapy process are needed to tease apart these issues—issues that are critical to understand if we are to plan more effective programs for optimizing family change.

Much of this article has emphasized the impact of a combined program of pharmaco- and family therapy on relapse rate over a 9-month to 1-year period after discharge for an episode of schizophrenia. It is obviously an important criterion for a successful maintenance program. But, relapse prevention is a minimal criterion for a treatment program. Can a family-intervention program extend beyond this defensive objective to faciliate improved social role functioning? The data here are far from complete. Findings from the Falloon *et al.* study do suggest that significantly greater improvements in social role functioning were observed in the family than in the individually treated group. Also, the recent report by Doane *et al.* (1985) indicates that a reduction in negative AS from pre- to 3-month assessment was associated with higher levels of social functioning than when this was not the case. So, it appears that modifications of the affective climate of the family go beyond relapse prevention to anticipate greater social improvement as well. Despite these encouraging findings, it still is not clear what level of social improvement is possible when such a multimodal program is continued beyond the 9-month point of active treatment used in the Leff *et al.* programs. Certainly, the optimistic results to date warrant continued efforts to test the limits of efficacy of such programs.

Along these lines, it would be very helpful to gather data concerning the long-term impact of these family-focused programs after they officially cease. Most of the controlled trials described in this article have offered drug and family interventions for roughly half of their sample for a fixed time period. At the end of the time period, these interventions typically cease or patients are transferred to some other clinical unit or service. What happens to those patients and their families at this point? Do they start to relapse rather rapidly or do they continue to hold the gains observed during the "official" treatment period? Evidence concerning maintenance or deterioration both in the patient and in intrafamilial relationships would in general be useful. If there is little retention of the gains observed during the controlled trials, this does not imply that these drug–family programs are without value. Instead, this could suggest that the treatment of schizophrenia requires a type of longer term commitment than most research studies can typically guarantee.

One final point, because the emphasis of this article has been upon the family of the schizophrenic and family-oriented treatment programs, we have not emphasized issues concerning the long-term pharmacotherapy of the patient. We should never forget that all of the successful family programs are built upon a foundation of regular and continuous pharmacotherapy. However, the successful addition of family-based intervention programs to regular pharmacotherapy raises the question of whether a potent social therapy permits alteration in the strategy of drug treatment in terms of dose level and pattern of treatment. Given the evidence that a comprehensive family-intervention program can produce some degree of stabilization of the stress level in the social environment, we now can consider whether this stabilization permits the use of lower dose levels of phenothiazine medication, or even more radical strategies such as intermittent or targeted use of medication. An ironic side effect of an effective family program may be that it permits greater latitude for experimentation in the complementary area of psychopharmacology.

ACKNOWLEDGMENTS

The UCLA research studies were supported by grants MH08744, MH30911, and MH14584. The authors are deeply indebted to Ian Falloon for his warm spirit of collaboration and to David Miklowitz, Karen Snyder, and Sibyl Zaden for their important contributions to various phases of this research.

REFERENCES

Anderson, C. M., Hogarty, G. E., & Reiss, D. (1981). The psychoeducational family treatment of schizophrenia. In M. J. Goldstein (Ed.), *New developments in interventions with families of schizophrenics* (pp. 79–94). San Francisco: Jossey-Bass.

Brown, G. W., Birley, J. L. T., & Wing, J. K. (1972). Influence of family life on the course of schizophrenic disorders: A replication. *British Journal of Psychiatry, 121*, 241–258.

Doane, J. A., Falloon, I. R. H., Goldstein, M. J., & Mintz, J. (1985). Parental affective style and the treatment of schizophrenia. *Archives of General Psychiatry, 42*, 34–42.

Doane, J. A., West, K. L., Goldstein, M. J., Rodnick, E. H., & Jones, J. E. (1981). Parental communication deviance and affective style: Predictors of subsequent schizophrenia spectrum disorders in vulnerable adolescents. *Archives of General Psychiatry, 38*, 679–685.

Falloon, I. R. H., Boyd, J. L., McGill, C. W., Razani, J., Moss, H. B., & Gilderman, A. M. (1982). Family management in the prevention of exacerbations of schizophrenia. *New England Journal of Medicine, 306*, 1437–1440.

Goldstein, M. J. (1978). Further data concerning the relation between premorbid adjustment and paranoid symptomatology. *Schizophrenia Bulletin, 4*, 236–243.

Goldstein, M. J., Judd, L. L., Rodnick, E. H., & Gould, E. (1968). A method for studying social influence and coping patterns within families of disturbed adolescents. *Journal of Nervous and Mental Disease, 147*, 233–251.

Leff, J. P. (1976). Schizophrenia and sensitivity to the family environment. *Schizophrenia Bulletin, 2*, 566–574.

Leff, J. P., Kuipers, L., Berkowitz, R., Eberlein-Vries, R., & Sturgeon, D. (1982). A controlled trial of social intervention in the families of schizophrenic patients. *British Journal of Psychiatry, 141*, 121–134.

Miklowitz, D. J., Goldstein, M. J., & Falloon, I. R. H. (1983). Premorbid and symptomatic characteristics of schizophrenics from families with high and low levels of expressed emotion. *Journal of Abnormal Psychology, 92*, 359–367.

Miklowitz, D. J., Goldstein, M. J., Falloon, I. R. H., & Doane, J. A. (1984). *British Journal of Psychiatry, 144*, 482–487.

Overall, J. E., & Gorham, D. R. (1962). The brief psychiatric rating scale. *Psychological Reports, 10*, 799.

Vaughn, C. E., & Leff, J. P. (1976). The influence of family and social factors on the course of psychiatric illness: A comparison of schizophrenic and neurotic patients. *British Journal of Psychiatry, 129*, 125–137.

Wing, J. K., Cooper, J. E., & Sartorius, N. (1974). *The description and classification of psychiatric symptoms: An instruction manual for the PSE and CATEGO system*. London & New York: Cambridge University Press.

General Discussion

Dr. Arthur Rifkin:* Let's take one or two questions specifically for Dr. Goldstein and then let's have all the participants come up for discussion.

Dr. John Cleghorn†: Could you tell me whether the patients in this study are all children in the families?

Dr. Michael J. Goldstein‡: Yes, they are.

Dr. Cleghorn: And what would be the mean age, roughly?

Dr. Goldstein: Mean age is, I believe, about 26.

Dr. Cleghorn: And could you elaborate on the notion that there are factors in the family therapy other than those producing increased compliance with drugs?

Dr. Goldstein: Well, there are many things that go on. I think the affective level may be a crude marker of many different subprocesses. For example, I think these family programs do a great deal to reduce the guilt of relatives about what's happened, their sense of having caused the illness. I believe they also play a big role in lowering expectations, quite frankly, of what you can get, how long it's going to take to get some kind of improvement in the patients. I think they establish new norms. I think they provide crisis-intervention services for families, so that when things heat up, there is somebody to call and intervene with them, even if over the telephone. So I think they are very important support systems, and they should not be seen as simply family-training modules. I think that is too narrow a view.

Dr. Cleghorn: Right, but is there much work to be done to separate out the saliency of these different factors?

Dr. Goldstein: Oh, I think there is. Remember, these are probes, as it were. The family is brought in, you tell them the purpose is to discuss some problems and that we'll leave them alone, and then we use this as a probe. But I think it is very important to have tapes of these family therapy and

* New York, New York.

† Toronto, Canada.

‡ Los Angeles, California.

individual therapy sessions to do more microanalyses of what transpires in them.

Dr. Ernest Gruenberg:* Am I correct in thinking that your criterion of relapse has to do with a decompensation in social-role functioning, a form of disability that is associated with whatever condition the patient has, and has something to do with respect for rehospitalization?

Dr. Goldstein: No. The criteria relapse was a clinical re-exacerbation of the very symptoms that the patient showed at the time he or she came into the study. There were a few cases that were marginal on this, but almost everybody had to show a major increase in the target symptoms that they showed at the time they came into the study.

Dr. Gruenberg: What are the target symptoms?

Dr. Goldstein: They were rated individually. These were schizophrenic symptoms on the PSE or DSM-III symptoms. Relapse was *not* defined on the basis of deterioration solely in social-role functioning. It had to be an increase in symptoms.

Dr. Gruenberg: In symptoms alone?

Dr. Goldstein: Symptoms, yes.

Dr. Gruenberg: No social-role criteria at all?

Dr. Goldstein: No, no, although they obviously would be correlated.

Dr. Gruenberg: No indications of disability?

Dr. Goldstein: Oh, there were many measures of disability taken on the patients, but that was not the criterion of relapse.

Dr. Gruenberg: Thank you.

Mr. Gerard E. Hogarty†: Mike, I want to congratulate you again. That was a tour de force. I wish you were in Pittsburgh or close to it. We do collaborate at a distance.

Dr. Goldstein: That's right.

Dr. Hogarty: It would be a terrific asset to have you in town. That was a wonderful presentation. I have two questions and another comment. Our own family study looks very much like yours at 9 months. However, in our own study and in Julian Leff's study, results are not looking as good in the second year, and a lot of relapse is due to drug noncompliance, which leads me to a question: Do you have any idea how many of the 10 relapses were actually off drug or noncomplying prior to their relapse?

Dr. Goldstein: In the relapses in general, half of them were compliant and half of them were noncompliant, and that did not differ with treatment condition.

Dr. Hogarty: There was only one relapse in the family therapy?

* Baltimore, Maryland.

† Pittsburgh, Pennsylvania.

Dr. Goldstein: Right. But there were equal numbers of compliant and noncompliant patients in both conditions.

Dr. Hogarty: That's not my question. My question is, how many of the patients who relapsed, relapsed off meds?

Dr. Goldstein: I would say half that were rated as noncompliant, which is different than being off meds, because that is a rating across the whole 9 months of treatment.

Dr. Hogarty: These are 3-month ratings? How many people had already relapsed by 3 months?

Dr. Goldstein: I believe that half of the cases had relapsed before the retesting had been done and half afterwards.

Dr. Hogarty: So it is conceivable that some of these affective responses are the result of a relapse and not necessarily the cause of it?

Dr. Goldstein: That's right.

Dr. Rifkin: Would the participants come up please? Let me start off with a question for Courtenay [Harding]. You found that you could not find predictors of outcome over that long period, and then you concluded that the person who recovered was active in his or her outcome. How did you arrive at that conclusion?

Dr. Courtenay M. Harding:* Well, in the first place, my comment about predictors is very, very premature and early on. What we did was to take a look at the Strauss outcome scale with the four items on it—work, social relations, hospitalization, and symptoms—and we looked at them at every 5-year milepost. What we found was that predictions began to fan out, so that by the 20th year, the predictions were very, very weak. It was like predicting tomorrow's weather from today's weather and then trying to predict next week's weather from today's weather, and the prediction just got weaker and weaker.

As far as the activity level to which I alluded in the presentation, we found it occurring in both the Yale and Vermont studies. These people began to actively participate in their own life and their own recovery, and so it is part of the process of recovery.

Dr. Rifkin: I guess it is a question of what is an outcome measure and what is a predictor.

Dr. Jack Durell†: I think this question is related to the one Dr. Rifkin just asked, but I have two questions dealing with the relationship of shorter-term course, that is several-year course, to longer-term course. The first is this: you were not able to see a relationship between the strictness of diagnosis and the longer-term outcome. I would ask, to what extent does it appear

* New Haven, Connecticut.

† Rockville, Maryland.

that shorter-term course, that is, 5-year course, predict 20-year course? The second, related question: There is a good deal of evidence that strictness of diagnostic criteria relates to the predictions of shorter-term course. That is, a schizoaffective will have a better shorter-term course than an RDC schizophrenic. How do you reconcile the issue of the failure of diagnosis, strictness of criteria, to predict longer-term course with the fact that it does predict shorter-term course?

Dr. Harding: There have been several studies, Manfred Bleuler's included, that said that what you were at 5 years was what you were for a long time thereafter, that the 5-year marker was quite predictive. Strauss and Carpenter also, I think, found that what you were at 2 years predicted fairly well what you would be at 5 years. I guess I would say two things to this: First of all, my data are 24 hours old, so I don't have my profiles drawn up yet, and I don't have my longitudinal patterns done yet. It seems, though, that what they were at 5 years, which looked fairly poor in our 5-year outcome, has changed dramatically, and therefore there are people who crossed over their predictors. We are also going to be looking at those people who had good premorbid status who crossed over their predictors to become poor-outcome people, and we have a group of people who were poor premorbids and who went to a good outcome status, and we will be reporting on that, too. It is a fascinating process.

As far as the diagnostic specificity for looking at their 5-year course, we could do that. We have what they were, and we have their 5-year outcome, and we have their 10-, their 15-, and their 20-year outcomes. It will be very interesting to find out what is going on there.

Dr. Hogarty: Could I try a response to that, too? I wouldn't readily accept your basic assumption. We did not say that schizoaffective disorders had a better outcome than the schizophrenic types. It was just that EE didn't predict it. There are a number of studies in recent years that would indicate that the course of schizoaffective disorders is a quite stormy one indeed, and not the good outcome described in studies in the 1940s, 1950s, and early 1960s, especially DSM-I, early DSM-II days, which might have included a number of major affective disorders in there.

I think in recent years it has become increasingly difficult to distinguish among subtypes of schizophrenia, including schizoaffective disorder, as different in their short-term outcome. I'm not aware of evidence.

Dr. Ming Tsuang:* I would like to stress a couple of points. Your data suggest very clearly at this point that family intervention is working. However, the finding was derived from short-term outcome, using criteria for measuring relapse. It will be important now to show how long the effect is going to continue to be sustained. Another point is that a successful intervention to

* Providence, Rhode Island.

prevent relapses, does not necessarily mean that the factor involved is always psychosocial. It is wrong to assume if it is biological, or even if it is genetic, that successful intervention cannot be done.

Dr. Hogarty: Well, you wear glasses, and that is a psychosocial intervention for myopia.

Dr. Tsuang: Let me finish. What I am stressing is that if one hopes that studies on the high-EE and low-EE families will have a great impact on the future research in schizophrenia, one should not be "myopic." One has to look into both biological and psychosocial aspects. By "biological," I mean that there are both environmental and genetic aspects, which should both be considered in future studies, to really make a significant impact. Though I am impressed with your results on the high-EE–low-EE, I still don't know what are the basic biological and psychosocial components. To quantify and to characterize, these will be very important aspects.

To tie this with Dr. Harding's studies, it is actually pretty much what we are now doing to really measure many, many points, and roughly speaking, our 40-year follow-up showed 20% free of symptoms using Feighner criteria 30 to 40 years later, meaning that at that point, 20% of the schizophrenics actually didn't show any specific symptoms, but it doesn't mean that. All of this 20% has been continuously free of symptoms. We are just checking at one point. If we checked the 5-year and short-term outcomes, it would be different.

So it is very important to look into many, many points, as long as NIMH is going to support this research. They always consider it very time consuming and give no money, and that is wrong. It is very important for the outcome study to concentrate on longitudinal aspects on many, many points. Bleuler also stressed that. His cases actually showed that some improved and some did not improve. If you take a point in time for schizophrenics, generally for patients and family, we talk about 25% of them, probably, at some point, being sure of remission. That is the literature.

Dr. Goldstein: Could I just say one thing: I have no conflict with genetic and biological interpretations of the data, and I think it is a very fruitful way to go, particularly if you have markers that can permit you to disentangle them beyond simply family history.

Dr. Sam Siris:* I want to comment about the way this session speaks to the session of yesterday afternoon. We have been talking about issues of outcome and issues of treatment strategy. I think it deserves emphasis that these two issues speak to each other. It is a point that has been emphasized in the past by Don Klein, that we can slice with a pharmocological knife to try to divide up the different syndromes at which we are looking. This is a particularly important issue to emphasize in studies of negative symptoms

* New York, New York.

and deficit states. Differences in neuroleptic dose may matter for these states as well as differences in drug. Differences in EPS and anti-Parkinsonian medication should not be neglected either. Additionally, it is necessary to examine differences in the affectivity of the schizophrenic episode and deficit state, because the patients are heterogeneous and the treatments are heterogeneous as well, and we certainly now have psychopharmacological tools to investigate some of these issues. Perhaps they will become less confusing if we look at them carefully along that dimension. Some of these symptoms may be side effects of the treatment, and, consequently, some of the "depressions" may be "side effects" of the treatment.

Dr. Hogarty: Sam [Siris], thanks to your work and your own exquisite reviews in the past, as well as our own observations we have learned that these patients with impaired affects, even after there is a remission of psychotic symptoms, have terrible courses. We note that 55% of our affectively impaired patients maintained on fluphenazine decanoate who resolve a psychosis go on to a relapse within 2 years, relative to about 26% without those impaired affects. That has led to a new series of investigations that will start soon. We and others are proceding systematically, using pharmacologic probes to try to sort this out.

Dr. Siris: Originally, a lot of affect in schizophrenia was thought to be associated with good outcome, and that probably is indeed the case if we are looking at the affect in the acute episode. But work that Nina Schooler has been involved in, and the work of others, has shown that the affective syndromes that occur later, that is, depressive-like syndromes that occur later in the course of the illness, are not necessarily associated with good outcomes at all.

Dr. Hogarty: It's a wasteland out there in terms of pharmacologic studies in recovered schizophrenic patients with residual impairments of affect—a wasteland.

Dr. Donald F. Klein:* I was interested in hearing over the past couple of days that a certain subgroup of the schizophrenics was referred to repeatedly. There is a certain interesting convergence there. These were the never-married, male, severe schizophrenics, and it comes out interestingly in terms of Sol Goldberg's paper and some of Dan Weinberger's stuff. This is a group of patients probably very heavy loaded for neurological, central-nervous-system damage. In Gerry Hogarty's work, they are the ones that seem to be the group that is sensitive to the EE variable. I think that makes a certain amount of sense.

I would like to talk about a couple of clinical observations. The never-married, male, severe schizophrenics, in my experience, have consisted largely of two groups of people. One is the people we referred to as childhood

* New York, New York.

asocials. They are the ones that have always been queer, friendless, peculiar people. They are the ones that Quitkin and his colleagues showed are high in neurological signs. You did some work with that, Arthur [Rifkin].

In my experience, those people have a uniformly disastrous outcome. It is not just a question that they do badly; they do terribly and continue to do terribly. Some patients that I have had personal contact with for over 20 years have shown not a flicker in terms of getting better.

The second group of schizophrenics are the chronic, fearful, paranoid schizophrenics, who usually develop their illness in the early teens, although their developmental history is not particularly peculiar. They are often quite ordinary children, but starting in their early teens, they become fearful, paranoid—fearful about their relationship with others—and easily make delusional misinterpretations.

Now, I submit that those two groups elicit in their families two quite contrasting types of adaptations: the asocials elicit overprotectiveness, and intrusiveness. The family is afraid to let them alone because they are afraid that they will somehow or other do something socially stupid or shameful, and they often have some legitimate ground for that fear.

On the other hand, the fearful paranoids elicit tremendous criticism. Further, the families themselves—at least we have the impression—often are themselves paranoid people (genetics?) and have a very high degree of criticism.

Now, the EE thing is all about criticism and intrusiveness and overprotection. I'm surprised to hear that there is no symptomatic difference between the low-EE and high-EE families in terms of the patient. My guess is that's a problem in the measuring devices. It is positively hard in the usual rating scales to make a real clear distinction between the transient, paranoid vocalization that occurs in all sorts of psychoses, and the fixed, systematic, anxious, fearful, paranoid state that I think is very likely the core of the bad response to EE.

One last point: There are studies that came largely out of Sol Goldberg's work, the whole NIMH group, as to what are the various things for which phenothiazines are good for and what are the various things for which they are no good. One of the things they are no good for is anxiety, and especially high degrees of anxiety in the paranoid schizophrenic sort of person. I submit that a lot of exacerbation that may be getting these people back into hospital may be an upwelling of anxious, fearfulness—"I just can't manage it; they are after me again"—without necessarily the development of a true delusional construction: "The Martians are after me." for instance. I think a refined analysis of the relapse data would be helpful.

Dr. Rifkin: Any comments by the panel?

Dr. Goldstein: Well, I think one of our sets of data definitely confirms Don [Klein's] point about the really poor premorbid cases who come from these emotionally overinvolved homes, and I do agree that a more refined analysis of the symptom syndromes along the lines that he suggests will probably reveal other connections as well.

Dr. Hogarty: I've been reluctant to go into any depth looking at the correlates of expressed emotion until I had some evidence that it had predictive validity. Now that we do for at least purer RDC schizophrenics, we will pursue that. We have noted that there are high correlations between EOI and poor premorbid history as well. I think, Don, your points are well taken. I will go back and take a look at paranoid subtype among those unmarried male patients, particularly.

I only want to point out that the interaction with severity of illness at hospital discharge does implicate the illness pattern in the patient at some level. Patients who do not recover from their episode and return to high-EE homes go on to have a further increase in symptoms, whereas high-EE patients that make a good recovery of symptoms have a more benign course and outcome. So maybe we didn't see that at the index episode, but we do see it at hospital discharge, which does implicate something in the symptom picture in subsequent course.

Dr. Rifkin: You know, in our Hillside Hospital sample, we were not able to show that severity of symptoms at discharge or dose at discharge were predictive of anything of long-term outcome.

Dr. Hogarty: No. There is no main effect for severity. Remember, no main effect for severity, only in interaction with EE.

Dr. John Nurnberger:* I have a comment and a question for Dr. Goldstein: With regard to the family-therapy data, I was very impressed with the affect that family interventions had in the studies that you cited. It's been my experience that family therapy for the families of these severely ill people can often be very painful for the family, even if it is done in a nonjudgmental, nonanalytic mode, and I wonder if there are families that are not suited for this kind of intervention? Can you say anything about drop-out rates and what kind of families tend to drop out or what kind of families tend to not respond?

Dr. Goldstein: I think the problem is connection rather than dropping-out. There are families who refuse entry into these programs, and I think we should really get together and collate them and find out how many they are. But my experience has been, once you get them in, they derive tremendous support and benefit from their participation and the drop-out rate is very low from that point on.

I think it is also important, even though I am a family therapist—you notice, I try not to use that word, "family therapy," because I think it has certain connotations of ways of relating to people, and objectives, and so

* Bethesda, Maryland.

forth—I think that these are really low-key programs with high support, tremendous morale building, and not confrontive or uncovering type of programs that we have been talking about, and I think that mostly families do not find that stressful and disturbing.

On the other hand, I think programs that attempt to focus on relational issues—and particularly past relational issues or even current relational issues that get too generalized from highly specific tasks of what people might want from each other in terms of taking out the garbage or things of this sort—can be very disruptive, because they tend to raise affect, and in these families, things that raise affect, raise EE. So you want a program that is a very low-EE, targeted program, whether it is done in a behavioral model or the more structural model that Carol Anderson uses.

Dr. Hogarty: We have a large program now. Probably, when everybody's in, we will have close to 100 patients in our trial. That's why our studies tend to be never-ending, but I think we have made the same observations that Mike [Goldstein] has made. We haven't, to my knowledge, lost any family that was able to show up early on to one of our workshops. And a workshop would not be considered to be analytically oriented at all, although listening to some of the audio tapes of these families later on, you may think that they went through a course in formal analytical psychotherapy.

What they do, I think, is to respond to the information that is provided, in a way that offers a cognitive mastery, and it is not at all indicting. I think one of the problems with prior attempts at family therapy with schizophrenic patients was a matter of communication, that somehow these families were causally implicated in the disease of their offspring, and these models now are radically, radically different. They are based on a psychosocial biological model, one that does not imply that the family caused the illness, but, rather, it has a role in its maintenance, as we have a role in its maintenance.

Dr. Joseph Zubin:* I want to make two brief comments. I want to go back to Courtenay Harding's contribution and to the opening of our session the first day. Seymour Kety quoted extensively from Kraepelin. Several people talked about Kurt Schneider and so on. I want to remind you that in that period in our history schizophrenia was a very malignant disorder. Kurt Schneider would tell the family of the schizophrenic, when he discovered their relative to be schizophrenic, "Go home and forget about your relative. He will never come back to you. He is gone forever."

This particular bias has persisted in our midst, even in some of our discussions yesterday and today. It seems to me, for example, to have cropped up when Bruce [Dohrenwend] asked the question, "Isn't it possible that the good results in Vermont are due to the fact that you had this very good system of treating the patients?" People ask me, isn't it possible that

* Pittsburgh, Pennsylvania.

Bleuler's outcome, the wonderful, more optimistic outcome, is not due to the fact that Bleuler was such a good clinician? But where in the world would you get the natural history of schizophrenia, if not under the best circumstances? You wouldn't want to go to the ghetto, where people are suffering from a lot of other sources of distress, to see whether the outcome is good there. You want to go to the best place, where the triggering mechanisms are at a minimum.

I want to make one final comment about the fact that Courtenay actually raised, namely, that chronicity may be a bias we have inherited culturally, which perhaps should be laid aside. We continually are surprised that a patient gets better. We try to explain it in a variety of ways. Maybe he wasn't even schizophrenic to begin with, and so on. I would put the shoe on the other foot. Let's now look at the chronics and say, "What is it about them that prevented them from becoming well?" What was it in their life story that perhaps made them persist in their condition, because in the long run, with very few exceptions, maybe 5%, everybody suffering from schizophrenia should get well!

Name Index

H

L

M

S

W

Subject Index